P9-DVV-807

DISEASE FREE

DISEASE FREE

How to Prevent, Treat and Cure
More Than 150 Illnesses
and Conditions

By MATTHEW HOFFMAN, WILLIAM LeGRO
and the Editors of **PREVENTION** Magazine Health Books

Rodale Press, Emmaus, Pennsylvania

Copyright © 1993 by Rodale Press, Inc.

All rights reserved. No part of this publication may be reproduced or transmitted in any form or by any means, electronic or mechanical, including photocopy, recording or any other information storage and retrieval system, without the written permission of the publisher.

Prevention is a registered trademark of Rodale Press, Inc.

Printed in the United States of America on acid-free ∞, recycled ♻ paper

Library of Congress Cataloging-in-Publication Data

Hoffman, Matthew.
    Disease free : how to prevent, treat and cure more than 150 illnesses and conditions / by Matthew Hoffman, William LeGro and the editors of Prevention Magazine Health Books.
        p.   cm.
    Includes index.
    ISBN 0–87596–149–5   hardcover
    1. Medicine, Popular.   I. LeGro, William.
II. Prevention Magazine Health Books. III. Title.
RC81.H685   1993
610—dc20   92–23249
                                                CIP

Distributed in the book trade by St. Martin's Press

        10 9   hardcover

OUR MISSION

We publish books that empower people's lives.

RODALE ❧ BOOKS

Executive Editor: Debora A. Tkac

Senior Editor: Russell Wild

Writers: Matthew Hoffman, William LeGro

Contributors: Douglas Dollemore, Stephanie Ebbert, Mark L. Fuerst, Marcia Holman, Gale Maleskey, Ellen Michaud, Leslie Nicholson, Cathy Perlmutter, Porter Shimer, Laura Stevens, Laura Wallace-Smith, Joe Wargo

Research Chief: Ann Yermish

Fact-Checking and Research: Susan E. Burdick, Christine Dreisbach, Melissa Dunford, Jewel Flegal, Dawn Horvath, Anne Imhoff, Karen Lombardi Ingle, Melissa Meyers, Paris Mihely-Muchanic, Cynthia Nickerson, Deborah Pedron, Sally Reith, Bernadette Sukley, Michele Toth

Production Editor: Jane Sherman

Cover and Book Designer: Stan Green

Copy Editor: Susan G. Berg

Office Staff: Roberta Mulliner, manager; Julie Kehs, Mary Lou Stephen

Contributing Advisory Board

Charles P. Kimmelman, M.D.
professor of otolaryngology at New York Medical College in Valhalla, New York, and attending surgeon at Manhattan Eye, Ear and Throat Hospital in New York City

Thomas Platts-Mills, M.D., Ph.D.
professor of medicine and head of the allergy and clinical immunology division at the University of Virginia Medical Center in Charlottesville

John Repke, M.D.
associate professor of obstetrics, gynecology and reproductive biology at Harvard Medical School and director of labor and delivery at Brigham and Women's Hospital in Weston, Massachusetts

David P. Rose, M.D., Ph.D., D.Sc.
chief of the division of nutrition and endocrinology at the Naylor Dana Institute of the American Health Foundation

William Ruderman, M.D.
chairman of the department of gastroenterology and chairman of the Investigational Review Board/Research Programs at Cleveland Clinic Florida in Fort Lauderdale

NOTICE

This book is intended as a reference volume only, not as a medical manual. The information here is designed to help you make informed decisions about your health. It is not a substitute for any treatment that may have been prescribed by your doctor. If you suspect that you have a medical problem, we urge you to seek competent medical help.

CONTENTS

ACNE

I n the beginning was the chin. The chin was pretty and without blemish, and the spirit of Woman was gay as she went from party to party. On the second day, a bump arose on her chin, and she worried. But when evening came, she dusted it with powder and went to the opera. On the third day, more bumps arose—on her brow, her cheeks and the very point of her nose. She scrubbed, she rubbed, she wished them away, but still they remained. Downcast and forlorn, she put away her paints, her powders, her ointments and creams. She even declined an invitation to tea. "Let there be darkness," she cried. "I sure as heck don't want anyone to see me looking like this!"

ADOLESCENCE REVISITED

You probably assumed maturity brought rewards—like wisdom, prosperity and a clear complexion. But as many adults have discovered, whiteheads, blackheads and pimples can surface at any age.

That's because the skin is packed with oil-producing glands called sebaceous glands. Most active on the face, chest and back, these glands manufacture the oil that keeps your skin soft and pliable. In adolescence, the new production of hormones stimulates the glands, making an oversupply of oils that back up and clog the pores. Since the oil can't get out, pressure builds. The walls of the ducts begin to swell, and pimples form. But adults can get acne, too. Emotional stress and the hormonal changes that occur during the menstrual cycle have been linked to adult acne. Acne is also believed to be inherited.

But acne isn't something you have to live with for the rest of your life. Whether you're young or old, have an occasional pimple or a full-blown case of acne, you may be able to help control the problem with simple skin care.

SAVING FACE

Most cases of acne involve more than one pimple, and doctors recommend more than one means of control.

Keep your nose clean. Gently washing your face once or twice a day is all you need, says Stephanie Pincus, M.D., professor and chairman of the Department of Dermatology at State University of New York at Buffalo. But don't overdo it. Overly vigorous scrubbing can compound the problem by irritating the skin. And forget about using abrasive or antibacterial soaps. They're no better than plain soap and water.

SMOOTHING OUT THE SCARS

The next time the movie camera closes in on your Hollywood heart-throb, ask yourself: Has this guy *ever* had a pimple?

Actually, many people have acne that disappears without a trace. Others aren't so lucky, and the deep, craterlike scars can leave a permanent record of the disease. The scars can rarely be eliminated, but they can be improved, says David W. Low, M.D., an assistant professor of plastic and reconstructive surgery at the University of Pennsylvania in Philadelphia.

The easiest technique is dermabrasion, in which your doctor planes the skin smooth with a high-speed brush or wheel. "What you're doing is sanding down the high spots," Dr. Low explains. The procedure isn't particularly painful, but there is significant postprocedure crusting and oozing. "Your face can look pretty bad during the first couple of weeks," he says.

Dermabrasion is effective only for shallow scars, he says. If you have deep, "ice pick" scars, your doctor may decide simply to cut out the scar, then stitch the skin back together. The trick, of course, is making the surgical scar less visible than the acne scar.

A third technique is called punch excision. First the scar is removed, then a plug of skin is taken from another part of the body and inserted in the hole. Once the graft takes, your doctor may use dermabrasion to make your skin even smoother.

Another option is to fill the scars with collagen, an absorbable gelatin protein. While collagen does improve the appearance of a scar, it will eventually be absorbed by the body. In most cases, the benefits will fade after six months to a year, Dr. Low says.

Regardless of the procedure, timing is important. Ideally, your doctor won't operate until new scars aren't being formed. It's also important to have realistic expectations, Dr. Low adds. "If someone has really severe acne scars, there's nothing you can do to remove all of the irregularities. You're not going to make the skin smooth. You're going to make it less rough."

Minimize the makeup. Women who regularly cover up with makeup can develop what doctors call *acne cosmetica*—cosmetic-clogged glands. To help keep your pores open, stick with water-based products that are easily removed with soap and water.

Listen to your blemishes. Even though there is little scientific evidence that foods such as chocolate, french fries and cheeseburgers cause acne, you should still let your face be your guide, Dr. Pincus suggests. If you are among those who *know* you break out every time you eat a hot fudge sundae, try splurging with yogurt instead. For some people, what they eat—or don't eat—may make a difference.

De-stress your life. When your hormones get riled up, as they typically do during times of stress, your skin gets excited, too.

Hands off. The next time a pimple blossoms on the tip of your nose, you might be tempted to give nature a little squeeze. Unfortunately, even gentle pressure can causes pimples to rupture, possibly causing a permanent scar. Time, not hands, can be the best medicine.

THE WORST-CASE BLUES

If you have a persistent, uncontrollable case of acne, your best bet is to see a dermatologist.

For mild cases, an over-the-counter drug called benzoyl peroxide will often do the trick. Benzoyl peroxide may cause your skin to peel and also alters the skin fats and bacteria. Here's how to use it. After washing, spread a thin layer of benzoyl peroxide over your entire face. Use it once a day at first, then as your face gets used to it, two or three times. Since you may not see improvements for six to eight weeks, try to be patient.

A prescription drug called tretinoin, a derivative of vitamin A, alters the growth of oil glands. Applied once a day, it can dry up current pimples and prevent others from forming. It may cause an uncomfortable burning or drying sensation, but most people soon get used to it, doctors say.

For acne that is inflamed, prescription antibiotics—taken orally or rubbed on the skin—can help, Dr. Pincus says. In most cases, these can be taken for months without causing side effects. Antibiotics such as tetracycline can make your skin more sensitive to sunlight, however, says Dr. Pincus, so you should be careful.

For acne that is out of control, your doctor may prescribe a drug called isotretinoin (Accutane). The most powerful acne remedy—in some cases, it will virtually eliminate the problem—it's also the most hazardous, sometimes causing itching, headaches, muscle pain and hair loss. When taken by a pregnant woman, it can cause birth defects. This drug isn't for everyone, but it can make a difference when nothing else seems to help.

Not everyone with acne needs to take medication, of course. But you should still get advice from your doctor. "Not everybody can be permanently cured, but everybody can be helped," Dr. Pincus says.

TREATMENT BREAKTHROUGH

CUTTING THE RISKS OF ACCUTANE

Doctors thought they had the perfect cure for acne in the early 1980s with the discovery of the drug isotretinoin (Accutane), a synthetic derivative of vitamin A.

Isotretinoin has the ability to eliminate even the most severe cases of acne for months or even years at a time. Unfortunately, there is a rub: untoward side effects. Accutane, while giving you smooth skin, can give you headaches, itching and muscle pain and can even cause your hair to shed. But most alarming, it can cause birth defects if taken by pregnant women.

But there are some researchers in Europe who still believe that Accutane can be the end-all for acne—without the bad side effects. They feel that lower doses of the drug taken for longer periods can produce the same benefits but cause fewer problems.

Doctors in this country disagree, says Alan R. Shalita, M.D., professor and chairman of the Department of Dermatology at State University of New York Health Science Center in Brooklyn. "It is conceivable that one could come up with a low enough dose that wouldn't cause birth defects, but this would be very difficult to prove," he says. "Who's going to take the chance of testing it?"

Another way to make the drug safer would be to simply limit the distance it travels, Dr. Shalita says. Today, isotretinoin is taken orally, which means it can reach—and perhaps cause problems in—many parts of the body. But researchers are investigating topical preparations that could be rubbed directly on the acne, putting the punch only where it's needed. "It would be safer this way, because the absorption into the body would be minuscule," he says.

AIDS

Yes, there is fear. Yes, there is confusion. But you should also know that AIDS can easily be prevented and there is hope for a cure.

"AIDS is absolutely preventable. There need not be another person who gets it," says F. Douglas Scutchfield, M.D., director of the Graduate School of Public Health at San Diego State University. "If you abstain from sex or are in a mutually monogamous relationship, and don't do intravenous drugs, you need not be worried about AIDS. It's that simple."

KNOWING THE ENEMY

Researchers have learned much about acquired immune deficiency syndrome (AIDS) since it first became a worldwide concern in 1981. They know that human immunodeficiency virus (HIV), the virus that causes AIDS, can invade the body through unprotected sexual intercourse, shared use of intravenous needles (a common practice among drug addicts) or blood transfusions. Cases of AIDS have also been passed between doctor (or dentist) and patient when there has been direct exposure to infected blood, but such cases are *extremely rare.*

There are at least two viruses, HIV-1 and HIV-2, that cause AIDS. The two are slightly different, but they are transmitted in the same ways and have the same deadly consequences. Worldwide, the two viruses infect an equal number of people. But for now, HIV-1 is much more prevalent in North America.

Once it enters the body, the AIDS virus attacks the immune system, specifically disabling the disease-fighting white blood cells. As the number of these cells decreases, the body's ability to combat illness withers. Initially, the body is able to fight back and develops antibodies to a portion of the virus (when a person tests HIV positive, it means those antibodies

are present in the blood). But for some reason that still puzzles researchers, the lethal portions of the virus remain invisible to the immune
system—much like a stealth bomber isn't detected by radar—and aren't
destroyed. Eventually the virus wins the battle, and the person is overwhelmed by a series of diseases such as pneumonia, tuberculosis and
Kaposi's sarcoma (a rare form of cancer) that take advantage of the body's
weakened defenses.

After infection, it can take years—perhaps up to ten years—for HIV
to paralyze the immune system and allow AIDS to develop a stranglehold
on the body. But occasionally symptoms of AIDS begin appearing within
one to two years after the person has been infected, Dr. Scutchfield says.

The federal Centers for Disease Control (CDC) in Atlanta estimates
that at least one million Americans are currently infected with HIV. Unfortunately, experts predict that number will grow significantly throughout
the 1990s. It's possible that 5 to 10 percent of the people who are infected
with HIV will never develop AIDS, says Daniel Hoth, M.D., director of the
Division of AIDS at the National Institute of Allergy and Infectious Diseases. But so far everyone who has been infected by the virus has later
developed the disease.

GETTING TESTED

One reason that AIDS is still spreading is that many people mistakenly
believe they can't get it, says Fred Kroger, director of the National AIDS
Information and Education Program at the CDC.

"The public still thinks AIDS is something that happens to other
people. They have this uncanny ability to disassociate themselves from
the individuals who get the disease," he says. "Whatever the group, whatever the risk behavior, it's not applicable to their situation. They think
things like 'I haven't had sex with 250 people, I've only had sex with 17, so
I can't be at risk.' The public's understanding of risk behavior is terribly
weak."

Intravenous drug users and homosexual and bisexual men account
for 75 percent of the AIDS cases in the United States, but a growing number
of heterosexual men and women are also contracting the disease. Worldwide, 80 percent of AIDS infections have been contracted through heterosexual intercourse, Dr. Hoth says.

If you have any reason to suspect that you may be infected, ask your
doctor to test your blood for AIDS. Not knowing if you have AIDS not only
puts your sex partners at risk, it also delays treatment that may extend
your life. "For most people, it's better to know than to not know," Dr. Hoth
says. "It's better not only for medical reasons but also for psychological
reasons. That way they can plan their life around this disease."

PLAYING IT SAFE

For now, AIDS is virtually 100 percent fatal. But it also is virtually 100 percent preventable. Here's how.

Practice safe sex. Abstinence or maintaining a mutually monogamous relationship is the best way to prevent AIDS. If that's not possible, use a condom and avoid promiscuous practices. Multiple partners and unprotected sex greatly increase your risk of contracting AIDS. Condoms—as long as they don't slip off or break during intercourse—effectively prevent the transmission of HIV from person to person.

Don't share needles or syringes. AIDS is transmitted through the blood and can easily be contracted by injecting yourself with a needle used by another person.

Don't get a blood transfusion just anywhere. Although steriliza-

---

TREATMENT BREAKTHROUGH

DOUSING THE AIDS FLAME

Finding a way to smother the raging wildfire called AIDS may be closer than you think. In fact, there is a good possibility that medications to both prevent and treat the deadly disease may be available by the year 2000.

"I'm not sure there will be a single vaccine. It's possible that there will be a cocktail of vaccines to help the immune system," says Jim Kahn, M.D., associate director of the AIDS program at San Francisco General Hospital.

Researchers are currently working to make it easier for white blood cells to detect and attack proteins attached to HIV, the culprit in AIDS. It's believed that the body may not be able to "see" these proteins, and as a result, the virus can do its deadly work unmolested by the immune system.

Several prototype vaccines are already under investigation. For example, investigators at Walter Reed Army Institute of Research in Rockville, Maryland, were the first to produce a genetically engineered vaccine that seems to stabilize and maybe even boost the immune systems of HIV-infected people.

In one study, 30 volunteers, all infected with the AIDS virus, received injections over ten months. Of the 30, 19 wound up with stable white blood cell counts and produced antibodies to the protein. In other words, in more than half the volunteers, the immune system began detecting an HIV protein that it previously didn't notice.

---

tion techniques and testing for HIV have virtually eliminated the risk of contracting AIDS through blood transfusion in the United States, that's not true elsewhere in the world. "I wouldn't get a blood transfusion in Africa if my life literally depended on it," Dr. Scutchfield says. If you're traveling, consider coming home before undergoing nonemergency surgery.

DESTROYING THE MYTHS

All the evidence about AIDS indicates that the virus can't be passed on by casual contact. But doctors worry that many people are being misled by false beliefs.

For example, some people think you can get AIDS by hugging, kissing or sharing food with someone who is infected. Others believe that having an infected person sneeze or cough at you will transmit the disease. Still others think that you can get the disease by being bitten by insects such as mosquitoes. In truth, there is no evidence that AIDS can be transmitted in any of those ways, Dr. Scutchfield says.

You also can't get AIDS by sitting on a toilet seat. In fact, the AIDS virus is so fragile that it dies almost immediately when exposed to open air, Dr. Scutchfield says. In addition, you can't get AIDS from donating blood, because the sterile needles used to extract blood from your body are only used on you, then discarded.

"That's been a big problem. People associated blood with HIV and stopped donating," Dr. Scutchfield says. "There is absolutely no way you can get AIDS from donating blood."

LOSING THE BATTLE, WINNING THE WAR

Fortunately, for those who do get AIDS, new drugs and improved treatments have increased life span significantly since the disease was first detected. "People who used to die within three months are now living for several years," Dr. Scutchfield says.

Drugs such as zidovudine (AZT), dideoxyinosine (ddI) and dideoxycytidine (ddC) can temporarily halt the replication of the virus in the body, but so far no drug or vaccine has been developed that will eradicate the virus completely. However, more than 88 drugs are in development, and researchers are working on a number of vaccines that may eventually turn the tide in this deadly war.

"I'm very optimistic that in the long run, we're going to find effective AIDS drugs," Dr. Hoth says. "We will get there. We will knock this disease out. But it's not going to happen overnight. It's going to take a while."

ALLERGIES

Can you imagine a world in which everything you thought was safe suddenly packed a potent, even dangerous, punch? For the approximately 40 million Americans who inhabit the world of allergies every day, the simplest things—trimming a tree, taking a walk or going out to dinner—can be rife with risks.

Fortunately, most allergies are mild. Hay fever, for example, the most common allergy of all, rarely causes anything worse than occasional sniffles, headaches or fatigue. But others aren't so harmless. If you're profoundly allergic to bees, for example, or to peanuts, seafood or antibiotics, a touch can be hazardous, even deadly.

There is one foolproof way to beat your allergies, doctors say: Stay away from whatever it is that gives you problems. Sometimes that's easy. If shrimp give you hives, order fish. If cats make you sneeze, buy a dog, a hamster or a goldfish. But what do you do when the very air makes you sick? You can't hold your breath all year! Fortunately, there are more practical ways to beat the allergy blues, as we'll discuss later. But first we'll take a look at the immune system. It's your body's first-line defense against intruders and, if you have allergies, the source of all your allergy woes.

MISTAKEN IDENTITY

Think of the immune system as an alert, powerful army that fights every day on your behalf. When foreign intruders—chemicals, for example, or parasites, viruses or bacteria—get inside your body, special proteins called antibodies evaluate the danger. If they sense that the intruder is harmless, nothing happens. If they sense danger, the immune system mobilizes for the kill.

When you have allergies, the immune system sets its sights on the wrong targets, says Howard J. Schwartz, M.D., a clinical professor of medicine at Case Western Reserve University in Cleveland. Instead of attacking only real enemies, it goes after harmless substances, called allergens, as well. And almost anything can be an allergen: Drugs, plant pollens, mold spores and cosmetics are some common offenders. When the immune system detects one or more allergens, it floods your body with defensive chemicals—histamine, for example—to fight the invaders. But the battle is counterproductive. These chemicals cause a more severe reaction than the allergen could. This reaction may include hives, congestion, inflammation and other irritating symptoms.

"It used to be thought that people with allergies had some sort of bizarre abnormality in their immune system, but that's not true," Dr. Schwartz explains. "It's part of the way that the body rids itself of foreign material. In a way, it's a 'normal' response—but the consequences can make somebody pretty darn sick."

Sometimes the immune system manages to correct itself, and children often lose their symptoms as they get older, Dr. Schwartz says. Unfortunately, allergies more often get worse, not better. In fact, the more you're exposed to a particular allergen, the more sensitive you're likely to become. And finding the source of the problem isn't always easy. This is particularly true of airborne allergens. After all, it's hard to spot something you can't even see.

HAY FEVER AND COMPANY

According to the American Academy of Allergy and Immunology, hay fever inflicts sniffles, headaches and itchy eyes on more than 14 million Americans every year. Of course, most people with hay fever are allergic not to hay at all but to pollens, mold spores and other airborne irritants.

Before your doctor can treat your hay fever, he'll have to know exactly what you're allergic to, says Robert G. Hamilton, Ph.D., associate professor of medicine at Johns Hopkins University School of Medicine in Baltimore and director of the school's Dermatology, Allergy and Clinical Immunology Reference Laboratory. The detective work usually starts with a skin test, in which various allergen extracts—cat pelt, ragweed pollen, even insect venom—are pricked into your skin one at a time to stimulate a response. When a red welt, called a wheal, appears, you'll know what the culprit is—and what to avoid in the future. Of course, you might be allergic to more than one thing, Dr. Hamilton adds.

"Probably the simplest and least expensive way to treat an allergy is to separate the individual from the allergen or the allergen from the individual," he says. It takes a bit of effort, but it can be done. Here's how.

CLEAN AIR ACTS

You can't stop trees and flowers from pollinating, but you can improve the air at home, especially in those rooms where you spend the most time—the bedroom, kitchen and living room. Here are some examples.

Cover your mattress. "We spend a lot of time in bed, where we slough off a lot of skin—and dust mites feed on flaked-off human skin," Dr. Hamilton says. While you can't eradicate these microscopic, and very potent, allergens entirely, you can reduce your exposure to them by topping your mattress with a washable cover.

If your mattress already is a few years old—and consequently is stuffed full of dust mites—it may be too late for a cover. Ask your doctor if a new mattress (with a cover) might be in order.

Vacuum them up. Dust mites flourish not only in bed but also on couches, curtains and carpets. If you vacuum frequently—some may need to do so daily—you can reduce their numbers, says professor of medicine Philip Norman, M.D., also of Johns Hopkins University School of Medicine.

Turn on the cooler. Although you can't see them, most pollen particles are relatively large, about two to three times the size of a red blood cell, Dr. Norman says. "Air conditioning, in both the home and the car, can help, because it filters the incoming air."

Mold spores are somewhat smaller than pollen particles, and they're harder to trap. If you have central heating and air conditioning, you can purchase superfine air filters that will help, Dr. Norman says. You can also buy a device called an electrostatic air purifier, which will trap large mold spores as well as pollen.

Shut the doors. The windows, too, if you want to keep allergy-causing pollen outside where it belongs. Of course, slamming the shutters won't help if every morning you walk the dog, work in the yard or for any other reason gulp the allergen-laden air. Many plants and trees do most of their pollinating early in the morning. It's a good idea to stay inside during those high-exposure times.

Beware of kitty. For some people, our feline friends are allergy-causing trouble, Dr. Norman says. "I don't know of any way to counteract it," he says. "Tabby has to go." But cat dander is tenacious, he adds. Even if you send Tabby to friends in the country, it may take several months before the air is clear again.

Keep things dry. Mold, and its allergy-causing spores, thrives in basements and garages, under sinks and on bathroom floors. You can fight back by repairing water leaks as soon as they occur.

Escapees always get caught. Some people get so tired of battling their allergies that they simply pack up and move. Moving can work—for a while. But people with hay fever commonly develop new sensitivities wherever they go, Dr. Norman says. So even if you escape birch pollen in the Southeast, you may get caught by Colorado sagebrush or Montana thistle. Even Arizona, long considered the country's allergy-free zone, is showing signs of infiltration.

ASSUAGING THE SNIFFLES

It's not always practical—or even possible—to eliminate from your world the allergens that make you sick. Besides, you don't want to run. You want to fight. Antihistamines are the surest way to go for the kill. These powerful drugs, available over the counter and by prescription, work by blocking the action of histamine, a key player in your allergic reactions. It's important to note that antihistamines are better at preventing symptoms than at relieving them, Dr. Norman says. To get the best results, take them *before* your allergies flare.

It's also important to remember that histamine isn't the only chemical your body releases that causes allergy symptoms, Dr. Norman adds. So even if you regularly take antihistamines, you still need to avoid whatever it is that's triggering your problems.

Antihistamines, however, are not without their side effects. They have the potential to knock *you* out, too—or at least make you logy. Although the newer antihistamines are less sedating than their predecessors, they can still cause fatigue, dryness of the mouth or digestive disturbances. If antihistamines aren't right for you, your doctor may instead prescribe a nose spray charged with steroids. "Steroids for hay fever are about the most useful medication after antihistamines," Dr. Norman says. "They're rapidly metabolized, so they're really quite safe."

If nothing else works for you, your doctor may recommend a three- to five-year series of shots called immunotherapy. The shots, which are often given once a week in the first few months, then usually once a month, contain minute amounts of the allergens you're allergic to. Of course, no one enjoys being a human pincushion year after year, but if you can endure the treatments, you will eventually get some relief, Dr. Norman says. (For more on immunotherapy, see "Immunotherapy and Beyond" on page 15.)

INSECT ATTACKS

If you are allergic to insect venom, a circling bee, wasp or fire ant can be as dangerous as a stranger with a loaded gun. At least 50 people die every year from insect stings, according to the American Academy of

JAMES SMITH: A SHOT SAVED HIS LIFE

James J. Smith of Voorhees, New Jersey, is a father, a private investigator and, at 6 feet 5 inches and 235 pounds, one heck of a big guy. So when he raked up a hornet's nest in his front yard and got stung three times on his hand, arm and face, he didn't worry too much. In fact, he just slapped at the bugs and went back to work. But 10 minutes later his face started swelling . . . and swelling . . . and swelling. After a while, he could barely get enough air to breathe.

"It felt like someone had a rope around my neck and was twisting it—not hard, but very gently—to stop me from breathing," Jim says. "I remember wondering how a little bug could have this great an effect on me." Even then, Jim wasn't particularly concerned. But his son, when he saw his dad's swollen face and hands, was very concerned. He convinced him to get to the emergency room—fast.

It was the right thing to do. When the doctor on duty heard his story, he quickly injected Jim with epinephrine, a powerful drug used to short-circuit the potentially lethal consequences of serious allergic reactions. The drug worked, and Jim quickly recovered. But his doctor gave him a warning: If he ever gets stung again, he could die. In the future, he said, Jim *must* carry his own epinephrine. "I bought one of those self-injectors, but I knew I'd never use it," Jim says. "I mean, how often do you get stung by three hornets at the same time?"

One year later, Jim was in his upstairs bedroom getting dressed for a town board meeting. It was a warm day, and the window was open to catch an afternoon breeze. It wasn't only fresh air that came inside. "When I put my underwear on, out came two bees. They nailed me on the rear end at the same time," he says.

This time, the dizziness and swelling hit almost immediately, and Jim felt as if he were going to pass out. He knew exactly what he had to do. First he swatted the bees. Then he shot a load of epinephrine into his thigh and rushed to the hospital. The doctor gave him yet another shot and the sobering news: If Jim had waited just a few more minutes, he wouldn't have made it.

Jim doesn't wonder anymore if a little bug can truly be so powerful; he knows the answer. That's why he keeps epinephrine injectors on the boat, in the house and in each of his cars. "This is not a drug that just gets rid of a little itching," he says. "This is something that can save your life."

Allergy and Immunology. A great many more deaths probably occur but aren't reported. What's worse, many of the victims may not have known they had an allergy until the message came, quite literally, out of the blue.

This doesn't necessarily mean you have to rush to the emergency room the first time you're stung, Dr. Schwartz says. For most people, it's normal to have some pain, swelling and itching where the stinger goes in. "It's only an allergy when you have a reaction that's remote from the place of the sting," he says.

If you do suspect an allergy—for example, if you get widespread itching or hives or you feel hot and dizzy and have trouble breathing—get to a doctor immediately, Dr. Schwartz says. After that, you need to think about the future, because second and third stings tend to be a lot more serious than the first one. To forestall problems, Dr. Schwartz recommends the following steps.

Keep your shoes on. Bees, wasps, yellow jackets and hornets don't spend their days plotting to nail you. But if you step on one with your bare feet, its reaction is sure to be quite pointed.

Blend in. Like you, insects are attracted to cologne, after-shave lotion and bright colors, Dr. Schwartz says. When you go camping, don't advertise your presence. Eschew fancy fragrances and wear subdued colors, he suggests.

Put away the food. "As you may have noticed when you put out a picnic table, they come from miles," Dr. Schwartz says. To keep hungry insects away from your buffet, cover the food as soon as you're done eating. Mop up spilled soft drinks and cookie crumbs as well.

If you have to spend a lot of time outdoors, you probably should consider immunotherapy, Dr. Schwartz says. "The protection rate has been very high. People who have been restung after completing the treatments don't seem to have any more trouble."

Of course, not all offenders lurk outside. Sometimes the worst enemy can be found right at home, at the same table, even on your plate.

FOOD ALLERGIES

Matt lives a thousand miles from the ocean, but he loves seafood. Crab, lobster, octopus, mackerel—he loves it all. But not scallops. He never, ever eats scallops. "If I eat them, I throw up," he explains. "It happens every time. Even if I only eat one, I'll be in the bathroom all night. I used to like them, but now I don't even like to be in the same room with them."

Actually, food allergies like this are uncommon, probably bothering only two or three people out of a hundred. Scallops and other shellfish are often to blame, although foods as varied as eggs, corn, milk, white fish

IMMUNOTHERAPY AND BEYOND

Many people can arm themselves against their allergies with tissues and antihistamines. Others have to go for the big guns: a series of injections called immunotherapy. If you know that a bee sting can put you in the hospital, or if every spring your symptoms keep you in and out of bed for two months while pollen fills the air, then immunotherapy (or immune therapy) might be the answer for you, says Howard J. Schwartz, M.D., a clinical professor of medicine at Case Western Reserve University in Cleveland.

Here's how it works. After your doctor identifies what you're allergic to—it might be ragweed pollen, insect venom or one of a hundred other things—he will inject you with minute, purified portions of the same substance, Dr. Schwartz says. As the weeks and months go by, he will gradually increase the doses. In time, your body will learn to live with these substances, and you'll start feeling a whole lot better.

But immunotherapy isn't without drawbacks. For one thing, the shots go on—and on and on—for years. They can be very dangerous as well. "You're giving graded doses of precisely that to which they are hypersensitive," Dr. Schwartz explains. "You have to do it very carefully, or you could provoke a bad allergy attack."

Today, researchers are trying to make immunotherapy not only safer but less uncomfortable as well. An obvious improvement would be to do away with the shots, says Philip Norman, M.D., professor of medicine at Johns Hopkins University School of Medicine in Baltimore. Unfortunately, the oral vaccines don't fare so well when they hit the stomach—it's a tough environment in there. For even small portions of the vaccines to survive, very large doses—up to 100 times the amounts normally injected—are needed. "People are paying $300 or more for a year's supply of insect venom," Dr. Norman says. "If you multiply that by 100, then the cost is out of sight." He speculates that the oral vaccines eventually will work, but it may take several more years to perfect them.

In the meantime, to make present treatments safer, researchers are tinkering with the actual molecules that constitute the vaccines. "If the molecules can be changed so that they will stimulate the immune system *without* stimulating the allergy side of it, that's good, that's real good," Dr. Schwartz says.

and peanuts also cause trouble. Some people break out in hives when they eat the wrong foods; others have headaches, diarrhea or nausea. Although it's rare, some people can die from eating the wrong foods.

As with hay fever, the best remedy—in fact, the *only* remedy—for food allergies is to stay away from foods that make you sick, Dr. Norman says. Of course, your doctor will want to be sure you really are allergic to something—that scrumptious, succulent shrimp, for example—before ordering you to give it up for good. Skin tests, this time with isolated food allergens, can usually nail it down.

TRIAL BY ELIMINATION

Unfortunately, people with food allergies are usually allergic not to one food but to whole groups of foods—shellfish, dairy products and certain grains, for example. It can be tricky knowing which food or group of foods is to blame. To find out which foods are friends and which are foes, your doctor may want to put you on an elimination diet.

The first thing he'll ask you to do is to keep a food diary, in which you will list *everything* you eat. (Be specific: Don't write "salad" when you really ate lettuce, tomatoes and onions.) At the same time, you'll keep a careful record of any physical symptoms that may be related to your diet.

Once your doctor narrows the list to a few suspects, you'll start the elimination process. This means that you'll give up, one at a time, the foods that might be causing you trouble. Suppose, for example, you see from your diary that every day you drank milk, you also got a stomachache. For the next week, you'll leave milk alone. If you don't get a stomachache (or whatever other symptoms you've been having), then you may have found the problem.

Of course, you might be allergic to other foods as well, so you may have to repeat this process several times. The only "cure" is to avoid the foods you're allergic to. Occasionally, however, people do become less sensitive. After a few months—or a few years—you can invite the banished foods, a little bit at a time, back to your table to see if things have changed.

Immunotherapy doesn't work for food allergies. If your symptoms are severe, you should wear a medical-alert bracelet identifying your condition, Dr. Norman says. Your doctor might also prescribe a self-injector loaded with epinephrine, a lifesaving drug commonly used for allergy-related emergencies, that you can carry with you.

ALTITUDE SICKNESS

U ntil recently, altitude sickness was something of a rarity. People didn't zip to Aspen for weekend ski trips. And serious climbers only ascended as fast as their feet would take them.

Things changed with modern transportation. Today's hikers, skiers and climbers can shoot from sea level to mountaintop in no time. They don't have time to adjust to changes in altitude, a process called acclimatization, says Benjamin D. Levine, M.D., an assistant professor of medicine at the University of Texas Southwestern Medical Center in Dallas and director of the Presbyterian Institute for Exercise and Environmental Medicine. "Anyone can get altitude sickness if they go up to high enough altitudes fast enough," he says.

HIGH ALTITUDE, LOW OXYGEN

Altitude sickness is caused by the low levels of oxygen available at high altitudes. Nearly 700 years ago, the explorer Marco Polo noted that high mountain air could be "so unwholesome and pestilential that it is death to any foreigner." The air at your favorite ski resort isn't so hazardous, of course. Indeed, says Dr. Levine, the vast majority of people who get sick at high altitudes will have only mild symptoms—headache, fatigue, nausea and loss of appetite.

Altitude sickness generally sets in within 12 to 48 hours of arrival at your high-altitude destination, gets worse during the night, then gradually improves as your body gets accustomed to the diminished oxygen stores. "For skiers going to Colorado, 25 or 30 percent of them will have some symptoms of altitude sickness, and some will lose skiing or vacation time because of it," Dr. Levine says. The risk is proportional to the altitude achieved. In studies in the Swiss Alps, researchers found that 13 percent of the people who climbed to 10,000 feet experienced altitude sickness. At 15,000 feet, the number jumped to 53 percent.

While the symptoms are usually mild, altitude sickness will occasionally cause disorientation, hallucinations and edema—the accumulation of fluid in the lungs or brain. Untreated, this edema can be fatal, Dr. Levine says. So don't take chances your first day on the slopes. You *can* protect yourself—if you follow the rules.

The Lowdown on Going High

To prevent altitude sickness, Dr. Levine says, you need to pace yourself. For starters:

Climb high, sleep low. The severity of altitude sickness largely depends upon the altitude at which you sleep. "If you can, spend your first night at lower altitudes—say, below 7,000 feet," Dr. Levine says. "For example, someone going to ski in Keystone, Colorado (9,000 feet), could spend the first night in Denver or Colorado Springs (5,000 feet)."

Ascend slowly. Above 8,000 to 10,000 feet, doctors say, you should allow one acclimatization day for each 2,000 feet you ascend. Indeed, going slowly is such an integral part of climbing that experienced mountaineers may take weeks to make a long ascent.

Pace yourself. Doing hard exercise soon after arriving at altitude often triggers symptoms. For example, people who ski hard their first day, then stay up dancing all night, are asking for trouble, Dr. Levine says. It's better to take it easy the first day, get a good night's sleep, then conquer the mountain the second or third day.

Bag the salt. Even mild cases of altitude sickness seem to be accompanied by slight edema, resulting in the swelling of tissues. You can fight edema by eating less salt and by drinking lots of water.

Can the beer. The sleeping pills, too. "Alcohol and sedatives, by slowing breathing, can aggravate the effects of altitude," says Dr. Levine.

Fill up on carbs. Unlike high-fat, high-protein foods, carbohydrates such as rice and potatoes help your metabolism work more efficiently, which can make it easier to get more oxygen at high altitudes.

Go down. This is the one sure cure for altitude sickness. Once people descend a few thousand feet, Dr. Levine says, they usually start feeling better within minutes or hours.

A Tip on Drugs

To prevent altitude sickness, prescription drugs such as acetazolamide and nifedipine work quite well, but they are not routinely recommended unless an individual has a previous history of altitude sickness.

For treatment, perhaps the most powerful drug is a steroid called dexamethasone, which can quickly relieve most symptoms. Because of possible side effects, however—ranging from high blood sugar to disorientation—dexamethasone is recommended only for emergencies, says Dr. Levine.

DISEASE
FREE

ALZHEIMER'S DISEASE

Were you to meet John Rawlings—67 years old, handsome, bright-eyed and athletic—you'd never suspect anything was wrong with him. But when he speaks, John hesitates, searching for the right words.

"Well," you might say, "he's a lawyer; he's trained to choose his words carefully." And you'd be right—but not totally right. The real reason for his hesitation is that sometimes John can't *find* the right words, and it's happening more and more often.

That's because John has Alzheimer's disease. And trouble with speech is one of the early symptoms.

THE DISEASE OF THE CENTURY

At age 67, John is a prime target for Alzheimer's. That's because it is a disease that strikes the aging. "We're seeing more people get the disease, partly because they're living longer and partly because it's easier to recognize, since we know more about it than we used to," says Rachelle Doody, M.D., assistant professor of neurology at Baylor College of Medicine in Houston. Unfortunately, the longer you live, the more likely it is you'll get Alzheimer's—one in ten if you're over age 65, up to almost one in two if you're 85 or older. These rates add up to four million Americans who, like John, increasingly can't find the right words.

But the disease doesn't end with forgetfulness. It also kills 100,000 Americans each year—often after reducing them to a vegetative state.

Alzheimer's ravages the brain. Some scientists theorize that brain cells are destroyed by beta amyloid, a splinter of protein that has no known function but is known to accumulate in the brain as years go by. This protein is found in greater amounts in the brains of people with Alzheimer's. Whatever causes this process of destruction, the cells involved in memory are usually the first to go.

That's why forgetfulness is a key symptom in the onset of this disease. Not the kind of forgetfulness in which you forget the name of an acquaintance you see twice a year or where you put the car keys, but the kind in which you forget your wife's name or what the car keys are for.

And because so much of our emotional state is controlled by chemicals in the brain, other symptoms may eventually include a change in personality: Restlessness and insomnia may set in, and there may be wild swings between tears and laughter, affection and paranoia, sweetness and rage. The deterioration may continue to the point where the person becomes mentally and physically incompetent.

THE ALL-IMPORTANT DIAGNOSIS

A correct diagnosis is always important. But a correct diagnosis is particularly important when Alzheimer's is suspected, because other *curable* illnesses can masquerade as this deadly disease, says Warren Strittmatter, M.D., associate professor of neurology at Duke University Medical Center. Small strokes, hormone insufficiencies, infections and nutritional deficiencies such as pernicious anemia can all cause symptoms that mimic Alzheimer's. But they can be cured, while Alzheimer's cannot.

Using brain scans, interviews with family members, physical and psychological examinations, lab tests and neurological testing, doctors have a 90 percent accuracy rate in diagnosing Alzheimer's. And they're expected to get even better, says neuroanatomist Creighton Phelps, Ph.D., vice president for medical and scientific affairs of the Alzheimer's Disease Association. "Our goal is to develop tests sensitive enough to detect the abnormal proteins associated with Alzheimer's in spinal fluid before the disease gets a real foothold."

An early diagnosis not only would reduce uncertainty for patients and their families but also would give patients a chance to slow or minimize symptom development by taking part in experimental treatments.

TAKING CONTROL

Despite his tragedy, John Rawlings is moving ahead with his life. He's gradually winding up his law practice. He's reaffirming ties of affection with family and friends. He's traveling to places he has always wanted to see. He's getting counseling. And he's avidly following the discoveries in the burgeoning field of Alzheimer's research, where there's always plenty going on.

Although there is no cure for Alzheimer's today, one experimental treatment that shows promise is the drug tetrahydroaminoacridine, or THA. By stopping the breakdown of the memory chemical acetylcholine, THA seems to produce a small but real improvement in some of the people who take it—especially in those in the early stages of Alzheimer's.

The drawbacks of THA? It can cause liver damage, which can be reversed only by reducing or stopping the drug, and it doesn't stop the progress of the disease—it simply slows it down.

On another research front, scientists are seeking medications to block an enzyme that helps make proteins that build up in the plaques and tangles left behind by beta amyloid's destructive trip through the brain. And other researchers are working with drugs that may be able to keep the brain cells from dying.

Experimental drugs aren't the only treatment available. Often supportive therapy for people with Alzheimer's and their families can also be helpful, says Lisa Gwyther, assistant professor of psychiatric social work at Duke University and director of the school's Alzheimer's Family Support Program. A caring professional may help ease the fear, uncertainty and depression that frequently overwhelm those with Alzheimer's—and may help them come to terms with the disease process.

YOU AS CAREGIVER

If a loved one has Alzheimer's, you may find yourself in the role of caregiver. You may get angry, depressed and anxious about your future and generally overwhelmed by the problems. You may rarely get a good night's sleep. "Taking care of a loved one with Alzheimer's can be like running a marathon without ever seeing the finish line," says Gwyther. But it can be a lot less frustrating, and you can be a more effective caregiver, once you learn how to do the job right.

Handling the initial diagnosis is a good place to start developing your new skills. The words "You have Alzheimer's disease" may be frightening, depressing and embarrassing to the person who hears them. How you react is all-important, Gwyther says. "You don't rub their nose in it. What frightens the person with Alzheimer's most is that they'll lose their value to their family. You have to constantly remind them of what they can still do, that they are loved and appreciated and that they won't be abandoned."

In some ways, a person with Alzheimer's may behave like a child, but Gwyther warns against seeing them that way. "You can't have the expectation that they'll grow up and become more independent like children do. The person with Alzheimer's remembers he's an adult and is very sensitive to put-downs and childlike treatment." *Never* talk about him like he's not there.

One common difficulty is dealing with your loved one's sometimes erratic behavior. "Often the person isn't even aware of how he's behaving or its effects on you," says Gwyther. "Always remember that it's brain damage and not ill will that causes the behavioral changes.

"Another hard thing to accept may be the loss of intimacy and conversation," she adds. You may have to change your expectations. Whenever you try to communicate with him, be sure to remember what he's going through, speak slowly, give one brief thought at a time and limit distracting or confusing noises. He can quickly forget anything; he may hear something yet not be able to act on it; or he may understand what you tell him in person but not what you say over the phone. Always be calm, reassuring and supportive.

SEEKING SUPPORT

A big problem for many families of people with Alzheimer's "is admitting their need for outside help or support," says Gwyther. "For many it may be the first time they've ever had to ask for help. They may be too proud. They may be embarrassed by their spouse's behavior. They may think 'No one can care as much as I.' They think they don't have the money. They want to do the right thing but may fight over what that is. They don't have enough information, or they may have too much *misin*formation."

Despite the vast increase in public awareness about Alzheimer's, Gwyther says, what hasn't changed is the use of outside services. "Most people use *no* outside help at all, even though they may be dealing with Alzheimer's for 10 to 15 years," she says. But help is there.

Nurses, for example, not only can help care for your loved one, they also can teach you the kind of practical tips that make care easier. A nurse or nutritionist can help you when feeding becomes a problem: Often a person with Alzheimer's forgets how or what to eat or may refuse to eat certain essential foods. Transportation services may take someone with Alzheimer's to and from adult day care or senior centers. A social worker can help you get the financial assistance available in your state. Day care staff can help the person with Alzheimer's enjoy life with supervised exercise, entertainment and social programs. Home care workers can help you with shopping, housework, bathing and cooking. Short-term residential care facilities can give you a few days' break from the stress.

And not all team players have to be pros. "Friends, relatives and neighbors are free," Gwyther says, even if it's just to relieve you long enough for a trip to the store or a movie. Groups you already belong to—churchs, clubs, work—can function as support groups. And of course, there are the many support groups devoted exclusively to Alzheimer's disease. Your local Alzheimer's Association—listed in the Yellow Pages under "Social Services" or in the Blue Pages under "Aging" or "Alzheimer's"—is the place to start.

Despite the strain of being a caregiver for a person with Alzheimer's, "heroism is much more common than defeat," Gwyther says. "Caregiving is a normal part of living. A lot of people do it all and do it well. But there are no saints caring for those with Alzheimer's. If you need help, ask."

ANAL AILMENTS

Poets have long praised the body. They praise the feet ("How beautiful are thy feet with shoes, O prince's daughter!"), the lips ("Thy lips are like a thread of scarlet") and nearly everything in between. Everything, that is, but the anus. Indeed, there's little about this strong little muscle that stirs the poetic soul. But the anus, most of the time, *is* worthy of praise.

Consider: The anus is the last link in your digestive chain. It prevents outside things from getting in. More important, it lets *inside* things out—and can do it on command. But the anus is also temperamental, prone to develop such ailments as fissures and abscesses. Sometimes, for no good reason, it'll itch like the dickens. While unpleasant, these problems are rarely serious. Better yet, they can often be prevented.

ANAL FISSURES

Even people who routinely forget lunches, birthdays and anniversaries can remember, years later, the exact *second* they got an anal fissure. "It can be excruciatingly painful when you move your bowels. People say that it feels like they're passing cut glass, or a knife, or something like that," says Scott D. Goldstein, M.D., an assistant professor of surgery at Jefferson Medical College in Philadelphia.

A CRUEL CUT

The lining of the anus is remarkably elastic, but it can stretch only so far. Should you pass an unusually large and hard stool, the lining can tear, Dr. Goldstein explains. The tears are rarely deep, but they can be painfully slow to heal. And until they do, each bowel movement will remind you that something below has gone terribly wrong.

The younger you are, and the narrower and more unyielding your anal canal is, the more likely you are to get fissures. As you age, your gastrointestinal tract gets progressively weaker—and your risk for fissures goes down. "The people who get fissures often are very young," says Steven D. Wexner, M.D., director of the Anorectal Physiology Laboratory at Cleveland Clinic Florida in Fort Lauderdale. "They often have a low-fiber, high-junk-food diet, they're always on the move and deferring the call of nature, and they end up getting constipated."

And constipated, when it comes to anal fissures, is the last thing you want to be. This is because constipation invariably is followed by the passage of one or more large, hard stools—precisely the type that cause fissures, Dr. Wexner says. When you already have a fissure, a hard stool can make the tear—and the pain—that much worse. If the fissure is deep enough, it can bleed, and when you see blood, Dr. Goldstein warns, it's time to see your doctor.

RELIEVING THE PAIN

Even though the bleeding that comes from a fissure is rarely serious, the bleeding caused by other problems—cancer, for example—is very serious. You can't be sure which it is until your doctor takes a look. Diagnosing a fissure is simple. In most cases, your doctor can make a visual diagnosis.

Treating a fissure is equally simple, Dr. Goldstein says. For most people, time, plus a high-fiber diet to soften the stool, will give the fissure a chance to heal—and prevent additional fissures from forming.

Fight fissures with fiber. A high-fiber diet swells, softens and moistens the stool, reducing friction as the stool makes its journey through the anal canal. Simply by eating several servings of fruit, vegetables and whole grains—doctors recommend you eat 20 to 35 grams of dietary fiber a day—you can ease the pain and prevent new fissures from forming.

Bring on the bran. Adding a little oat, wheat or rice bran to your diet by sprinkling it over food or stirring it into water or juice is a quick way to boost your fiber power. Bran was once sold only in health food stores, but it is now available in grocery stores, too. Two tablespoons of oat bran, for example, contains 11.75 grams of fiber—about one-third of your recommended daily amount. Another way to boost your fiber is with a psyllium seed preparation. Be warned, however, that large amounts of fiber, when you're not used to it, can cause gas, cramping and diarrhea. To be on the safe side—and to protect your social life—start with 1 teaspoon of bran per meal, and work up from there.

Water it down. Of course, all of that fiber, like so much sawdust, will soak up lots of water in your intestine. To keep yourself—and your stools—lubricated, drink at least six to eight glasses of fluid a day.

Try an OTC. If you can't seem to get enough fiber in your diet, an over-the-counter stool softener containing docusate sodium can help, Dr. Goldstein suggests.

Lube the tube. If you already have a fissure, an emollient can lubricate the anal canal, helping stools slide smoothly past. Some emollients come in suppository form, but as Dr. Wexner points out, "suppositories immediately go up above the anus (where the fissure is) and into the rectum." You're better off applying a dab of emollient, such as petroleum jelly, with the tip of your finger.

Take a sitz bath. Sitting in a tub of shallow, warm water won't make your fissure go away, but many people find it does have a soothing effect on their bottom, Dr. Goldstein says.

As much as your bottom hurts, resist the temptation to apply anesthetic creams, Dr. Goldstein adds. While local anesthetics can deliver short-term relief, "we don't like to use them, because some people can get a reaction that can be much worse than the original problem," he says.

FISSURE FIXERS

In most cases, anal fissures will heal on their own after a few days or weeks. But sometimes they don't heal, and the pain goes on and on. If after a month your bowel movements still feel like cut glass, your doctor may recommend alternative remedies to ease the ache.

The sphincterotomy—the suffix *-tomy* comes from the Greek and means "incision"—is a relatively simple surgical procedure in which the anal canal is cut and slightly enlarged. This allows more room for passing stool, thus reducing the risk for damage. "It's imperceptible to the patient, but it takes the pressure off the fissure and allows it to heal," Dr. Goldstein explains.

Another surgical procedure is called excision. Basically, the surgeon cuts out the old fissure, then sutures the newly cut ends together so that they can heal. Despite some postoperative discomfort, excision works quite well, relieving pain in up to 90 percent of cases.

Although rarely practiced in this country, a procedure called anal stretching has also been known to help. The procedure is simple. Under general anesthesia, the doctor inserts his fingers, one at a time, into the anus. Then for 5 minutes, he dilates—stretches—the anus, which can help "break" the contractions that cause the pain. It also, unfortunately, sometimes results in uncontrolled sphincter muscle damage and consequently in a significant degree of postoperative incontinence. "It's still used to a degree in England and some other countries, but by and large it has been replaced with sphincterotomy, which is a much more controlled way to decrease the pressure," Dr. Wexner explains.

ANAL ABSCESS

You've had boils before, but a zit where you sit? You can't see it, you can't feel it, but . . . owww! It's darned painful! What can you do?

"An anal abscess is on a part of the body that doesn't lend itself to self-examination—although people, believe me, do try!" Dr. Wexner says. But even with mirrors cleverly arranged, you can't tell if an abscess is big or little, mild or serious. Most abscesses are mild, he says, but others can be quite serious.

A PAINFUL PROBLEM

An anal abscess, Dr. Goldstein explains, is very much like a boil. "It doesn't start on the surface of the skin, it starts underneath and then comes to the surface," he says. In other words, by the time you know something is wrong, that abscess already has a head start. Here's what happens.

The anus is surrounded by 6 to 12 glands that secrete the mucus that keeps the anus lubricated. But sometimes—after a bout with diarrhea, for example—the glands become infected. The resulting infection can cause the glands to swell, fester and fill with pus. At the same time, you start looking for excuses not to sit down.

Untreated, an abscess will often "point" within a few days, then rupture on its own. But the waiting, Dr. Wexner says, can be painful. It can also be dangerous, because there's no guarantee that an abscess will only move toward your skin. While you wait for it to point, it may be burrowing in the *reverse* direction, toward the inside of your rectum.

ENDING AN ABSCESS

The pain is what drives people to seek help as soon as possible. "An abscess hurts all the time," Dr. Wexner says. "It's going to hurt when you sit on it, and it's going to hurt when you're not sitting on it." The solution? "You have it drained," he says. "Usually your doctor can drain it right then and there in the office."

The relief, he adds, is instantaneous. When the pus drains away, the pain drains away, too. And in most cases, the only drug needed is a local anesthetic, although your doctor may recommend an antibiotic as well.

Occasionally an abscess will continue to spread, burrowing a hole right through the anal tissue. Eventually it can form a fistula, a tunnel that can extend from inside the anus to the skin outside. The result can be a constant—and painful—flow of pus, blood and even stool. "If the gland is chronically infected, you're going to need surgery to clean it out," Dr. Goldstein says.

While as many as half of all abscesses will eventually form fistulas, you may help prevent this by seeing a doctor promptly, he adds.

ANAL ITCHING

Every day, your anus takes a beating. It's constantly exposed to stool and to the many chemicals and irritants that the stool contains. It's rubbed with paper—white and colored, perfumed and plain—scrubbed with soap and wrapped in tight underwear. No wonder it sometimes gets a little itchy.

GLITCHES THAT ITCH

Pruritus ani is a fancy name for one of nature's more common disorders. It means "itchy anus," and it can strike any time the skin's normally protective barriers collapse, letting itchy things in. "Anything that causes a breakdown in the normal skin surface can set up an irritation that results in itching," Dr. Goldstein says.

But pruritus ani is only a symptom. Some of the causes include skin disorders (eczema, psoriasis), parasites (pinworms), inappropriate hygiene (either too vigorous or too lax) or diet (too much coffee or spicy foods). Prolonged diarrhea can also irritate the anal area, as can some of the over-the-counter products people use to treat itching.

Anal itching can be relieved, Dr. Goldstein says, but first you have to know what's *causing* it. Your doctor can help.

ELIMINATE THE ITCH

Perhaps the most common cause of anal itching is diet, says Dr. Goldstein. To get relief:

Cut the coffee. "What I see most frequently is coffee abuse," Dr. Goldstein says. "People sit at work and drink mug after mug of coffee. The oil in the coffee coats the skin around the anal opening, and that's very irritating."

Douse the culinary flames. Avoid spicy foods or foods that are highly acidic, such as tomatoes and citrus fruits, Dr. Wexner suggests.

Change papers. "A lot of toilet tissues contain formaldehyde, which holds the pattern on," he says. Formaldehyde is fine for laboratory frogs, but your bottom doesn't need preserving. If you like patterns, change the wallpaper—but stick with white toilet paper.

Keep the suds simple. As with toilet paper, try to avoid scented or colored soaps, Dr. Wexner says. Also use only one brand of laundry detergent at a time. If one detergent is causing trouble, switch to another.

Turn on the air. After you've washed yourself, dry the area with a hair dryer. Set it on *cool,* naturally.

Dress light. Tight, binding clothes—particularly those made from synthetic fabrics—can trap moisture, which often makes the itch worse. So nix the nylon and wear loose-fitting cotton instead.

Be clean. But don't get carried away. After every bowel movement, give a final wipe with a cotton puff moistened with water. You can follow this with a light dusting of nonmedicated talc to keep the area dry. Whatever you do, don't wipe too hard. "You don't want to do anything to hurt the skin," Dr. Goldstein warns.

Use cream to soothe. Your itch should gradually disappear. In the meantime, an over-the-counter hydrocortisone cream, applied several times a day, is an excellent short-term remedy for itchy inflammation, says Dr. Goldstein. "Most people will experience a great deal of relief, and within a few weeks everything should be back to normal."

ANEMIA

Karen was a dynamo, juggling family outings, work assignments and out-of-town trips with seemingly boundless energy. But sometime around last summer, she noticed, her get-up-and-go had gotten up and gone. She even slipped away from work sometimes to grab a quick nap at home. "I was afraid of getting caught, but I couldn't help it," she says.

Finally, fearing the worst, Karen dragged herself to the doctor. First he took a blood sample. Then he gave her the good news. "You have a touch of iron-deficiency anemia," he said, "and a little boost of iron should do the trick."

LOW OXYGEN, LOW ENERGY

People with anemia have a shortage of red blood cells and hemoglobin, the protein that carries oxygen to cells throughout the body, says Allan Jacob Erslev, M.D., professor of medicine at Thomas Jefferson University Hospital in Philadelphia. In other words, the body doesn't have enough oxygen to work at peak efficiency. The result can be fatigue, mood changes, headaches and heart palpitations.

There are many disorders that can cause anemia, but having too little iron in the blood is the most common cause. This kind of anemia often comes on so slowly that people get used to it and don't even know something's wrong. "But when I give them iron, they suddenly discover they feel so much better," Dr. Erslev says. "The difference can be quite striking."

Are you at risk for iron-poor blood? Let's see.

PEOPLE AT RISK

"In women, iron-deficiency anemia almost always is due to excessive menstrual flow," Dr. Erslev says. Menstruating women typically lose twice as much iron as either men or nonmenstruating women do. And during the nine months of pregnancy, when a baby is growing and sharing the mother's nutrients, they can lose even more.

Although men don't menstruate or give birth, they aren't immune to iron-deficiency anemia. Gastrointestinal bleeding—caused by ulcers, parasites or cancer, for example—can very quickly deplete a man's iron stores. For obvious reasons, doctors of male patients with iron-deficiency anemia tend to be less concerned about the anemia itself than about the underlying problem that's causing it.

It's also possible to become anemic by not eating enough iron-rich foods. Rapidly growing children, particularly fussy eaters, may have difficulty meeting their body's needs. And since the type of iron found in fruit and vegetables is not as readily absorbed as the iron in meat, strict vegetarians who don't take supplements may be slightly more prone to iron-deficiency anemia than meat-eaters.

This doesn't mean you should start taking loads of iron supplements because you *think* you're anemic. Too much iron can cause as many problems as too little. So if you suspect something's wrong, see your doctor. He can tell you how much—or how little—iron you really need.

ANIMAL AND VEGETABLE KNOW-HOW

Before we talk about treating iron-deficiency anemia, let's take a quick look at the two types of iron—heme and nonheme. Although each is absorbed in different ways by your body, both can help you prevent iron-deficiency anemia.

Meats contain a type of iron called heme (pronounced *heem*) iron. Because heme iron is easily absorbed by the body, doctors used to recommend liver as a quick-acting answer to low iron stores. That's because liver is an iron mine, containing as much as 15 milligrams of iron—the Recommended Dietary Allowance (RDA) for women—per 3-ounce serving. But liver is also loaded with cholesterol, an unwelcome addition at today's heart-conscious tables.

Fortunately, there are healthier sources for heme iron than liver and hamburgers, says Elaine McDonnell, staff nutritionist at Pennsylvania State University's Nutrition Center. Lean meats such as chicken, turkey and top round steak (trimmed of fat) all can help you boost your iron stores without contributing unhealthy amounts of fat and cholesterol to your diet.

The second type of iron, nonheme iron, is found primarily in plant foods. Unlike heme iron, it isn't as easily absorbed by the body. Generally, you can expect to absorb 23 percent of heme iron but only 2 to 10 percent of nonheme iron.

However, there's a trick to boosting your absorption of nonheme iron,

McDonnell says. "When you eat foods that have only nonheme iron, try to eat another food at the same meal that's high in vitamin C," she suggests. Vitamin C has been shown to help enhance absorption of nonheme iron. In fact, meat also improves the absorption of nonheme iron, so combining meat and vegetables at mealtimes is an excellent way to put extra iron in the bank.

As you might expect, there are also foods that can block iron absorption. The best examples are tea and coffee. Does this mean you have to give up your favorite brew if you have iron-deficiency anemia? Not necessarily, McDonnell says. Just avoid them within 1 hour after a meal.

Iron Out Anemia

If your blood tests have revealed you're low in iron, there's a good chance you have the medicine you need right at home. Your kitchen is loaded with iron—in the pantry, the freezer and the refrigerator. To stay healthy, men and postmenopausal women need to consume approximately 10 milligrams of iron a day. For women of childbearing age, the RDA is 15 milligrams a day, although pregnant women may need more. Here are some ways to make sure you get enough iron *and* save some up for a rainy day.

Bone up on red meat. It really is a good source of heme iron. Still, you don't want the fat and cholesterol that sometimes go with it. To get the benefits of red meat without the risks, shop for *lean* meats. A lean

---

PICA: THE WORST KIND OF CRAVING

Have you ever had a food craving so powerful that you couldn't resist it? Well, people with a rare condition called pica also have compulsive cravings—not for foods but for unsavory substances such as laundry starch, clay, cigarette ashes or dirt. These bizarre cravings may be caused by iron-deficiency anemia, says Allan Jacob Erslev, M.D., professor of medicine at Thomas Jefferson University Hospital in Philadelphia.

Paradoxically, the cravings of those lacking in iron are not necessarily for substances rich in iron. And it's not always iron-deficiency anemia that causes pica—sometimes pica *causes* iron deficiency. People may eat so much laundry starch, for example, that they're simply too full to consume more normal (and more nutritious) foods.

But pica, when caused by iron deficiency, is easily treated, Dr. Erslev says. Once people with pica are given supplemental iron, the cravings will usually disappear, often within 24 hours.

shoulder-cut pork chop, for example, contains 1.3 milligrams of iron. A 3-ounce serving of chicken breast or turkey breast (without the skin) has about 1 milligram of iron.

As we've learned, the heme iron in meats can boost the absorption of the nonheme iron in cereals, salads and vegetables. So while you're preparing that chicken breast:

Pop a potato in the oven. One tasty, high-iron spud with the skin contains almost 3 milligrams of iron—20 percent of a young woman's RDA.

IRON: GOING TO THE SOURCE

Without sufficient iron, the body can't manufacture enough new blood cells packed with hemoglobin, the red-cell protein that transports oxygen in the blood. Meat is the best source of iron because it contains heme iron, which is readily absorbed by the body. Approximately 50 to 60 percent of the iron in beef, lamb and chicken, as well as approximately 30 to 40 percent of the iron in pork, liver and fish, is

FOOD	PORTION	TOTAL IRON (mg.)
Heme Iron Sources		
Clams, cooked, moist heat	1 doz.	15.10
Oysters, cooked, moist heat	6 med.	5.63
Deer, game meat, roasted	3 oz.	3.80
Tuna, light, canned in water	3 oz.	2.72
Shrimp, cooked, moist heat	3 oz.	2.62
Top round, lean, broiled	3 oz.	2.34
Lamb loin, lean, roasted	3 oz.	2.07
Ground beef, extra lean, broiled	3 oz.	2.00
Chicken leg, roasted	3 oz.	1.31
Pork tenderloin, lean, roasted	3 oz.	1.31
Turkey, light meat without skin, roasted	3 oz.	1.31
Haddock, cooked, moist heat	3 oz.	1.14
Chicken breast, roasted	3 oz.	1.04
Veal loin, roasted	3 oz.	0.73
Salmon, sockeye, cooked, dry heat	3 oz.	0.47

Don't forget the beans. "Beans are a great source of iron," Mc-Donnell says. One serving of navy beans contains 2.3 milligrams of iron, while lentils pack an iron punch of 3.3 milligrams.

Try some chard. This leafy green contains 2 milligrams of iron per 1/2-cup serving. Or for an iron whammy, have some spinach (3.2 milligrams) or beet greens (1.4 milligrams).

Cook it in iron. Those trusty cast-iron pots are more than just versatile kitchen tools. Foods that are cooked in cast-iron pans actually

heme iron. The remainder is nonheme iron, a less readily absorbed form.

Plant foods, such as carrots, potatoes, beets, pumpkin, broccoli, tomatoes, cauliflower, cabbage and turnips, are also good sources of iron, although it's in nonheme form. Absorption of the nonheme iron in legumes (like soybeans) and iron-fortified cereals can be enhanced by combining them with either meat or vitamin C.

Here are your best sources of both heme and nonheme iron.

FOOD	PORTION	TOTAL IRON (mg.)
Nonheme Iron Sources		
Tofu, raw, regular	1/2 cup	6.65
Blackstrap molasses	1 Tbsp.	5.05
Potato, baked with skin	1	2.75
Kidney beans, cooked	1/2 cup	2.58
Lima beans, cooked	1/2 cup	2.08
Spaghetti, enriched, cooked	1 cup	1.96
Hummus	1/2 cup	1.94
Artichoke, cooked	1 med.	1.62
Oatmeal, cooked	1 cup	1.59
Edible-podded peas, cooked	1/2 cup	1.58
Kidney beans, canned	1/2 cup	1.57
Figs, dried	3	1.25
Pearled barley, cooked	1/2 cup	1.05
Prunes, dried	5	1.04
Whole-wheat bread	1 slice	1.00
Raisins	1/4 cup	0.93
Broccoli, cooked	1/2 cup	0.89
Apricots, dried	5	0.83
Romaine lettuce, shredded	1 cup	0.62
Brown rice, medium grain, cooked	1/2 cup	0.52

absorb some of the iron, passing it along to you, McDonnell says.

Fill up on cereals. They're quick to prepare and good to eat, and they can boost your iron. In fact, some 85 percent of ready-to-eat breakfast cereals are fortified—enriched with *added* nutrients. So while a cup of regular oatmeal contains 1.6 milligrams of iron, a cup of fortified instant oatmeal contains 8.3 milligrams. Other fortified cereals contain anywhere from 1.8 to 18 milligrams of iron per serving.

PERNICIOUS ANEMIA: NOW THERE'S A CURE

To have healthy blood cells, you need not only iron but also vitamin B_{12}, a nutrient found in meats, eggs and dairy products. It doesn't take much: Most people need only 2 micrograms (a microgram is one-millionth of a gram) a day. And because B_{12} is so durable—it can remain active in your body for up to three years—a little goes a very long way.

But vegetarians who abstain from eggs and dairy products may be deficient in this essential nutrient. And if you have a condition called pernicious anemia—doctors estimate it affects approximately 1 percent of people over 65—your body can't extract the B_{12} it needs from your diet, says Michael L. Freedman, M.D., professor of internal medicine and director of geriatrics at New York University Medical School. Here's what happens.

There is a protein in your stomach called intrinsic factor (IF) that transports vitamin B_{12} from your stomach to the lining of the small intestine. There the vitamin gets absorbed into your bloodstream. But as people age, they begin producing less IF. The result, Dr. Freedman says, is pernicious anemia, which can cause fatigue, infections, neurological damage and, if left untreated, death.

But pernicious anemia isn't as pernicious as it used to be. "It's one of the most treatable things we have," Dr. Freedman says. For people who don't produce IF, supplemental doses of B_{12}—usually given by injection—will "cure" the disease. (Vegetarians can protect themselves merely by taking B_{12} supplements.) And in the future, some people may not need shots at all, he adds. "Some studies show that if you take massive doses of B_{12}, you can get enough of it even without the injections."

As with iron-deficiency anemia, pernicious anemia isn't a condition you can diagnose yourself. Do not take large doses of vitamin B_{12}—or any other vitamin—without checking with your doctor.

Enjoy some dried fruit. Dried apricots, along with figs, prunes and raisins, also contain healthy amounts of blood-building nonheme iron.

Wash them down with OJ. Taking vitamin C along with your meals can boost your absorption of nonheme iron, McDonnell says. So have some orange juice with your breakfast cereal, or slice a ripe tomato to garnish a leafy lunchtime salad.

Consider a supplement. "When your iron stores get depleted, it can be very difficult to build them up just with a good diet," Dr. Erslev says. Consequently, your doctor may recommend that you take iron supplements along with your high-iron diet. Indeed, some people routinely take iron supplements—during menstruation, for example—to keep pace with normal losses.

While iron supplements are most effective when taken on an empty stomach, they occasionally cause stomach irritation. For this reason, your doctor may suggest you take your supplement with meals, particularly if you have a temperamental tummy.

It's important to remember that taking too much iron can be dangerous. In very large doses, it can cause vomiting, diarrhea, even convulsions. In addition, as many as 1 in 300 people suffers from hemochromatosis, a genetic defect that can lead to iron overload. So don't take iron supplements without checking with your doctor first.

ANXIETY

D o you feel like something horrible is about to happen, but you're not sure what? Do you feel apprehension and dread even when everything around you is peaceful and calm? Do you feel a knot in your gut at the thought of making a speech, catching an airplane or going to dinner with your spouse's boss? If so, you're suffering from an all-too-common condition known as anxiety.

Everyone feels some anxiety. To a certain degree it's natural—even good. But too much anxiety can crush you—mentally and physically. Some of the common symptoms of anxiety are clammy hands, dry mouth, trembling, rapid heartbeat or breathing, headaches and drug or alcohol abuse. Serious cases can bring nausea, vomiting or diarrhea.

For some people, anxiety comes at the drop of a hat, while others feel anxiety only at the drop of a bomb. "Each person has a threshold of sensitivity," says psychiatrist Alexander Bystritsky, M.D., director of the Anxiety Disorders Program at the University of California, Los Angeles. If your threshold is too low, if you're one who gets anxiety at the drop of a hat, you can learn to keep your head on. You can control anxiety.

ERASING YEARS OF FEARS

When it comes to anxiety, you have many treatment options. There's no reason for you to live in fear anymore! The simplest treatments can even be done on your own.

Banish catastrophic thinking. Anxiety can transform ordinary life into a string of catastrophes. But the string can be cut by asking yourself some key questions, says Michelle Craske, Ph.D., assistant professor of psychology at the University of California, Los Angeles. Ask yourself: Am I inflating events and situations, making them into something they're not? Where's the real evidence of impending danger and doom?

Take this scenario: You're an accountant's wife worrying that he's in some danger at the office, so you call him 15 times a day—making him lose all track of his debits and credits. The calls threaten his career and your marriage; they obviously have to stop. Ask yourself: What kind of danger could my husband possibly be in at the office? Has he ever been endangered there before? What are the real odds that he's in danger? If something did happen—say he got smothered in red tape—how bad could it be?

Tape your catastrophe. An excellent way to get a handle on your catastrophic thinking is to make a tape recording of it: Talk into the microphone about the scenario that worries you, all the terrible things you imagine could happen. Then play it back over and over again and discover how you're overworrying, turning the normal into a catastrophe. "When you listen to something repeatedly," Dr. Craske says, "you get used to it, the emotion lessens, and then you're much better able to analyze it rationally."

Learn a relaxation technique. Controlled breathing, progressive muscle relaxation and meditation can all help to alleviate anxiety. Controlled breathing works by taking a deep breath, holding it for a few seconds, then exhaling slowly. Try it three times when you're feeling anxiety, suggests Carol Lindemann, Ph.D., director of the Anxiety Disorders Center of the New York Psychological Center.

Progressive muscle relaxation is simply tensing, then relaxing, every muscle in your body, beginning with your head and neck and continuing on down to your feet—one at a time.

Meditation can be as simple as repeating in your head a "cue" word, like *peace* or *calm,* over and over (perhaps while you do controlled breathing). With practice, you should be able to relax within seconds merely by repeating your cue word to yourself.

Set a goal. Each day you should set a goal—no matter how small—and do your best to achieve it, says Meg McGarrah, former director of the Anxiety Disorders' Self-Help Group Network. Suppose that every time you need to drive, you start to perspire and shake. "One day you might just make yourself sit in the car in the garage," McGarrah says. "When you're comfortable enough with that—it doesn't mean you have lost all fear—back the car down the driveway. Next day, drive around the block. Then to the store. Then on the freeway." Before you start, you may want to practice your muscle relaxation exercises. If it helps, take along a buddy.

Lose control. Most people with anxiety disorders have a control problem, Dr. Craske says. They're perfectionists, they can't delegate responsibility, they're afraid things won't work if they don't do it themselves.

(continued on page 40)

WHEN FRETTING TURNS TO PHOBIA

Frank Hughes is terrified of dogs. The 84-year-old man is convinced that their sole purpose on this earth is to bite him. Large or small, black or white, Doberman or Chihuahua, it doesn't matter. Deep in the heart of every mutt is a secret determination to bite, tear, mutilate or otherwise take a chunk out of Frank Hughes.

That's why Frank makes sure he steers clear of anything on four legs that barks. If he sees a neighbor walking down the street with something attached to a leash, Frank will cross to the other side. If he visits a relative whose dog comes prancing up to the car, Frank will stay in the car until the dog is politely removed.

You could say Frank is afraid of dogs. But Michael Kozak, Ph.D., a psychologist at the Medical College of Pennsylvania's Center for the Treatment and Study of Anxiety, is more likely to say that Frank has a phobia.

Beyond Normal Fear

There are three indications that what you're feeling is a phobia rather than an everyday, run-of-the-mill fear, says Dr. Kozak.

One is that the fear is unrealistic. If you're afraid of ladybugs, for example, your fear just doesn't make any sense.

The second indication is that the fear persists even after you've been given good evidence that you shouldn't be afraid, says Dr. Kozak. Say you walk up to a house with a big dog in the yard. You're afraid the dog bites, so you stop. But the owner comes out and tells you that the dog never bites. He loves people, especially people who look like you.

That information should enable you to change your perception of the dog and go into the yard, says Dr. Kozak. If it doesn't, then your fear may very well be a phobia.

The third indication that you have a phobia is that your fear disrupts your life. If you don't visit your mom because you have to cross a bridge to get to her house, or if you can't take a new job on the 16th floor because you're afraid of elevators, says Dr. Kozak, that's a phobia.

Scientists aren't sure how phobias develop. One theory is that a phobia is a learned response: A dog bites you, and after that, you're afraid of dogs.

Another theory is that since many of us have the same phobias—snakes, small animals and insects are the top three—a phobia may actually be leftover genetics. It may be, says Dr. Kozak, that at some time in our distant past, it was beneficial for us to fear something like a snake so intensely that we avoided it like the plague. We didn't inherit the fear itself, he emphasizes, but we may very well have been biologically programmed to learn it.

Halting the Terror

Should you try to overcome a phobia? Well, that depends on how severely it affects your life, says Dr. Kozak. "I've got a friend who's afraid of bats, for example, but she lives in an urban area. So the only way her phobia disrupts her life is that she won't go into the small animal house at the zoo." Her phobia doesn't disrupt her life in any big way, so she does nothing about it.

When the disruptions are significant, however, you might want to use a simple behavioral technique to get rid of them, suggests Dr. Kozak. The technique is called exposure. All you have to do is periodically expose yourself to whatever it is you're afraid of for an hour or two at a time.

Now walking out into the middle of a bridge high over the water and standing there for a couple of hours might not sound like much to you. But to someone who's afraid of bridges, the thought alone is terrifying.

That's why it's also a good idea to have a friend along during exposure. Friends are helpful in providing a reality check, urging you to stay with it and uncurling your fingers from any railings to which you may become attached.

"What I do is park my car and walk with the patient to the middle of the bridge," says Dr. Kozak. "We stand there for a while, then walk back and forth repeatedly."

It generally doesn't take too many sessions to eliminate the phobia, he adds. But the total number of hours it does take will vary from person to person. There's no magic formula that says this particular fear needs this particular number of hours of exposure.

So what about Frank Hughes? Well, if Frank really wants to get over his fear of dogs, says Dr. Kozak, he should start spending some time around fluffy little puppies.

"Well, you *can't* do everything yourself," she says. "Stop grasping for control. Learn how to say no to people. Set short-term and long-term goals to manage your time, and stick to those goals." Let the world take care of its own problems.

Work it out. When you're feeling anxious, take a fast walk, a jog or a bicycle ride. "Exercise is extremely helpful," Dr. Lindemann says. "Anxiety and panic increase your stress levels, and exercise works off the excess."

Listen to the calm. There are many relaxation audiotapes on the market, and "they're about the easiest and cheapest way to learn to relax," says Dr. Lindemann.

DESPERATELY SEEKING SUPPORT

If you've tried the above tips, yet you're still feeling anxiety, and if that anxiety lasts for a month or longer, then you have a serious case. Mental health experts often refer to such long-term, serious anxiety as "generalized anxiety disorder." If that's not what you have, you may be experiencing a specific kind of anxiety disorder, such as panic attacks (they're just what they sound like) or a phobia. In any case, you'd be doing yourself a big favor if you were to stop trying to cope with the problem alone.

Dr. Bystritsky suggests that you find a therapist who has experience in dealing with anxiety disorders and with whom you feel comfortable. The right kind of therapy may restore your calm in little time. For instance, therapists who use cognitive-behavioral therapy (ask a prospective therapist if he does) can often deal with certain cases of anxiety, such as phobias (wildly irrational fears), in as few as 20 to 30 sessions.

One option you might wish to discuss with your therapist or family doctor is medication. Treating anxiety with drugs has come a long way in recent years. Most anxiety-battling prescriptions belong to a family of drugs called benzodiazepines. "These drugs are intended to eliminate anxiety that is counterproductive, not to create an imaginary world in which tragedy ceases to be tragic," says North Carolina family physician Joseph Talley, M.D. They are designed to relieve the acute anxiety that makes it impossible for you to help yourself or to benefit from therapy.

You might also want to consider joining a support group. If you can't find one, start one. The point of such groups is empowerment, says McGarrah. "It can provide companionship and information. Knowledge is power. A group helps you take charge of your recovery," she says. As a person who has recovered from anxiety symptoms, McGarrah has literally written the book on self-help groups—*Help Yourself: A Guide to Organizing a Phobia Self-Help Group,* available from the Anxiety Disorders Association of America, 6000 Executive Boulevard, Suite 513, Rockville, MD 20852.

APPENDICITIS

Whether you're working in the yard, eating a gourmet meal or just sleeping the night away, your bones, muscles and organs all are working together to get the job done right. All except one, that is. Deep inside your gut, jutting off the end of the large intestine like a small worm, is the appendix.

As far as doctors can determine, this useless organ does only one thing: It gets infected, causing appendicitis.

A DANGEROUS TRAP

Treating appendicitis is pretty straightforward. But before we talk about that, let's take a look at the appendix and see why it causes so much trouble.

We said that the only thing the appendix does is get infected, but that isn't entirely true. As part of the colon, it oozes a steady supply of mucus. Unlike the colon, however, the appendix is quite narrow. This means it readily becomes clogged—from small kinks, swollen tissue or wayward bits of hardened fecal matter called fecaliths.

But even a blocked appendix continues to produce fluids, and that's what makes for trouble, says John Schaffner, M.D., an associate professor of medicine and director of clinical gastroenterology at Rush Presbyterian Hospital–St. Luke's Medical Center in Chicago. Since the fluids can't escape, pressure inside the appendix begins to rise. "This balloon [the appendix] fills up with more and more fluid. Then bacteria invade and cause the infection," he says.

This infection, called appendicitis, can cause fever, nausea and loss of appetite. It also causes pain on the lower right side, between the navel and hipbone. If it's not treated, an infected appendix can rupture, spilling bacteria into the abdominal cavity. This in turn can cause peritonitis, a potentially fatal complication in which the peritoneum, the membrane that lines the abdominal cavity and covers the stomach and intestines, gets inflamed, says William F. Nowlin, M.D., a clinical assistant professor of surgery at Indiana University Medical School.

THE RISE AND FALL OF APPENDICITIS

In antiquity, appendicitis was quite rare. But about 100 years ago it began to occur with increasing frequency in the United States and other Western countries. Then in recent years, it began slipping into decline again.

Some researchers have suggested that dietary fiber is responsible. In countries where much fiber is eaten, people seem to get fewer cases of appendicitis. In this country, where appendicitis is more common, it is *most* common in young people, particularly younger males—and they're typically the ones who eat the least fiber, says Dr. Nowlin.

But the fiber connection is far from conclusive. In a British study, researchers found that children with appendicitis ate approximately the same amounts of dietary fiber—about 19 to 20 grams a day—as did their healthier classmates. So while dietary fiber may play a role in appendicitis, it doesn't seem to be the lead player.

THE KINDEST CUT

Preventing appendicitis may still be a mystery, but how to treat it is not. Doctors treat approximately 250,000 cases of appendicitis every year, and removing the appendix, a procedure called an appendectomy, is one of the most frequently performed operations in the United States. So don't panic when you hear the word *surgery*. Your doctor has had plenty of practice!

It's very important that you see a doctor *before* your infected appendix has had time to rupture. "There is a fair window of opportunity—usually a good 24 to 36 hours after symptoms begin—to get help. It's not like all of a sudden it's going to blow up," says Dr. Schaffner.

In fact, some 15 to 20 percent of the people operated on for appendicitis turn out to have a *normal* appendix. This doesn't mean that surgeons are careless, though. On the contrary, they're eminently careful. But it's a lot safer to remove a healthy appendix than to miss the one that might later prove to be fatal, Dr. Nowlin explains.

ARTHRITIS

When 80 percent of Americans develop some degree of arthritis by the age of 60, you have to wonder why the condition is even considered a disease. Maybe we should just think of it as a natural consequence of aging, like wrinkles and gray hair.

But then young children sometimes get arthritis, as do teenagers and athletes in their prime. In fact, the average age at which arthritis is diagnosed is only 47—hardly over the hill.

Arthritis is a disease all right, and it can strike in many forms. When most people talk of "arthritis," however, they're talking about either osteoarthritis or rheumatoid arthritis—by far the two most common. Both disrupt the normal functioning of the body's joints or the tissue surrounding those joints (as do all forms of arthritis). Osteoarthritis does damage in a wear-and-tear, "degenerative" way. Rheumatoid arthritis does its harm by causing inflammation.

The good news is that research is beginning to show that much can be done to discourage certain types of arthritis from occurring in the first place—osteoarthritis especially, says Harris McIlwain, M.D., a member of the rheumatology group McIlwain, Silverfield and Burnette in Tampa, Florida, and coauthor of *Winning with Arthritis.*

OSTEOARTHRITIS: NOTHING INEVITABLE ABOUT IT

Osteoarthritis, the number one offender, causes pain that tends to be made worse by strenuous activity and relieved by rest. Morning stiffness may occur, but it generally lasts no longer than about a half hour. The pain tends to be localized to one or several joints usually of a weight-bearing type—for example, the hips, knees, ankles, feet or back.

"Osteo" causes deterioration of the cartilage (padding) between bones of weight-bearing joints. This, in turn, can cause bones to rub together, which causes the body to respond by putting out more calcium for the growth of new bone. Whammo—joints begin to find themselves with more bone than they can handle. Some of it ends up forming fingerlike "spurs" called osteophytes. These osteophytes can inhibit joint movement or can chip and leave deposits within joints to aggravate joint movement even further.

What sets this destructive scenario into motion?

"We used to think that osteoarthritis was strictly a wear-and-tear disease brought on by high levels of physical activity or simply age," Dr. McIlwain says. "But now it seems there's often a precipitating factor, either an injury or the chronic overuse of a joint. The joints are like any other part of the body in that there are right and wrong ways to treat them. If more of us could learn to use rather than abuse our joints, osteoarthritis might not be such a widespread problem."

USE VERSUS ABUSE

Here are some tips for being kinder and gentler to your joints, all of which may help prevent osteoarthritis. Even if you already have the disease, these strategies can help minimize your discomfort.

Be active—but not insane. Just because some physical activity is good doesn't mean more is better. Learn to respect your body's limitations in terms of both the frequency and the intensity with which you exercise. Three 20- to 30-minute periods of exercise a week are enough to maintain good cardiovascular health, experts say. If you go beyond that, pay close attention to your joints to be sure they're not complaining about going along with you.

"Regard pain not as the path to success but rather as a roadblock telling you to ease up," says James M. Fox, M.D., medical director of the Center for Disorders of the Knee in Van Nuys, California. It's common to feel some muscular soreness after you've exercised, but it should disappear within a few days. Pain that persists is the kind to watch out for. It means that you're overexerting or that you've got a problem in a joint that repeated activity is only going to make worse. Cut back or change to a less stressful activity such as swimming, Dr. Fox suggests.

Learn the right ways, not the wrong. Proper technique is crucial, whether you're playing tennis, lifting weights or jogging around the block, Dr. McIlwain says. "An activity that is not unduly stressful to a joint if done properly can be downright abusive if done improperly. It's well worth it to get proper instruction. You'll be more successful in your sporting activities, and also more durable."

Don't defeat your feet. Most sporting activities start with the feet, so cushion them well. By wearing properly cushioned, shock-absorbent shoes, you can reduce stress on your weight-bearing joints, Dr. McIlwain says. It's also important to wear shoes that fit well and are specifically designed for the activity for which they're being worn. No deck shoes on the tennis court, please.

Maintain a reasonable body weight. Research shows that excess weight can attack the weight-bearing joints in two ways. Not only do those extra pounds put undue stress on joints directly, they also discourage the kind of active lifestyle needed to strengthen the muscles responsible for protecting the joints.

RHEUMATOID ARTHRITIS: THE UNPREDICTABLE ONE

Rheumatoid arthritis, the number two offender, dishes out pain that tends to worsen following periods of inactivity and to lessen after moderate exercise. Morning stiffness generally lasts longer than a half hour. Pain affects not just one or two joints but numerous joints, and usually on both sides of the body. And the joint pain may be accompanied by other, more generalized discomforts.

Rheumatoid arthritis can be especially problematic because it tends to be a "whole body" disease, capable of causing not just painful joints but also fever, weight loss, fatigue, anemia and even depression.

Precisely why this happens remains unclear, although the prevailing suspicion is that rheumatoid arthritis in some way causes the body's immune system to turn on itself. Harmful substances are released within the joints that not only harm the silklike sheathing (synovial membrane) responsible for keeping joints free-moving but also spark toxic reactions elsewhere in the body.

Also characteristic of rheumatoid arthritis is the youthfulness of its target audience. The disease tends to strike people in their twenties through forties. For reasons unknown, it is three times more likely to strike women than men.

"We're making advances, but rheumatoid arthritis remains a mysterious disease," Dr. McIlwain says. "Sometimes it goes no farther than causing joint pain, but other times it's more problematic. Unlike osteoarthritis, which is fairly predictable, rheumatoid arthritis is not."

Rheumatoid arthritis, because it is such a mystery, is also difficult to know how to prevent. But we *can* tell you how to prevent many of the symptoms.

FOR GENERAL ARTHRITIS RELIEF: GET MOVING

Whether it's osteo, rheumatoid or almost any other form of arthritis, the best way to achieve relief can be summarized in a single word: you.

This is not to say that medication or perhaps even surgery may not also be required, but "how much personal responsibility you take for management of your condition is the key to success," Dr. McIlwain says. "Applications of moist heat, daily exercise and appropriate rest periods can make the difference between controlling arthritis and having it control you."

Let's look at that prescription one element at a time.

Apply a touch of heat. Heat gives relief by helping to loosen the muscles, ligaments and tendons that surround a joint. "This facilitates joint movement and is especially advisable prior to exercising an arthritic joint," Dr. McIlwain says. "It's a little like warming the honey before trying to pour it. Not just the muscles and connective tissue but the lubricative fluids within a joint operate more smoothly when warm."

Moist heat works best—a shower, a bath, wet towels, a whirlpool or a moist heating pad. Heat should be applied for 10 to 15 minutes at least twice daily.

TREATMENT BREAKTHROUGH

BONING UP OUR DEFENSES

Considering the number of people affected by arthritis, you can bet that any medical breakthroughs in treating this disease will be greeted with much enthusiasm. Talk to researchers in the field, and you can sense *their* enthusiasm.

The progress being made in understanding arthritis is "very encouraging," says Steven Friedman, M.D., professor of medicine at the Hospital for Special Surgery and Cornell University Medical College in New York City. "Research at the most basic molecular level is now showing us the processes by which many types of arthritis work. Hence it should only be a matter of time before drugs can be developed that safely alter selective processes."

In most inflammatory types of arthritis, such as rheumatoid arthritis, inflammation appears to be the result of an attempt by certain well-meaning T-cells (key players of our immune system) to wage war against what they perceive to be a foreign invader—which is, in fact, your own joint tissue. "It's as though the T-cells call in the army, the navy, the marines and even the air force when just the army might do," Dr. Friedman says. "This creates a kind of molecular chaos, resulting in inflammation that winds up doing more harm than good. The new drugs being worked on attempt to reduce this hypervigilance."

Particularly effective for arthritic hands or feet is a "paraffin bath," a mixture of paraffin (a waxy substance) and mineral oil into which hands or feet are dipped, thus receiving a warm coating. A towel can then be wrapped around the hand or foot to insulate it further. (Check with your doctor for the device that prepares the paraffin/mineral oil mixture, available at most medical supply stores.)

"The form of heat that works best and is easiest to apply is the method to use," Dr. McIlwain says. "Let your comfort and convenience be your guide."

Add a little cold. For added benefit, ice can be applied in conjunction with heat therapy—10 to 15 minutes of heat followed by 10 to 15 minutes of ice. Put the ice in a plastic food bag or a standard ice bag, available at most pharmacies. Never apply ice to skin directly. "The hot/cold alternation can be especially effective during flare-ups when pain is unusually bad," Dr. McIlwain says.

Other types of inflammatory arthritis are caused by direct infection of the joints. Here early intervention with antibiotics will continue to be the mode of cure, Dr. Friedman says. The future, however, is sure to bring antibiotics more fine-tuned to specific infecting organisms.

Also promising is research into drugs capable not just of protecting but of actually helping to rebuild cartilage worn away by osteoarthritis. Surgical techniques for replacing joints destroyed by osteoarthritis also continue to be improved. "The most exciting development in this area is the success being achieved with artificial joints," says Paul Lotke, M.D., professor of orthopedic surgery at the University of Pennsylvania School of Medicine. "The joints are designed with tiny holes on their surface, so that the bone to which they're being attached can actually grow into them, thus eliminating the need for cement, which over time can lose its grip."

Also progressing by leaps and bounds is the use of computer technology to custom-design joints if necessary to be exact replicas of those being replaced, Dr. Lotke says. A computerized series of x-rays (CAT scan) is done of the existing joint, which then becomes the blueprint for its precise duplicate. "You get a much better fit for the most complicated problems this way, and a much better chance for success," says Dr. Lotke.

Work up a little sweat. Earlier you learned that exercise is one of the best ways to prevent arthritis. It's also good treatment.

Many doctors used to tell those with arthritis not to exercise. Not anymore. Accumulating research shows that aerobic exercise—the kind that gives the heart a workout—helps people with arthritis.

Aerobic exercise actually reduces joint pain. It also increases strength and aerobic capacity (our ability to take in air and circulate blood). And it may improve more subjective concerns, such as mood and social activity.

If your doctor approves, try walking, dancing, swimming or, if knee disease isn't severe, bicycling. (Stationary bikes are best unless you ride on flat terrain.)

A good place to start is with the Arthritis Foundation's PACE (People with Arthritis Can Exercise) program. You can get the program's home videotapes, or you can participate in a class taught by trained instructors. Contact your local foundation chapter or write to P.O. Box 19000, Atlanta, GA 30326. Ask for brochure number 9763, which tells how to do exercise safely. The brochure is free.

Pump a little iron. While you're working out aerobically, you should also get some pump into your routine. "For years we thought that exercises that improve flexibility and range of motion were enough, but now it appears that building strength around a joint may be just as important," says Dr. McIlwain. Adding weight lifting to your exercise program is the way to do it. Be sure to see your doctor first, however, to be sure your condition would benefit. It may also be advisable to begin your weight lifting under the guidance of a physical therapist, who can prescribe a variety of exercises specific to your particular case.

Rest deeply. Aha! So the game plan against arthritis is not one of all work after all. "There are times to exercise joints and times to rest them," Dr. McIlwain says. "If a joint is going through a period of especially acute inflammation or pain, it should be rested. If many joints are involved, a brief period of bed rest may even be required."

Short of that, however, even just 15- to 30-minute periods of lying down (once in the morning and once in the afternoon) can help during especially painful times. It's also wise to learn to pace yourself when doing chores, taking short rest periods intermittently during an activity rather than pushing through to finish uninterrupted. Proper rest is also important at night, Dr. McIlwain says. He recommends up to 10 hours' bed rest a night during times when pain and fatigue are especially severe.

Don't say no to sex. According to at least one study, 70 percent of those with arthritis may experience up to 6 hours of pain relief following sex. "Two reasons have been suggested to explain this phenomenon," says Warren A. Katz, M.D., chief of the Division of Rheumatology and chairman of the Department of Medicine at Presbyterian Medical Center in Philadelphia. "One is that sexual intercourse triggers a surge of cortisone that helps reduce the inflammation and pain in a joint. It's also possible that brain chemicals called beta-endorphins, released during orgasm, help reduce pain." Dr. Katz suggests not going into a bout of romance cold, however. "Allow time for a warm shower or bath beforehand," he says.

ANTI-ARTHRITIS MEDICATIONS

Along with daily heat treatments, exercise sessions and appropriate rest, getting on the right regimen of medication can also combat arthritis. "Drugs shouldn't be relied on solely, but they can serve as a helpful adjunct to the other modes of therapy," Dr. McIlwain says. "It's important to find the medication that works best for a particular condition, however, and has the fewest side effects."

Medications most effective against arthritis fall into three basic categories—those that fight the inflammation of arthritis (called anti-inflammatories), those that attack primarily the pain (analgesics) and those that combat muscular tension. In extreme cases, combinations of the three types may be used, but it's always best to seek the simplest treatment plan possible to reduce the risk of side effects, Dr. McIlwain says.

ANTI-INFLAMMATORIES. These come in two basic forms. The powerful but also potentially dangerous cortisone derivatives are available by prescription only (generic names include prednisone, methylprednisolone, triamcinolone and dexamethasone). The much safer though less potent noncortisones are generally available over the counter. Ibuprofen is among this group, as is aspirin, although these medications have pain-reducing and anti-inflammatory capabilities combined.

ANALGESICS. These treat primarily the pain caused by arthritis and can be especially helpful during flare-ups, when pain may be severe. Many are available over the counter (acetaminophen sold as Tylenol, Datril, Panadol or Anacin-3, for example), while the more potent ones require a doctor's prescription. Codeine is in this group, as is propoxyphene.

MUSCLE RELAXANTS. These can be helpful when arthritis causes muscle spasms that produce pain separate from the arthritis itself, which occurs in cases usually involving the back or neck. Caution must be used when taking muscle relaxants, however, as dependency can develop rather quickly. Available by prescription only, diazepam (Valium) and cyclobenzaprine (Flexeril) are two common types.

THE ANTI-ARTHRITIS DIET

Can dietary changes alter the course of arthritis?

After years of skepticism, scientists finally seem to be looking positively at that question. "What you eat may make a difference in quenching the fires of both kinds of arthritis," says George L. Blackburn, M.D., Ph.D., an associate professor of surgery at Harvard Medical School and chief of the Nutrition/Metabolism Laboratory with the Cancer Research Institute at New England Deaconess Hospital in Boston.

Most encouraging has been research into the effects of a class of fatty acids called omega-3's, prevalent in oil-rich fish such as salmon, tuna, halibut, herring, mackerel, whiting and sardines. One study using fish-oil capsules found that sufferers of rheumatoid arthritis experienced reductions in joint stiffness of 33 percent after taking 15 capsules daily for 14 weeks. They also reported being free of fatigue for 2½ hours longer each day. Omega-3's work, researchers speculate, by helping to reduce inflammation caused by a hormonelike substance called leukotriene, the same culprit that anti-inflammatory drugs such as aspirin work to counteract.

But might the same effects be achieved by eating fish instead of taking fish-oil capsules?

Yes, says Dr. Blackburn. The key seems to be in reducing another

---

PROFILE IN HEALING

PETER GATEWOOD: GETTING A LEG UP ON ARTHRITIS

He had excelled in soccer, football, basketball, baseball and tennis in both high school and college. But at the age of 22, Peter Gatewood suddenly found that he could barely crawl to the bathroom.

"That's how much pain I was in," Peter recalls of the rapid onset of arthritis in his feet. "It started as a feeling of stiffness, but within a few weeks I could barely walk."

So severe was Peter's condition that he was forced to break off his studies at Pennsylvania State University, where he was just a semester away from receiving his bachelor of arts degree in English literature. "The pain was most concentrated in my feet, but my whole body felt drained," he says.

When Peter returned to his hometown of Philadelphia for an examination, he was told he had osteoarthritis concentrated mainly in the joints of his large toes, a condition that his doctor felt was the result of heredity plus years of athletic abuse. Both of Peter's parents suffered from arthritis, and the rock 'em, sock 'em sporting life Peter had led probably created an overload that his predisposition was unable to handle.

Peter's treatment involved injections of cortisone directly into the

class of fatty acids called omega-6's (prevalent in fried foods, most vegetable oils and margarine) while increasing intake of omega-3's at the same time. "If you pay close attention to your diet, reducing vegetable oils and eating fresh or canned fish several times a week, you'll probably achieve good results without having to take fish-oil supplements," Dr. Blackburn says. Note that two vegetable oils *low* in omega-6's are canola oil and olive oil, so use these for your cooking and salad dressing needs. Note, too, that good nonfish sources of omega-3's are soybeans and tofu; include these in your diet for an additional pain-relieving boost.

But the benefits of a fish-rich diet don't stop at omega-3's, Dr. McIlwain points out; there's the calorie advantage. "Not only can people help reduce their inflammation, they can help reduce excess weight that may be contributing to their pain. Most fish, even the type rich in oil, is considerably lower in calories than equivalent amounts of beef or pork."

For best results, fish should be baked, broiled or poached—not fried—and canned fish should always be purchased packed in water rather than vegetable oil, when possible.

---

affected joints—"certainly not a pleasant experience," he recalls, and one that would be a temporary solution at best. "The injections helped relieve the pain and swelling, but I knew they were only masking the symptoms. I wanted to do something that could improve my condition more directly, and something that could give me the control rather than my doctor."

So Peter decided to get physical. He had done a lot of reading about cases where the right kind of exercise had been helpful, and since exercise had always been such a big part of his life, he decided to give a milder approach a try. He decided to try the oriental martial art of slow, rhythmic movements known as t'ai chi.

"I experienced some pain at first," he recalls, "but within just a few sessions it began to disappear. The movements allowed me to shift my weight over my painful joints slowly, without a lot of jarring force, and soon the movements started to actually feel good."

In addition to his martial arts classes, Peter is now cycling, swimming and lifting weights. "Keeping active in ways that are respectful of my condition has been the key," he says. "As long as I can avoid the jarring and pounding, I feel great. All things considered, I'm probably in better overall shape now at 27 than I was in college before my arthritis struck."

ASTHMA

Ahhhhh, a bright, crisp day in winter. Warmly bundled in coat and hat, you pause on the doorstep to savor one of the delights of the season. Inhaling deeply, you set off on that brisk, health-promoting walk. The rush of cold air into your lungs sends a sparkle of well-being throughout your system . . . right?

If you're one of the approximately 15 million Americans with asthma, unfortunately . . . wrong. For many people with asthma, cold air is just one item in a depressingly long list of triggers for bronchial spasms that can make breathing a frightening struggle.

Well then, let's change the scene. The air's as warm as toast, and it's spring. Flowers nod on their green stalks, urging you out into the gentle sunshine . . . right? Wrong again. Part of the mystery of asthma is its close relation to allergy. Those innocent trees and grasses may be pumping out pollens that could trigger a nasty asthma attack.

Does this mean that if you have asthma, you're doomed to a severely restricted life, cut off from normal activities? Only if Olympic athlete Jackie Joyner-Kersee, actor Christopher Reeve (Superman) or former vice president Walter Mondale seems "cut off" to you. All of these famous folks have done battle with asthma and gone on to live healthy, fulfilling lives—and so can you.

But first let's take a look at the disease itself—how it works and how you can work to win the battle for breath.

LABORING LUNGS

Easily irritated or "twitchy" lungs are the central feature in all cases of asthma—which can range from merely inconvenient to life-threatening, if not properly treated. During an asthma attack, the bronchi and smaller bronchioles—the tubes through which oxygen passes into the lungs—

become swollen and inflamed. As if that weren't enough, the glands that lie within these passages produce excess mucus, which congests the airways even further. A person who is having an asthma attack struggles for air, often feeling as though he or she were trying to suck it in through a narrow straw.

Besides difficulty in breathing, other common signs of asthma are a tight feeling in the chest and chronic coughing. Not all of these symptoms occur in every case, however, so careful diagnosis by a physician is essential.

A major change in understanding asthma has happened in recent years. Traditionally, asthma had been thought to result primarily from the spasming muscles in the lungs. Although the muscles surrounding the bronchial tubes do clench down during the first phase of an attack, it's a persistent *inflammation* of the lungs that causes attacks to recur.

"It's as though people with asthma have a case of poison ivy in the lungs," says Thomas Platts-Mills, M.D., Ph.D., professor of medicine at the University of Virginia Health Sciences Center in Charlottesville.

Although major strides have been taken in the treatment of asthma, the disease remains a serious health threat. Death rates virtually doubled between 1970 and 1989, and the overall prevalence of asthma may have been underdiagnosed previously. A large increase in asthma deaths has been in children aged 5 to 14. Researchers speculate that causes of the increase include air pollution, inadequate physician visits and inappropriate treatment. Sometimes asthma is missed in adolescents who show symptoms only after cold-weather workouts or in adults who never exercise because they always feel too out of shape.

Doctors estimate that 12 percent of adults have some degree of asthma. If you're in that 12 percent, it's easy to panic during those suffocating moments, but bear in mind that asthma is primarily characterized by *reversible* airway obstruction. Once you've weathered an asthma attack, its negative effects on the body generally subside. In the great majority of cases, asthma does not cause serious, permanent damage to the lungs or heart.

TRIGGERS EVERYWHERE

What can cause the wheeze? Asthma has multiple triggers, some easy to understand and manage, others tough to decipher. Exercise can induce asthma attacks in many persons with the disease (more later on why you *don't* have to become sedentary, though!). A viral infection or bout with sinusitis can also bring it on.

But the biggie is allergens—substances from both the indoor and outdoor environments that can induce inflammation in the lungs and trigger allergic reaction. Indoor culprits can range from microscopic bugs called house dust mites, or *(shudder)* cockroaches, to the family dog or cat, says Dr. Platts-Mills.

Small comfort if Tabby is your best friend. But there are a number of simple and very effective things you can do to protect yourself, short of packing the cat off to the shelter.

Wash the cat. Really. "It's not easy to do with adult cats but very easy

---

PROFILE IN HEALING

KURT GROTE: SWIMMING IS A BREEZE

Even when he was a toddler, life was not a breeze for top Stanford University swimmer Kurt Grote. At 18 months, he was coughing a lot at night and had chapped, red cheeks from a constantly streaming nose.

The family pediatrician diagnosed his condition as asthmatic bronchitis, but he assured Kurt's parents that it didn't necessarily mean that Kurt had chronic asthma.

After testing Kurt for allergies at age three, the doctor prescribed a couple of oral medications, including Quibron. But as Kurt grew, so did his symptoms. He was having daily asthma attacks, missing day after day of school and waking up nights with wheezing. At age five, he had a bout with pneumonia.

"He was in the hospital for five days, and his mother, Peggy, stayed with him the whole time," his father, Philip, recalls. "I'm pretty sure that without the administration of modern medicine, he would have been gone."

Kurt's mother, Peggy, remembers another scare: "One particular evening I should have gotten him to the hospital, but I couldn't. He almost didn't come around, and I recognized then that asthma is nothing that you play around with."

Kurt didn't play around with asthma—he played right *through* it. From those breathless beginnings has come a serious student and star athlete who's now a freshman at Stanford. And while he's at it, he has overcome the asthma enough to become the fourth all-time best breaststroker in the history of the university. So far.

Looking back, Kurt remembers when things started looking up. Once he got started on an inhaler, life changed for the better. At first,

if you start them young," says Dr. Platts-Mills. He suggests "once a week in the shower with Mom."

Roll up the rugs. Carpets are notorious dust collectors. Polished wood or linoleum floors can go a long way toward reducing both dust mite and cat allergens in the home and keeping your airways clear, says Dr. Platts-Mills. If you have wall-to-wall throughout your house, at least consider removing it in the bedroom.

Love that leather. Buy leather or vinyl rather than upholstered furniture.

---

the Grotes felt some uncertainty about the use of inhalers. The pediatrician hadn't recommended one, and anyway, since it didn't cure the problem, wouldn't it become a sort of crutch?

But in their search for answers to their son's frustrating condition, they joined a San Diego asthma support group and learned from other parents of children with asthma. When they brought up the idea of an inhaler to their pediatrician, he agreed that Kurt was now at an age when he could benefit from its use.

"The first time I used it, it was like a miracle," Kurt says. "It cleared up my asthma attack in about 15 seconds."

When Kurt was in seventh grade, the Grotes turned to Eli Meltzer, M.D., a San Diego asthma specialist.

"That was the first time we felt like we were getting some control over the illness," Philip says. "Kurt took a battery of medications—he was on about four medications, and still is."

At first when Kurt wanted to go out for swimming, his parents hesitated. But Dr. Meltzer assured them that for asthma, swimming was an excellent sport. "He said that above the surface of the water, there's a lot of spray moisture, which tends to remove the pollens from the air and also moisturize the lungs," says Philip.

Careful medication, a supportive family and an athlete's determination have had a lot to do with Kurt's success. In spite of a regimen including two types of pills and two inhalers (Intal and Ventolin), Kurt is a winner.

"I think it's really important to have the right attitude and not use it as a crutch," says the aquatic 18-year-old. "I know that I have asthma, but I try to think of it as something that's not going to stop me from what I want to do."

Filter your furnace. The hot blast from a forced air furnace spreads more than heat. Mold, dust and other problematic substances are sent flying throughout the house every time that fan kicks on. It's a good idea to replace the filter frequently.

Ban the butts. Not only should people with asthma not smoke, they should avoid contact with sidestream smoke from other people's cigarettes as well. Tobacco smoke should come nowhere *near* a person who has asthma.

Go undercover. Or rather, put your mattresses and pillows in plastic covers to protect yourself from exposure to tiny, invisible dust mites. And you *do* have dust mites in your bedding—they take up residence in even the finest homes.

Ban stuffed toys. Depriving your asthma-prone child of her teddy bear may sound mean, but that innocent-looking bear body is probably stuffed with dust mites as well as cotton.

Turn up the heat. Be sure everything is washed in the hot cycle. Some may like it hot, but dust mites don't.

Once you've made appropriate changes in your house, it's relatively easy to keep down the dust, dander and mites, says Dr. Platts-Mills. "The primary anti-inflammatory treatment for asthma," he emphasizes, "is to avoid exposure to the allergen in the first place."

GRASPING THE ANTIGASPING STRATEGIES

So you've created a safe haven at home. Venturing outside—be it a walk through the woods, a fancy evening at your favorite restaurant or a day at the office—brings you in contact with a whole new set of problematic substances. A few precautions should help protect you.

Open those airways. Just as they do before exercising, many people with asthma use a bronchodilator inhaler before an unavoidable encounter with a trigger outdoors.

Monitor that menu. Metabisulfite—a preservative sometimes sprayed on fresh fruits and vegetables or found in wine and other foods—may trigger an asthma attack in sensitive individuals. If you're not sure whether a particular item is safe, don't hesitate to ask the waiter to look into it.

Minimize hazards at work. Occupational asthma can be a challenge to deal with. Certain fumes, gases, dust and vapors in the workplace can bring on an attack—although it usually takes repeated exposures before a problem develops. Be on the alert for problem substances and strive to minimize your exposure.

THE ONE-TWO PUNCH

Once you understand the nature and treatment of asthma, you can often manage your treatment yourself. But when you need some help, there's plenty to be had.

Your family physician or asthma specialist may teach you to use a peak flow meter, a simple device that measures the flow of air coming out of your lungs. Monitoring your own symptoms and carefully following

---

TREATMENT BREAKTHROUGH

EVERYONE WILL BE BREATHING EASY

People with asthma should find it a little easier to breathe in the 21st century. Because for all practical purposes, says researcher Malcolm Blumenthal, M.D., the disease is heading for a cure.

Dr. Blumenthal, director of the Allergy Center at the University of Minnesota, is one of a handful of researchers who have found evidence of a gene or genes that control an allergic response associated with asthma.

The gene has been linked to a part of a chromosome called HLA-B7, SC31, DR2. This may look like the formula for a household cleaner, but to scientists, it's actually pretty close to a mailing label. It may contain enough information to identify exactly where in the body the asthma gene is located, and with the painstaking research now being conducted by Dr. Blumenthal and his colleagues, the gene's exact location will hopefully be identified.

What will happen then? First, doctors will probably have to redefine asthma, says Dr. Blumenthal, because if what he suspects is true, asthma is not a single disease but actually several different diseases with a few common characteristics.

Second, doctors will diagnose the disease differently. Instead of having you inhale something that triggers an attack and then waiting to see if you react, doctors will be able to detect the gene through a simple blood test. They'll even be able to identify it before birth. If one parent is asthmatic, for example, doctors will be able to check the fetus for the gene—and then possibly reprogram it—before a baby draws its first breath. The whole area of genetic engineering is in the future.

For those who are already walking the streets with asthma, adds Dr. Blumenthal, once scientists have located the disease's genetic address, new forms of treatment will be possible.

---

your medication regimen will go a long way toward easing your symptoms.

Even in mild asthma, treatment must be aimed at controlling lung inflammation as well as the bronchial spasms characteristic of the disease. The lowest effective dose of an effective drug, or frequently a combination of drugs, is likely to be prescribed. The most widely used method of getting the medicine to the problem is with a metered-dose inhaler.

The inhaler may seem tricky to use at first, since you want to blast your lungs rather than the back of your throat. But with a little practice, you'll soon be a practiced puffer. If the inhaler gives you a problem, your doctor can prescribe a spacer device, which makes the inhaler a lot easier to aim.

Prescription drugs used in asthma therapy include inhaled anti-inflammatory agents (usually steroids) followed by beta-adrenergic stimulants or other bronchodilators.

Recent publicity about the adverse effects of overusing beta-adrenergic (beta-2 agonist) inhalers has alarmed some people with asthma, but an expert offers assurance.

"There is cause for concern, but one should not forget that beta-2 agonists are a lifesaving drug," says Raja Ogirala, M.D., assistant professor of medicine at the Albert Einstein College of Medicine in New York City. "It is the most important drug, because it gives immediate relief.

"At our center we tell patients, use your steroid inhaler every day, regularly, at the dose prescribed by your doctor, and if you occasionally still have symptoms, then use your beta-2 agonist."

If a tough case of asthma doesn't respond to anti-inflammatory agents or bronchodilators, doctors sometimes prescribe oral steroids. Antihistamines may help to control allergic symptoms, which can precipitate asthma attacks. Immunotherapy, or allergy injections, has recently been shown to also be effective.

WARM UP TO EXERCISE

One of the best weapons in your own arsenal of asthma fighters is regular aerobic exercise, such as walking, running or bicycling. Doctors say that such exercise helps people with asthma because it makes breathing more efficient. Some sports, like tennis or swimming, are easier to tolerate because they take place in a warm, humid environment or involve short bursts of activity, but many others are also within your reach.

The keys to a wheeze-free workout? Warm up and pretreat. Doctors recommend 5 to 10 minutes of moderate exercise before you pour on the effort and a similar cool-down period afterward. And a pre-exercise burst from your inhaler before you swing that racket will serve you well.

BACK PROBLEMS

C hris sighed as she climbed into bed. After three trips to the mall, two grocery expeditions and one weekend clean-a-thon, she was ready to call it quits. And so was her back—it ached like crazy. "Well, a good night's sleep and a hot morning bath will take the kinks out," Chris thought as she drifted off to sleep.

But her back had different ideas, and by morning the damage was done. When Chris awoke, all she felt was pain—terrible, clamorous waves of pain. She felt as though someone were beating her back with a hammer. When she tried to roll over, the pain instantly doubled; she couldn't even move her legs. Chris cried out: "Will someone *please* call the doctor!"

But her doctor, to her great relief, said not to worry. "It's probably just a muscle spasm, and the best thing you can do is stay in bed," he reassured her. "You can get up to use the bathroom, but that's it." "The way I feel now," Chris thought, "I couldn't get out of bed if the house was on fire!"

However, just a few hours later, she actually did sit up. That evening, she walked downstairs for dinner, and three days later the pain was nearly all gone. A week later, Chris waited in her doctor's office. She had just one question: "What the heck happened?"

THE OMNIPRESENT OUCH

"For the most part, back problems are caused by some type of sprain in the muscles or tendons," says Augustus A. White III, M.D., professor of orthopedic surgery at Harvard Medical School and chief of the Spine Surgery Division at Boston's Beth Israel Hospital. "It may hurt like crazy for two or three days. Then it hurts moderately for maybe two weeks. Then after four or five weeks, you'll probably be more or less normal."

Of course, the long journey from "Ouch!" to "more or less normal" isn't something to sneeze at. (Sneezes and coughs, as back pain veterans will attest, can momentarily double your pain.) And you're not likely to avoid the situation, either. It doesn't take six rounds with a heavyweight to wrack your back. Just sleeping wrong can do it—or taking out the trash, or bending over to pick up a paper clip. In fact, backache, aside from sore throats, is the most common condition doctors treat. To put this in perspective, take a look at ten of your friends: At least *eight* of them will eventually have back problems.

Make that expensive back problems. Doctors estimate that the nation's bad backs—counting lost wages, doctors' fees and other expenses—cost more than $16 billion each year. But the good news, according to Dr. White, author of *Your Aching Back: A Doctor's Guide to Relief,* is that serious back problems—for example, ruptured disks—are quite rare. Sure, backaches hurt, but surgery and long-term pain rarely belong in the picture.

Of course, this is hardly reassuring for people like Chris who find themselves, with little warning, flat on their back and "paralyzed" with pain. But when you look at all the places your back can go wrong—there are 33 vertebrae between the bottom of your head and the top of your tail—you may be surprised it doesn't trouble you more often.

SPINAL ARCHITECTURE

Imagine your spine—better yet, reach behind and feel it—as a tall, curved stack of doughnuts. (The hole in the middle is for your spinal cord.) Your spine may feel solid, but it's not. In fact, it's eminently flexible. Every time you nod your head, brush your teeth or lumber through the limbo, your spine's muscles, ligaments and vertebrae bend along with you.

But everything that moves can also *stop* moving. That's what happened to Chris. While she slept, her stressed muscles called a labor strike—their way of taking the day off. But her muscles didn't merely put up their feet and relax. In fact, they did the opposite and bunched themselves into powerful, painful contractions called spasms.

But muscle spasms rarely *cause* back problems, Dr. White says. They're simply a response to other things—strained ligaments, for example, or simply too much hard work.

Malfunctioning facet joints can also cause back pain, Dr. White says. The facet joints are the gliding surfaces between vertebrae. Partially coated with slick cartilage, they allow you to twist your hips when you dance the twist. That is, until they get sore. Then your twist gets twisted, and you sit out the next 10.

Perhaps the most famous—or infamous—back problems are caused by faulty spinal disks—ruptured disks, slipped disks and herniated disks. Actually, these terms all mean pretty much the same thing: trouble! Because many people will eventually have disk trouble, and a great many more will *think* they do, we'll talk a bit more about disks—what they're supposed to do and what happens when they don't do it.

SHOCK ABSORBERS WEAR OUT

You probably aren't aware of it, but every time you jump out of bed, run to the store or pirouette past the petunias, your back takes a heck of a lot of pounding. That's why your vertebrae have their very own shock absorbers, the spinal disks. Remember the doughnuts we stacked up earlier? Well, your disks really are like jelly doughnuts: flexible outsides wrapped around a soft, gelatinous middle. When you squeeze a doughnut (or a disk), it *absorbs* the pressure; release the pressure, it springs right back.

But as your disks age, they can become as dry and brittle as day-old doughnuts. In some cases, the flexible outside will crack open—herniate—allowing the soft middle to ooze right out. Essentially, the spine loses the use of one of its shock absorbers.

That's not always a problem, Dr. White says. There are plenty of healthy, pain-free people walking around with moderately herniated disks. In most cases, they don't even know anything happened. (However, they do get slightly shorter!) But when the disk begins to push against nearby nerves, the pain can be excruciating. In fact, a "pinched" nerve can send shooting pains into both arms and legs. It can cause muscle weakness or even paralysis. In some cases, it can cause the bladder to lose control.

If you're beginning to worry about your own disks (*and* the jelly doughnuts you bought last week), relax. For one thing, disks dry out all the time without causing problems. Even when they do rupture, the pain often goes away on its own. On the other hand, a bush-league backache can still cause major-league pain. It's always better to prevent a backache, Dr. White says, than to wait for it to go away.

WATCH YOUR BACK

As you might expect, much of the advice doctors give for avoiding back pain begins with "don't": don't lift too much, don't work too hard and so on. But first, to begin on a more positive note, we'll discuss some "do's."

Work on your trunk. No, put the keys away—it's *your* trunk that's important. Doctors agree that strong trunk muscles—particularly the *psoas* (which connect the lower back to the inside of the hips) and the *erector spinae* (which are parallel to the spine)—can help keep backs feeling good. Think of your back as a building. When the foundation is strong, it stands up; take away the foundation, and the only way it can go is *down*.

SURGICAL PRECISION WITHOUT INCISION

Back surgery has always been tough stuff. To get a good view, surgeons have always preferred large incisions—4 or even 5 painful inches—right up the middle of your back.

But incisions are getting smaller all the time, says Oheneba Boachie-Adjei, M.D., associate medical director of the Southern California Complex Spine and Scoliosis Center in Whittier. This is because surgeons are learning, with the aid of magnification, to perform complicated surgery with minute instruments inside relatively small cuts, Dr. Boachie-Adjei says.

If smaller is better, then a new, still-evolving technique called percutaneous diskectomy may someday revolutionize back surgery, Dr. Boachie-Adjei says. Instead of making incisions, the surgeon inserts a hollow tube—about one-half the diameter of a pencil—into a small hole in the back. Into this tube go even *smaller* instruments. The surgeon never sees the spine directly; the whole operation is seen through a fluoroscope, a type of x-ray machine. "If it can be proven to be as successful as conventional surgery, the advantages will be tremendous," Dr. Boachie-Adjei says.

In addition, lasers may someday replace some of the surgical instruments now used for back surgery, he says. Lasers can focus their beams with incredible precision and may help surgeons reach, through tiny incisions, hard-to-reach parts of the spine. Eventually, Dr. Boachie-Adjei says, people may have laser back surgery and return home the same day.

As you might expect, these new techniques aren't without controversy or limitations. Some surgeons believe the small incisions simply are too small to ensure thorough operations. For example, they ask, how is a surgeon to remove disk fragments that are *bigger* than the incision? How will he locate detached fragments that float *beyond* the tiny surgical field?

These concerns are valid, Dr. Boachie-Adjei says, and it may be many years before doctors know for sure if microsurgery really can replace—or supplement—the traditional techniques. In the meantime, he says, many surgeons now believe that starting small often is the best approach. "Then if they encounter large disk fragments, all they have to do is perform traditional surgery," Dr. Boachie-Adjei says. "They've left their options open."

Swimming is an excellent way to strengthen these muscles, doctors say. And because swimming, in effect, reduces gravity, it's the ideal exercise for people with arthritis or other joint problems. Don't know how to swim? No problem: *Walking* in waist-high water also does the trick.

Put on your walking shoes. Or your running shoes, aerobics shoes or any-exercise-you-want shoes. (If you're a swimmer, of course, you can leave the shoes at home.) The more you exercise, the less your chances for spending painful weekends inspecting ceiling tiles, says Richard Plummer, D.C., director of Springfield Chiropractic Services in Inman, South Carolina. Aerobic exercise, by improving circulation, helps keep your spinal disks supple, Dr. Plummer explains.

"For most people, walking is the simplest, easiest exercise, and all you need is a pair of sneakers," he says. "People can walk every day of the week—in their neighborhood, up and down stairs or inside shopping malls when the weather's bad. Walking, when you're upright and your arms are swinging, is one of the best exercises for your lower back."

But if you're getting ready for a strenuous workout, Dr. White warns, plan it for later in the day. Your disks take on extra fluid at night and, like most tipplers, are a bit unruly in the mornings. Let them wake up before dragging them to the gym.

Have you hugged your garbage can today? Try to hold things close to your body when you pick them up, doctors advise. The temptation, when you lift a bag stuffed with garbage, is to hold it at arm's length. But what's good for your nose isn't always good for your spine.

Take a stretch. You're looking for trouble when your pants wear fastest at the seat. Long-term sitting is extremely hard on your spine—not to mention parts of your anatomy a little farther south. Actually, sitting puts about 50 percent more stress on your spine than standing does. All that extra pressure, Dr. White says, may irritate various structures in the spine, including the disks. So give your back—and your bottom—a break. Walk around. Take a stretch. Or do something really radical: Work standing up.

Pull those shoulders back. You probably argued when Mom told you to stand up straight. Well, you apologize right now! Even though good posture doesn't *guarantee* healthy backs, people who slump (when they sit, stand or talk on the telephone) are just asking for trouble.

Smooth the sway. When you look in the mirror, you'll see that your back naturally has some curve to it. But if you stand around flat-footed for long periods, a little curve can feel like a sharp hook—right into your lower back! Lifting one foot onto a step or stool will reduce the curve, doctors say, and that eases the strain. No matter where you are, there's probably a step somewhere. At the store, for example, rest your foot on the shopping cart. At an art gallery, look for a foot-level piece of modern sculpture. (Just kidding!)

SOME DISK DEMOLISHERS

Naturally, all your good habits won't save your back if you persist in lifting pianos, wrestling alligators and jumping off the roof. They won't even save you from life's minor, but very risky, transgressions. To keep your back healthy, you should:

Drop some weight. Your back already has to carry you—and whatever you're wearing, carrying or lifting—every day. When you start adding on the pounds, your back will b-e-n-d under the extra weight, Dr. White says. Give it a break, and put that spare tire back in the car where it belongs.

Pause before you pitch. One of the worst things people do to their backs, Dr. Plummer says, is push them into action on a moment's notice. "They've been sitting at work all day in their three-piece suit. Then they change their clothes, rush to the park and start playing softball, and their

---

PROFILE IN HEALING

PATRICIA AMBROSINI: SHE PUT PAIN BEHIND HER

The worst part wasn't the pain, although there was plenty of that. It wasn't even the lost wages, or the suspicious bosses, or the resentment her family couldn't quite hide. The thing that really hurt, says Patricia Ambrosini of Helmetta, New Jersey, was watching entire seasons pass her by.

"I love to do things," cries Patricia, her voice packed with excitement. "I love to rake leaves, but I had to watch the fall come and go, and I couldn't rake leaves. I used to manage a ski shop, but I went that whole winter without skiing—not once!"

Until she got hurt, Patricia worked in the East Coast retail store for more than a year. She loved her job and made good money. Also, she and her fiancé were eagerly making plans for a spring wedding. Then on a Sunday afternoon, Patricia lost her balance while hefting boxes at the store. "At that moment, I felt like somebody shot me in the back," she remembers. "Everything locked up from my shoulders right down to my hips—it was a horrible feeling."

"Okay," Patricia told herself, "I've just strained my back, and I'll be better soon." But that night, "I started getting numbness in my fingers and radiating pains down my arms," she says. "My legs felt like they weren't there, and my feet were tingling."

---

muscles can't take that," he says. You don't have to stretch all day just to pitch a few strikes, Dr. Plummer adds. Just limber up before you mount the mound.

Shake it up. Even if you're the office workhorse, you should occasionally remove your nose from the company grindstone, advises Dr. Plummer. "People sit at their desks day in and day out, and it gets to the point where the pain is just too much," he says. "When you feel tightness or tension in your back or neck, get up and move around a little bit, even if it's only for 30 seconds." Your back—not to mention your nose—will thank you for it.

Bad vibrations. It's not really road bumps that bash bad backs, Dr. White says, but car vibrations. Most cars vibrate at frequencies between 4 and 5 cycles per second—precisely the frequencies that can put your spine in park. Limit your driving time to 2 hours a day, he advises. If you have to drive more than that, consider buying a car that vibrates at different—and safer—frequencies.

Patricia's doctor gave her painkillers, inflammation-fighting drugs and orders to take it easy. It might be just a sprain, he told her. But when she wasn't improved a week later, he enrolled her in daily physical therapy sessions. The therapy seemed to work, and Patricia was back at work two weeks later. She lasted two days before the pain, worse than before, overwhelmed her.

Her doctor said it was time to run several tests. When the results came back, his suspicions were confirmed. Patricia appeared to have two herniated disks, and they were putting uncomfortable pressure on her spinal nerves—in layman's language, pinched nerves. He recommended back surgery to remove the pressure. Full of fear, she agreed.

"When I woke up after the surgery, I didn't have that pain in my ankle, that pain in the side of my shin and in my knee and that pain in my hip," Patricia says. "I knew I was better." As it turned out, Patricia's problem was caused not by a ruptured disk but by "knots" of damaged ligaments. When her surgeon removed the ligaments, the pressure—and the pain—was gone.

Her back is recovered, but one thing still hurts, Patricia says. "Until I actually had the surgery, a lot of people seemed to think that this whole thing was in my mind," she says. "I just felt awful, because people didn't have any idea what I was going through."

Snuff the butts. "Smoking is a vasoconstrictor, which means it limits the supply of blood to some parts of your body," Dr. White says. "When you interfere with the nutrition of the disks, that can cause problems."

SAVING YOUR BACK

Even if you do good things for your back and avoid all the dangers, you could *still* get hurt, Dr. White says. In fact, back injuries are so common that few people never experience a back problem. Fortunately, doctors agree that there are things you can do both to beat the pain and to hasten your recovery.

The word *cure,* says Alan S. Bensman, M.D., medical director of the Minnesota Center for Health and Rehabilitation in Minneapolis, really doesn't belong in conversations about back pain. "The word *rehabilitation* is more accurate," Dr. Bensman insists. "Rehabilitation doesn't mean your problems have gone away. It means you've learned to do the very best with the body you've got." So whether you've had back pain all your life or you just pulled a muscle in Sunday's game, some of the following probably can help.

Find your position of comfort. Everyone with back problems has at least one posture or position that puts the *least* strain on their back. Some people might be most comfortable when they stand with their back bent slightly forward; others will feel better when they're ramrod straight.

Naturally, there's a catch, Dr. Bensman says. Your favorite position has to be *functional* as well. "I have people who come in here all bent over like pretzels, and they say, 'It's comfortable for me.' Well, it might be comfortable, but it's not functional," he says.

Put it to bed. Doctors agree that lying in bed can take painful pressure off that sensitive spine. People who have ruptured disks often feel better after two or three days of bed rest. "Most back injuries will resolve when the pressure is removed," Dr. Bensman says.

In the past, doctors advised people with acute back pain to spend at least 20 hours a day—for up to ten days—between the sheets. But studies suggest that two days, for most people, probably is enough. Of course, this doesn't mean you should hoist refrigerators on the third day. Give yourself a few weeks to recover.

Catch some ZZZs. Since you're in bed anyway, you may as well get some sleep—relaxing, healing sleep. "Deep sleep has been identified as a time when muscle healing occurs," Dr. Bensman says. When you're not sleeping, he adds, find positions in bed that don't hurt your back. Most people find that lying on their stomach is out—it puts too much pressure on the spine. Lying on your back with your knees slightly bent may be the best position. If you usually sleep on your side, curl up and tuck a pillow between your knees.

Open the medicine chest. For most people, aspirin is the drug of choice for fighting pain and inflammation, Dr. White says. If you can't take aspirin, other over-the-counter drugs such as acetaminophen or ibuprofen can help. (However, acetaminophen only fights pain; it does not attack inflammation.) Or ask your doctor about the more potent nonsteroidal anti-inflammatory drugs. They sometimes work when over-the-counter remedies don't. If your pain is really ferocious, your doctor might recommend stronger prescription drugs—codeine, for example, or other narcotics. But these drugs can delay recovery, so they're rarely recommended for long-term use.

Finally, your doctor may suggest another kind of prescription if he thinks that a lack of deep sleep might be hindering your body's ability to heal itself. "Amitriptyline (Elavil), an antidepressant with sedative effects, taken in low doses (10 to 15 milligrams) 1 to 2 hours before bedtime, may be useful for just this reason," says Dr. Bensman.

Ice is nice. Like aspirin, ice cubes are a simple (and inexpensive) way to relieve muscle strains and ligament pains, Dr. Bensman says. Because cold reduces the swelling and helps the muscle relax, it can help reduce painful inflammation. Before you lay on the ice, first wrap it in pillowcases or washcloths, Dr. Bensman advises. You want to chill your back, not freeze it solid.

Some like it hot. After a few days of ice, if you feel like a change, go ahead and warm things up. Heating your back with a heating pad and a hot bath (*not* at the same time) can help relax muscle spasms, Dr. Bensman says. Follow treatment with some light stretching. Remember, however, that applying heat soon after an injury can increase pain and inflammation.

Rub it out. After a few days of chilly compresses, reward yourself with a long, leisurely, luxurious massage. It won't cure your backache, Dr. Plummer says, but it should make you feel better—and not only on the outside. "Massage stimulates the circulatory system and the lymphatic system, and that helps bring fluid and nutrients into the muscles," he says. "It also helps remove the lactic acid, a painful by-product of damaged tissue."

Hit the switch. Transcutaneous electrical nerve stimulation, or TENS, is a new type of therapy for back pain. Small electrodes are placed on the skin near the injury, and electrical currents are shot into the body. Some researchers believe these currents interrupt the passage of pain signals from your hurt back to your brain. TENS may also raise the body's production of painkilling endorphins.

Some doctors, however, aren't convinced. A study published in the

New England Journal of Medicine, for example, found that people treated with TENS units improved about as much as those treated with placebo (inactive) machines. If it doesn't seem to help, however, Dr. White says to stop using it.

Take a deep breath. But first close your mouth. "When you take a slow, deep breath through your nose, you're helping yourself relax, and you're stimulating the production of endorphins, your body's natural pain reducers," Dr. Bensman says. (If you have a stuffy nose, this technique isn't for you!)

Stretch it out. Stretching is one of the best things you can do for a bad back, Dr. Bensman says. You don't need a fancy program, and you don't have to spend a dime. In fact, you can do your morning stretches before your feet even hit the floor. Stretch your legs, your arms, your neck and your back. Do this for a few minutes every morning, he says, and you will just naturally be a lot more mobile—and less prone to back pain. Abdominal exercises, such as sit-ups, also help strengthen the back.

The secret, Dr. Bensman says, is *daily* care—whether your back's hurting or not. "You can't stop taking care of your back just because you're feeling better," he warns. "The biggest mistake people make is to think their back problems are just going to end. They are not."

BELL'S PALSY

It may begin with a feeling of dryness in one of your eyes and, over the next few hours, evolve into a paralysis that creeps down your face, eradicating your flirtatious wink and dazzling smile.

A stroke? Probably not, unless you also have hearing loss, speech difficulties or weakness or paralysis in your arms or legs. More likely, it's a less serious but equally terrifying condition called Bell's palsy.

"Bell's palsy is more gradual than a stroke," says James Stankiewicz, M.D., professor and vice chairman of the Head and Neck Surgery Department at Loyola University Medical Center in Maywood, Illinois. "A stroke would be like one minute you're fine, the next minute your face is contorted. Bell's palsy is more progressive. The person will develop a gradual weakness in the face over several hours or a day that may cause complete paralysis of one side of the face. It's not dangerous. You're not going to die from it. But it is a terrible thing to wake up and find your face contorted."

The good news is that Bell's palsy has nothing to do with a stroke, and 70 to 85 percent of people who get it fully recover within one to two months. And although a recurrence can happen without warning, only one in ten people who are stricken by the ailment ever suffers from it again.

Still, doctors know that offers little reassurance to many people afflicted by this puzzling disease. "Eight weeks may seem like a lifetime if your face isn't moving," says Kedar Adour, M.D., of the Facial Cranial Nerve Research Center in Oakland, California.

BELL'S MANY FACES

Bell's palsy, described by Sir Charles Bell in 1821, is the most common cause of facial paralysis in this country, striking 20 out of every 100,000 people each year. It can completely paralyze one side of the face but more commonly results in a temporary partial paralysis of the mouth or eyelid. The affliction can also cause pain on the face or behind the ears that may be as bad as an intense earache, says Dr. Adour.

Doctors aren't sure what causes Bell's palsy, but they suspect that it is a viral infection that may be linked to herpes simplex, the same virus that causes cold sores.

In fact, many of the same triggers that produce cold sores—stress, pregnancy, menstruation, exposure to sunlight or cold drafts—are also implicated in the onset of Bell's palsy.

Doctors say nothing can be done to prevent it, and often it gives no clues that it is about to attack. "Typically, the patient will go to sleep feeling fine, and when he wakes up, he has a facial paralysis," says Ronald Amedee, M.D., assistant professor of otolaryngology/head and neck surgery at Tulane University in New Orleans. "In most patients, there really is no tip-off in the days preceding that this paralysis is going to happen."

In most cases, the paralysis gradually recedes as mysteriously as it strikes. When it does occur, however, you should see your doctor immediately, because there are many other causes of facial paralysis, including tumor, head trauma, central nervous system diseases and medication.

GETTING BACK CONTROL

Most likely, your doctor will write you a prescription. Steroid drugs such as prednisone may help relieve inflammation around facial nerves and speed recovery. The majority of physicians would consider prescribing steroids, even though there are no studies proving the drugs' effectiveness for Bell's palsy, Dr. Amedee says.

But taking your medication isn't the only thing you can do. While waiting for the ailment to run its course, you must do some vital things to prevent complications, say the experts.

Keep the eye moist. "In the Bell's palsy patient, the worst complication that can occur is that the eye remains open and the cornea dries out. That can lead to blindness," Dr. Amedee says. If you have Bell's palsy, wear dark glasses in daylight. Your doctor likely will also prescribe eyedrops and antibiotic ointments to keep your eyes moisturized.

Massage your face. "Massaging helps keep muscle tone," Dr. Amedee says. "One of the problems when the face isn't working is that some of the muscle tissue can die or become filled with scar tissue. By exercising those muscles with your fingers, you can minimize that process."

Massaging may also give you an emotional lift. "It gets the patient back in touch with himself. He touches his face and realizes that it's coming back to life," Dr. Amedee says.

Massage your face at least twice a day for 10 to 15 minutes, Dr. Stankiewicz suggests.

Keep an eye on pain. "If a particle of dust blows into a Bell's palsy patient's eye, they may not feel it for a long time, and when they do, they're not going to be able to naturally rinse it out with their own tears," Dr. Amedee says. "I always tell patients with any kind of facial paralysis to get in touch with me immediately if they feel any pain in the eye."

SURGERY: A LAST RESORT

In extremely rare cases, the paralysis is permanent, and surgery may be needed to compensate for it.

"After a suitable amount of time—a year to 18 months—there are some surgical procedures that can give the face symmetry from side to side," Dr. Amedee says. "One is called a facial sling. It's actually a mini-facelift that gets rid of sagging muscle tissue and makes it harder for someone to see that there is a problem."

Another operation that implants gold weights in the eyelids may help some people regain the ability to blink.

But Dr. Amedee says these drastic surgical procedures are seldom needed. "I'd say 90 percent of Bell's palsy patients get better without surgery."

BRONCHITIS

Friends, Romans, countrymen *(clears throat)*, lend me your ears! I come to bury Caesar *(harumph)*, not to praise him. *(clears throat)* The evil that men do *(takes drink of water)* lives after them *(harumph)*, the good is oft interred with their bones *(HARUMPH, HARUMPH, HARUMPH)*; so let it be *(clears throat)* with Caesar. . . ."

Had Mark Antony in Shakespeare's *Julius Caesar* been suffering from bronchitis, this is what his rousing send-off might have sounded like. Bronchitis makes people cough, and once they start coughing, they can be hard-pressed to stop. Antony's audience, instead of cheering, might have thrown cough drops instead.

COUGHS THAT WON'T QUIT

As the name suggests, bronchitis is an inflammation of the bronchi, air passages in your chest that carry oxygen to the lungs. To soothe this inflammation, your body churns out protective secretions to coat the airways. At the same time, its mechanism for removing mucus slows down. The result is a buildup of, well, gunk. Your body responds with coughs, its mechanism for clearing surplus mucus.

"The symptom of bronchitis is a productive cough, usually with discolored sputum. You may have a wheeze and shortness of breath as well," says James K. Stoller, M.D., head of the Section of Respiratory Therapy at Cleveland Clinic, Cleveland.

Bronchitis is a common problem, doctors say, affecting 10 to 25 percent of all adults. If you have *acute* (short-term) bronchitis, a viral infection often caused by colds or flu, it will probably clear up in a week or two. *Chronic* (long-term) bronchitis, on the other hand, can last for years. It's typically caused by breathing airborne irritants such as cigarette smoke, dust or air pollutants.

SIMPLE PREVENTION

The best way to prevent acute bronchitis is to prevent colds and flu. As for chronic bronchitis, the best way to both treat it *and* prevent it is—you guessed it—to quit smoking.

Chronic bronchitis is extremely common among smokers, particularly those 45 and older. In fact, doctors have estimated that approximately *90 percent* of the people with chronic bronchitis got it from smoking. No wonder bronchitis is sometimes referred to as "smoker's cough."

To make things worse, smoker's cough isn't limited to smokers. Because of the secondhand effects of cigarette smoke, people who live, work and play with smokers also are at risk. This can be particularly troublesome for children, whose natural defenses aren't yet fully developed. Among children whose parents smoke, the risk for developing respiratory problems can actually double.

However, there is some good news. The sooner you give up cigarettes, Dr. Stoller says, the better your chances for improving bronchitis.

FINDING FAST RELIEF

Apart from steering clear of cigarette smoke and other pollutants, there is really no way to "cure" the cough of chronic bronchitis. Nor would you want to. Coughing is an essential mechanism for clearing accumulated mucus from your airways. But by thinning the mucus, you can help your cough work more efficiently and cause less discomfort. For starters:

Swig some water. Particularly if you have a viral infection, which can dry you out and make your mucus thick and gummy. By staying well hydrated—six to eight glasses of water a day should be enough—you can help liquefy the mucus, making it easier to cough up.

Savor some hot soup. Doctors agree that hot liquids—Grandma's chicken soup is an excellent example—are even better than plain water for relieving chest congestion. But if Grandma isn't cooking this week, brew some tea instead. Or sip some hot water—*any* hot liquid can help, doctors say.

Feast on fire. At the supper table, that is. When you eat fiery foods—hot red peppers or horseradish, for example, or flaming Indian curries—your mucous membranes respond by secreting a profusion of fire-fighting liquids. These liquids can help liquefy thick phlegm, making it easier to cough up.

Try licorice lozenges. Along with the expectorant herbs horehound, peppermint and eucalyptus, this sweet-tasting substance may help stimulate the breakdown of accumulated mucus, says herbal expert Varro E. Tyler, Ph.D., professor of pharmacognosy at Purdue University.

Plug in the vaporizer. Winter air may dry your airways, making them more susceptible to bronchitis. A humidifier or vaporizer may help keep your pipes lubricated, Dr. Stoller says. To prevent molds from growing, however, vaporizers must be kept scrupulously clean.

DRUGS TO THE RESCUE

As long as your coughs are "productive"—that is, they're bringing up phlegm—they should be encouraged, Dr. Stoller says. In fact, there are dozens of drugs you can take that will make them even more productive. These drugs, called expectorants or mucolytics, make the phlegm less sticky and hence easier to cough up. Many over-the-counter cold remedies contain expectorants (along with other ingredients). Ask your pharmacist for recommendations.

Unlike productive coughs, *non*productive coughs, which also can accompany bronchitis, offer no benefits whatsoever. Caused by tickles deep inside the throat, a nonproductive, "dry" cough can be terribly uncomfortable, Dr. Stoller says. In fact, people have fractured ribs during cough attacks. To stop a dry cough, your doctor may recommend lozenges or cough syrups to help calm the tickle. Drinking fluids can also help. So can drugs that actually inhibit the cough reflex. "We might use cough suppressants when people are up all night coughing," Dr. Stoller says. "That type of cough can be quite incapacitating."

If you've been coughing for more than a week or two, and the resulting phlegm is foul-tasting and discolored, then you may have a bacterial infection called, naturally, bacterial bronchitis. To knock out the infection, your doctor may prescribe antibiotics such as tetracycline or ampicillin. Once the bacterial infection clears up, your bronchitis may disappear as well.

Should you have bronchitis *and* asthma, your doctor may recommend you use a bronchodilator to relieve airway spasms. If you're still having problems, he may give you a prescription for steroids as well. These powerful drugs can often relieve the airway congestion associated with asthma in about a week, usually without causing any side effects.

For acute bronchitis, "tincture of time" often is the best medicine, Dr. Stoller says. For chronic bronchitis, however, time will work against you unless you remove yourself, and your lungs, from the source of the problem. "So much of bronchitis is caused by smoking," Dr. Stoller says. "People finally are quitting, but discouragingly slowly."

BURSITIS

With names like miner's elbow, housemaid's knee and weaver's bottom, it sounds more like a wildflower from a seed catalog than an uncomfortable, bumpy inflammation. But once you've had bursitis, you won't mistake this annoying condition for a bed of roses.

There are approximately 150 fluid-filled *bursae* distributed throughout your body. Essentially, each bursa is a cushion that helps facilitate movement between adjoining parts of your body. On the back of your hand, for example, bursae help the skin glide freely back and forth. You also have bursae on your elbows, knees and the sides of your body, explains Joseph D. Zuckerman, M.D., vice chairman of the Department of Orthopedic Surgery and chief of the shoulder service at the Hospital for Joint Diseases Orthopaedic Institute in New York City.

When bursae get injured, whether from injuries, overuse or even poor posture, they become inflamed and begin to swell. That's bursitis. Naturally, the bursae that get the most abuse and are nearest the surface—those on the knees, elbows and hips—are the ones most likely to get inflamed. "People who spend a lot of time on their knees—maids, for example, or carpet layers—can have a golfball-size or larger swelling on the front of their knee," says Dr. Zuckerman.

But those in other professions may also get bursitis, says W. Ben Kibler, M.D., medical director of Lexington Clinic Sports Medicine Center in Lexington, Kentucky. "One of my patients is a judge, and he listens to a lot of cases by resting his elbows on the bench," Dr. Kibler says. "The right one was swollen a couple of months ago, and now the left one is swollen."

While unsightly, bursitis isn't always painful. But an infected bursa can prevent you from moving, walking or doing anything at all, according to Clifton S. Mereday, Ph.D., chairman of the physical therapy program at the State University of New York at Stony Brook. "It can be excruciatingly painful," he says.

JOINT EFFORTS

It's not always clear why bursae get inflamed, or why some people get bursitis more often than others. Still, there are things you can do to dump the bumps—*before* they occur.

Change your game. Since bursitis is often caused by repetitive motions—throwing a baseball, for example, or kneeling in a garden—a change of pace can be a joint-saver. So occasionally swap the baseball for a croquet mallet. Work in the house instead of the garden. Hang up your running shoes and take a long walk instead.

Give your knees a break. People who spend their days laying carpet, fixing plumbing or digging up tulips are particularly prone to bursitis. And because bursae on the knee are so near the surface, they're easily pricked and sometimes get infected, Dr. Zuckerman says. Try to spend more time on your feet than on your knees. Or if your job requires frequent kneeling, invest in a well-padded cushion or some good knee pads. A little protection today can prevent a lot of pain tomorrow.

Straighten up. People who slump in their seats, slouch at parties or inadvertently look for pennies when they walk put all sorts of pressure on bursae in their backs and shoulders. "By walking more erect, your chances of developing bursitis are reduced," Dr. Mereday says.

Keep yourself strong. Weak muscles lead to poor posture, and poor posture, as we've seen, can cause bursitis. A little exercise—lifting weights, having a swim or just taking regular walks—can prevent both these problems, Dr. Mereday says.

Have a good stretch. Because bursae and tendons are so close together, what affects one can also affect the other. So before you hit the track—or the tennis court or soccer field—take a few minutes to warm up and stretch.

SWELL TREATMENTS

You *tried* to stay off your knees, but the geraniums beckoned you thither—and now you have bursitis. What do you do now?

Try the pharmacy. Over-the-counter drugs such as aspirin and ibuprofen can ease bursitis pain and reduce swelling. In some cases, doctors say, this will be the only medical treatment you'll need. Take daily, as directed, for two to three weeks until the pain and swelling are gone. If there's no improvement, see your doctor.

Chill out. While you're resting, go ahead and put the swollen bursa on ice, says Dr. Mereday. Applying cold helps reduce the pain and swelling. Wrap ice packs or cubes in a towel or washcloth and place on the injury for 10 minutes, several times a day.

Now get moving. Once the pain subsides—this should happen in a day or two—try to get the injured part moving again, Dr. Mereday adds. "Not moving is how you develop frozen shoulder, for instance. It's not the bursitis that causes it but the adhesions [scar tissue] you get later. So you want to get it moving as soon as possible."

BIG-LEAGUE HELP

Most cases of bursitis can be treated at home. But when the pain gets bad, or you suspect you have an infection, it's time to see your doctor, Dr. Zuckerman says.

When you have red, painful swelling that doesn't go away, you probably have an infected bursa, Dr. Zuckerman says. For this you need antibiotics, which in most cases will quickly eliminate the infection. To relieve painful swelling, however, your doctor may drain the bursa as well.

In some situations, when the pain of bursitis has not improved with rest, ice or anti-inflammatory medications, a steroid injection can be beneficial. This approach is used very sparingly, and it's important that there be no infection present, Dr. Zuckerman says.

Occasionally bursitis will be so painful and long-lived that your doctor will recommend surgery to remove the swollen bursa. But this is rare, Dr. Kibler says. Most of the time, self-care—and perhaps drugs—will do the trick.

CANCER

Cancer. "The Big C." The indiscriminate slayer. Cancer is so sinister that it was made the target of an all-out "war" when President Nixon signed the Federal Cancer Act in 1971. Scientists have been going tooth and nail against the dreaded disease ever since, standing over microscopes looking for causes, bombarding tumors with radiation and high-powered drugs, devising new techniques in hopes of stopping the killer.

Yet the war against cancer drags on. Some even argue it's being lost. Yes, individual battles are being won as advances in both the diagnosis and treatment of cancer are being made—but cancer's list of casualties rises. Cancer has yet to pass heart disease as our number one killer, but while death rates from heart disease have been declining in recent years, death rates from cancer have been on the rise—up by roughly 10 percent over the past 30 years. If it proliferates at its present rate, cancer could overtake heart disease as the number one cause of death by the year 2000.

Which means what for the future of our efforts against this loathsome disease?

Simply that we're going to have to bring more of the war against cancer closer to home. We're going to have to start fighting The Big C in our kitchens, dining rooms, backyards and barrooms, *in addition* to the hospitals, operating rooms and labs.

"Each and every one of us needs to start taking more personal responsibility for the disease," says John Laszlo, M.D., the American Cancer Society's (ACS) senior vice president for research and the author of *Understanding Cancer*. "We're going to have to stop waiting for scientists to cure what may be easier to prevent."

GETTING CANCER BEFORE IT GETS US

As much as we tend to think of cancer as a disease that can strike anyone at any time and in any place, the experts now feel that as much as

70 percent of all cancers may be due to factors within our control. We, in a sense, may "ask" for the disease by leading the lifestyles that we do.

"More than 80 percent of people who get lung cancer, for example, are smokers," says Dr. Laszlo. "And more and more, we're seeing how the effects of dietary fat, alcohol abuse, obesity and excessive exposure to the sun can increase cancer risks."

In short, we need to start thinking of The Big C as standing for *control.* "If we did everything possible to prevent cancer and also followed the latest recommendations for early detection, we might be able to reduce cancer deaths substantially over the next generation," says Clark Heath, M.D., ACS vice president of epidemiology and statistics.

The victory against cancer is going to have to come from us as much as from doctors and scientists. But that doesn't mean we have to live the lifestyle of a monk or wear a space suit to protect against environmental hazards. A lifestyle of moderation and common sense is all that's needed, says Dr. Laszlo. Here's a list, based on a survey of leading cancer experts, of the ten strategies thought to be the best cancer fighters. They're things you can do starting right now, things that touch your everyday life, things that can give *you* the margin of control over this largely preventable disease.

Break the tobacco habit. Roughly 90 percent of all lung cancer deaths in men, and 79 percent in women, are caused by smoking. The habit also increases risks of cancers of the mouth, pharynx, larynx, esophagus, pancreas, uterus, cervix, kidney and bladder—the bottom line being that smoking is thought to be responsible for about 30 percent of cancer deaths overall. Add the risks posed by chewing tobacco and snuff (which contribute to cancers of the mouth, larynx, esophagus and throat), and it becomes clear why avoiding tobacco is so important to a cancer-free life. "The list of chemicals in tobacco includes some of the most potent cancer causers known," says Dr. Laszlo.

If you've got a pack of cigarettes in your hand right now—drop them! They won't be the only thing to drop. "The odds of getting lung cancer drop steadily and dramatically when people quit," says Dr. Laszlo. "Natural repair of the cells that line the air passages begins almost immediately. In many cases, precancerous changes that have been caused by smoking can be totally reversed."

Are pipe and cigar smokers exempt from smoking's risks? No, because some passive inhalation of smoke is unavoidable, even if you think you don't inhale. Regardless of whether you inhale or not, you're subject to increased risks of lip, mouth and tongue cancer, says Dr. Laszlo.

Avoid passive smoking. Breathing smoke from someone else's cigarette may be more harmful than we previously thought. Some studies suggest that "sidestream" or "passive" smoke may even be worse than smoke directly inhaled, because it has not had its tar content reduced by traveling through the cigarette's filter. "Living with a smoker may increase a nonsmoker's risks of cancer by as much as 50 percent," says William Shingleton, M.D., former director of the Cancer Center at the Duke University Medical School. Working in a smoky environment for 8 hours a day also can substantially elevate your risks. So if you find yourself confronting either of those situations—stand up for your rights.

Limit exposure to the sun. A suntan may make you look good, but looks can be deceiving. Nearly all of the 600,000 cases of skin cancer diagnosed each year are thought to be sun related. Just as tobacco smoke

VITAMIN C PROTECTION

Can vitamin C fight cancer? A growing number of studies indicate the answer is yes.

For example, a study of over 10,000 women worldwide found a significant relationship between higher dietary vitamin C intake and

FOOD	PORTION	VITAMIN C (mg.)
Orange juice, unsweetened, from concentrate	1 cup	392
Pummelo, raw	1	371
Papaya, raw	1	188
Guava, raw	1	165
Tomato soup, condensed	1 cup	133
Orange juice, raw	1 cup	124
Peaches, frozen, sliced, sweetened	1/2 cup	118
Red chili peppers, raw	1	109
Orange juice, frozen, unsweetened, from concentrate	1 cup	97
Cranberry juice cocktail, bottled	1 cup	89
Grapefruit juice, unsweetened frozen concentrate	1 cup	83
Kiwifruit, fresh, raw	1	74
Orange, raw	1	70

can disrupt the genetic mechanisms responsible for keeping cellular division orderly, so can the ultraviolet rays of the sun. And once out of control, skin cells can be among the most unruly of them all. The most serious form of skin cancer, called melanoma, can spread with fatal speed if not treated early.

But if there's anything good to say about skin cancer, it's that it can easily be prevented, says Dr. Laszlo. Prevention is as easy as avoiding prolonged exposure to direct sunlight between the hours of 10:00 A.M. and 3:00 P.M., wearing protective clothing when out in the sun and applying sunscreen. Be especially careful to protect yourself from the sun's rays at high altitudes and in areas near the equator, says Dr. Laszlo. And don't

lower risk of breast cancer. They say that boosting your intake of vitamin C to around 380 milligrams may help provide protection against certain types of cancers.

The following high-C foods should be part of your anticancer arsenal.

FOOD	PORTION	VITAMIN C (mg.)
Grape juice, sweetened from concentrate	1 cup	60
Strawberries, frozen, sweetened, sliced	1/2 cup	53
Sweet green peppers, raw, chopped	1/2 cup	45
Tomato juice, canned	1 cup	45
Edible-podded peas, raw	1/2 cup	43
Kohlrabi, raw, slices	1/2 cup	43
Strawberries, raw	1/2 cup	42
Broccoli, raw, chopped	1/2 cup	41
Broccoli, frozen spears, boiled, drained	1/2 cup	37
Brussels sprouts, frozen, boiled	1/2 cup	36
Cauliflower, boiled, drained	1/2 cup	34
Sweet potatoes, boiled, skinless, mashed	1/2 cup	28
Asparagus, boiled, drained	1/2 cup	24
Cabbage, fresh, shredded	1/2 cup	18
Fruit cocktail, canned, light syrup	1/2 cup	2

think that getting a suntan at a tanning parlor is without hazard. Despite advertising claims that may tell you otherwise, rays from a bulb that tan you are just as much of a risk for cancer (and wrinkles) as rays from the sun.

Go easy on alcohol. Studies of people who imbibe leave little doubt: As the drinks go down, cancer risks go up. One study found that heavy drinkers have a 2- to 6-fold greater-than-average risk of cancers of the throat and mouth. Some studies, but not all, suggest that the risk of breast cancer may double for women who drink. Even bigger trouble appears to be in store for heavy drinkers who also smoke: Risks of throat and mouth cancer skyrocket to 15-fold, and risks of esophageal cancer may increase by as much as 25-fold, when cigarettes and alcohol are combined.

How does alcohol do its damage?

Researchers can only guess at this point, but several theories look plausible. By overburdening the liver, heavy drinking may compromise that vital organ's ability to detoxify potentially cancer-causing substances, especially those resulting from smoking. Heavy drinking—of hard liquor particularly—may also irritate tissues of the mouth, throat and esophagus in a way that makes them more susceptible to cancer. Or certain drinks, particularly darker liquors such as rum, bourbon and scotch, may produce cancer-causing by-products in the distillation process.

Whatever the biological mechanisms involved, the statistics don't lie. More than a few drinks a day increases your risks of cancer of the mouth, throat, pancreas, esophagus and liver. And according to some studies, heavy drinking may also boost your risks of cancer of the breast, stomach and rectum. "If you're going to drink," says Dr. Laszlo, "you should keep your intake to no more than two or three drinks a day, and avoid drinking the hard stuff straight." The less diluted the drink, the more irritating to the gullet, and the greater the risk of cancer to the upper gastrointestinal tract, he says.

Cut down on dietary fat. Scientists aren't yet certain why, but a diet high in fat seems to increase risks of cancers of the breast and colon, and perhaps of the prostate and ovary as well. Whether by inciting cancer-causing hormones or cancer-causing digestive enzymes or by feeding cancer cells directly, dietary fat may be what scientists call a cancer "promoter," a substance that does not instigate cancerous changes in cells initially but does encourage continuation of already existing changes by providing a favorable environment. In the case of breast cancer, for example, a diet high in fat seems to elevate levels of the hormone estrogen, which is suspected of feeding tumor growth. With colon cancer, a high-fat diet may do its harm by causing the excessive release of bile acids, which in large amounts act as promoters on the lining of the intestine.

"We're just not sure yet of the exact mechanisms involved in the cancer/dietary fat link, but population studies leave little doubt that the connection exists," says the ACS statistics expert Dr. Heath. "In countries where less fat is consumed, we find fewer cancers."

PROFILE IN HEALING

JUNE ADLER: BEATING BREAST CANCER

It's best prevented, yes, but cancer also is a disease that in many cases can be cured—if discovered and treated in time. Just ask June Adler. At age 44, she discovered a lump the size of a grape in her right breast. The diagnosis: cancer.

She was "devastated," and the news hit even harder when her doctor said a modified radical mastectomy—complete removal of her breast—would be required.

"That's when I called the self-help group Y-Me," she says. "I wanted to know all my options, and they were extremely helpful. They told me that a less radical procedure known as a lumpectomy, which removes the lump without removing the breast, might be possible and that I should get a second opinion to see if it might work in my case."

June did more than get a second opinion. She got a second and a third, and both were in agreement that she was a good lumpectomy candidate. Radiation treatments in combination with chemotherapy would be required to supplement the lumpectomy, but it was a sacrifice June was willing to make.

The lumpectomy was performed in March 1986 and was followed by 11 months of radiation and chemotherapy treatments. "The cancer had spread to my lymph nodes, so they wanted to be sure they got it all," June says.

But they did not. In March 1988 a small tumor was discovered on June's left lung. "That's when I really had to gather my strength," she says. "I was just beginning to feel my ordeal was over. But I wasn't going to give up. After the surgery, I enrolled in a course that taught me how to use visualization to combat cancer. I was going to fight my disease in every way possible."

Today, thanks to continued follow-up care and a fighting spirit, June is cancer-free. She has also gone on to direct one of Y-Me's regional offices in Northbrook, Illinois. "Their help was invaluable to me," she says. "They helped me make the right decisions at the right time, decisions that helped me save not just my breast but my life."

That being the case, the American Health Foundation recommends that total fat in the diet not comprise more than 20 to 25 percent of total calories. If you're an average American, that means you should be eating about *half* the fat you eat now. A good way to start cutting back is to add more fruits and vegetables to your diet and to go easy on animal products, such as meat and cheese.

Bulk up on dietary fiber. If it helps to think of fiber as your body's scrub brush, go right ahead. Fiber's unique dietary talent is that it doesn't

BRIMMING WITH BETA-CAROTENE

More and more studies are showing that people who eat foods rich in beta-carotene have a lower risk of developing cancer than those who eat these foods less frequently. Beta-carotene is a nutrient found in dark yellow and green fruits and vegetables that is converted to vitamin A in your body.

Although vitamin A is toxic in large doses, beta-carotene is not. But you can overdo beta-carotene, which usually becomes apparent

FOOD	PORTION	VITAMIN A (IU)	BETA-CAROTENE (mg.)
Carrot juice, canned	1 cup	63,347	25
Sweet potatoes, canned, mashed	1/2 cup	19,286	12
Pumpkin, canned	1/2 cup	26,908	8
Carrot, raw	1	20,253	8
Carrots, frozen, boiled, drained, sliced	1/2 cup	12,922	8
Carrots, raw, shredded	1/2 cup	15,471	6
Mango	1	8,061	5
Spinach, boiled, drained	1/2 cup	7,371	4
Butternut squash, baked	1/2 cup	7,141	4
Turnip greens, frozen, boiled, drained	1/2 cup	6,540	4
Dandelion greens, boiled, drained, chopped	1/2 cup	6,084	4

get digested. Rather, it passes right through you, often escorting potential carcinogens along with it.

In the case of colon cancer, fiber is thought to help dilute and remove potentially cancer-promoting bile acids. In the case of breast cancer, some fiber may reduce levels of cancer-promoting excess estrogen.

The Department of Health and Human Services says that if Americans would eat more fiber and less fat, colon cancer could be reduced by 30 percent. Researchers from the National Cancer Institute are even more

by the skin taking on an orange glow. Cutting back on beta-carotene-rich foods, however, should solve the problem.

There is no Recommended Dietary Allowance for beta-carotene, but any single food serving containing over 1.8 milligrams (or over 3,000 international units [IU] of vitamin A) is considered to be a rich source.

Below are the foods richest in this nutrient, beginning with the very best.

FOOD	PORTION	VITAMIN A (IU)	BETA-CAROTENE (mg.)
Passion fruit juice, yellow	1 cup	5,953	4
Cantaloupe, raw	1 cup	5,158	3
Collards, frozen, boiled, drained, chopped	1/2 cup	5,084	3
Kale, boiled, drained, chopped	1/2 cup	4,810	3
Hubbard squash, boiled, mashed	1/2 cup	4,726	3
Beet greens, boiled, drained	1/2 cup	3,672	2
Vegetable juice cocktail, canned	1 cup	2,831	2
Swiss chard, boiled, drained, chopped	1/2 cup	2,762	2
Broccoli, frozen, boiled, drained, chopped	1/2 cup	1,741	1

optimistic. They feel that a daily intake of 20 to 30 grams of fiber could cut rates of colon cancer in half.

What are the best sources of cancer-fighting fiber?

Insoluble fiber—the kind most prevalent in wheat bran, whole-grain cereals and breads, vegetables and fruits—seems to speed things through the intestines best. Wheat bran has also been shown to reduce estrogen in the blood. But soluble fibers—the kind prevalent in oat bran and beans—also seem to have cancer-fighting effects. Authorities agree that it's probably best to get a good mix of both types.

How do you get adequate fiber in your diet?

One combination that would give you at least 20 grams of fiber is one bowl of wheat bran cereal with a tablespoon of raisins and an apple for breakfast and, for lunch, a bowl of baked beans with a large salad and a slice of pumpernickel bread. But there are many possible combinations.

Splurge on fruits and vegetables. "Population studies leave little doubt that a varied diet containing plenty of fruits and vegetables can reduce risks for a wide range of cancers," says Dr. Heath. Not only are fruits and vegetables rich in fiber, most are extremely low in fat as well as veritable treasure chests of potential cancer-fighting nutrients—vitamins A and C, beta-carotene and bioflavonoids.

Scientists speculate that these nutrients may exert their protective effect by guarding cells from free radicals, molecules in the body that are thought to encourage cancer by altering the genetic makeup of cells.

Other nutrients prevalent in the pulpy portions of citrus fruits are thought to enhance the anticancer activity of naturally occurring enzymes in the body. A similar enzyme boost may also be exerted by cruciferous—cabbage family—vegetables (broccoli, brussels sprouts, cauliflower and cabbage) in a way that helps the liver break down and eliminate potential carcinogens from the body.

To help fruits and vegetables do their best work, eat them as fresh as possible, cook to a minimum and include their skins and peels (well washed) when feasible to maximize fiber and nutrient content. Your goal should be to consume at least two servings of vegetables and two servings of fruit each day.

Stay slim. Cancer and fat—whether the fat is on your plate or your waist—don't seem to make a healthy pair. Obesity (measured as being 40 percent or more above one's ideal weight) was found in an ACS study to increase cancer deaths in women by 55 percent and in men by 33 percent. Overweight women had higher rates of death from cancer of the endometrium, uterus, gallbladder, cervix, ovaries and breast. Overweight men had higher rates of death from colon, rectal and prostate cancer.

Some theories on the cancer/obesity link include the speculation that eating a lot of calories boosts metabolism, resulting in more frequent cellular divisions that could increase cancer risks. "One very important point is that the type of diet that tends to produce obesity in the first place may be a factor—one high in dietary fat and low in fiber," says Dr. Heath.

Whatever the reason, as body weight rises above normal, so do risks of cancer. Maybe that's the logic to pin to your refrigerator door.

Avoid environmental hazards. "Allow for plenty of ventilation when painting, varnishing or using any chemical product indoors," says John Vena, Ph.D., a professor with the Department of Social and Preventive Medicine at the State University of New York at Buffalo. Also be careful with pesticides and herbicides around the home—read the labels carefully. Wash fruits and vegetables before eating to remove any chemical residue. And have your house checked for high levels of radon, a naturally occurring gas that has been linked to lung cancer.

Beyond that, there's often not a lot you *can* do about environmental hazards, Dr. Vena says. "There are certain work-related substances some people may need to worry about—nickel, chromates, asbestos and vinyl chloride, for example—but most industries now control these substances fairly well. It would still be a good idea to learn about the substances you are working with. Also for anyone who has had a history of working with chemicals or dusts, it's important to let their doctor know, so that any complications could be detected as early as possible."

As for recent speculations on the cancer risks posed by electromagnetic fields, the research is still very preliminary, says Dr. Vena. "It does make sense to update certain appliances that could be showing wear, however—things like electric blankets or hair dryers that involve very close contact. This would offer as much protection against fire and electrocution as against cancer," he says.

Get regular exercise. Exercise seems to give certain cancers a run for their money. "Exercise might be underrated as a cancer-fighting strategy," Dr. Vena says. One study looked at former female college athletes and found they had lower rates of breast and reproductive organ cancers than women who had not been athletic in college. Dr. Vena's own research has found risks of colon cancer to be twice as great in sedentary people as opposed to those in physically active occupations.

"We're still speculating as to why exercise seems to have a protective effect," Dr. Vena says. "Stress reduction could be a factor, as could improved bowel regularity. It's also possible that people who exercise regularly tend to eat more healthfully and take better care of themselves generally." Exercise, of course, also helps to combat obesity; this in itself can have a protective effect.

Whatever the reason, cancer seems to have a tougher time hitting a moving target. Try to get at least 30 minutes of some sort of physical activity—even if it's as moderate as a brisk walk, washing windows or weeding the garden—at least three times a week. That may be all it takes to keep cancer defenses in good shape.

THE IMPORTANCE OF EARLY DETECTION

If someone wanted to give you a penny this year, two next year, and double the sum every year for 30 years, would your first reaction be "Thanks, but don't waste my time"?

A penny doubled every year for 30 years would produce the decidedly handsome sum of $5,368,709.12. And yet it's this kind of *Ripley's Believe It or Not* arithmetic, unfortunately, that lies behind the importance of early detection of most types of cancer.

"There are mitigating circumstances, such as the strength of a person's immune system, but most tumors will do their best to grow in what's known as an exponential fashion," says Michael Bookman, M.D., of the Department of Medical Oncology (the study of tumors) at the Fox Chase Cancer Center in Philadelphia. "This means that one cell becomes two,

---

TREATMENT BREAKTHROUGH

"SUPERFOODS" TO THE RESCUE

Eat your fruits and vegetables and decrease your chances of getting certain kinds of cancer. Doctors have been saying it for years. Now the National Cancer Institute (NCI) is poised to go one step better. The Designer Foods Research Project has one aim in mind: to hunt down nutrients known as phytochemicals locked inside common foods and to find some way to concentrate them and manufacture new foods—superfoods with super cancer-fighting potential.

Imagine a future in which even *desserts* might become edible medical missiles aimed at preventing cancer! That future may become a reality. Here's the NCI's strategy.

1. Identify the most powerful cancer-fighting substances found in fruits, vegetables, herbs and other edible plants.
2. Calculate their ideal concentrations and most potent forms.
3. Then test them in studies with high-risk or cancer patients to see if they really can stop the disease.

The cancer-fighting nutrients targeted in this program would be

two becomes four, four becomes eight and so on. As with the example of the pennies, it doesn't take long for the numbers to become huge."

Hence the importance of catching and arresting the spread of most cancers as early as possible. Not only is treatment of the initial tumor more likely to be successful, there's less chance that it will have metastasized— spread to other sites.

The ACS recommends a general cancer-related checkup every three years for people 20 to 40 years of age, and then one every year after that. The checkup can be done by most family physicians and should include examinations of the thyroid, testes, prostate, mouth, ovaries, lymph nodes and skin.

In addition to these general checkups, women should be routinely checked for breast and cervical cancer every year after the age of 20, and men should be checked for colon and rectal cancer every year after the age of 40.

TRIED-AND-TRUE TREATMENTS

So prevention is job one in the fight against cancer, and early detection is job two. That leaves job three, should it be necessary: getting the best and most appropriate treatment should a cancer be found. Many experts

engineered into their purest and most powerful form. "We're going after common foods plus some ingredients that people don't know much about but have been eating for years," says Herbert F. Pierson, Ph.D., a toxicologist at the Diet and Cancer Branch of the NCI.

The Designer Foods Research Project is still in the diaper stage— researchers are busy trying to find and fingerprint the phytochemicals while attempting to understand how they work. "There's an awful lot of research that has to be done, but the future certainly looks bright," says Dr. Pierson. Looking ahead, he says that someday—with the right addition of phytochemicals and subtraction of fat—it may be possible that even potato chips and other "junk" foods will be man-ufactured so as to be good for our health!

"Studies say that about half of all chronic diseases like cancer may be linked to diet," says Dr. Pierson. "If that's true, then making foods healthier, by taking advantage of what Mother Nature has already given us to work with, may lead to a significant reduction in cancer."

recommend getting opinions from at least two experts before deciding on a course of treatment. You want to be as informed as possible, because the first shot at curing cancer is always the best shot. Cancers that recur become progressively more difficult to treat.

Here's a brief description of the major types of treatment being used today. Sometimes these treatments are used by themselves, but more often in combination.

SURGERY. Surgery to remove the cancerous growth, or as much as possible, is the oldest form of treatment for cancer, dating back to the Middle Ages. Often surgery is used in conjunction with chemotherapy or radiation therapy in cases where all of a tumor is not removed or if the cancer is thought to have spread.

RADIATION THERAPY. Radiation is sometimes an alternative to surgery and works by killing cancer cells through exposure to high doses of x-rays. Since cancer cells exist around and among normal cells, however, a drawback to radiation therapy is that it cannot be highly selective in sparing healthy tissue. This can make the therapy inadvisable for treating certain cancers involving major organs. On the plus side, however, radiation therapy is painless. Treatments take only a few minutes daily and are usually done on an outpatient basis.

CHEMOTHERAPY. Chemotherapy involves introducing drugs, usually through injection, that kill cancer cells by interfering with the way they reproduce. Often a variety of drugs is used to combat the uncanny ability of cancer cells to adapt in ways that can make them resistant to chemotherapy's effects. But if the right combination is used, results can be dramatic. Also dramatic, however, can be chemotherapy's side effects: nausea, vomiting, hair loss, sores in the mouth, diarrhea and increased susceptibility to infection. Fortunately, new drugs are bringing some of these side effects under control.

ANTIHORMONE THERAPY. In the treatment of both breast cancer and prostate cancer, drugs to keep troublemaking hormones under control have been quite successful. Tamoxifen, the antihormone drug most commonly used to treat breast cancer, has few side effects. Those drugs used for prostate cancer, however, may cause troublesome nausea and breast tenderness.

IMMUNOTHERAPY. In this technique, drugs are given to boost the body's own abilities to fight cancer naturally. Interferon has been the most publicized of these drugs. "Interferon has been highly successful in treating one rare type of leukemia but has been considerably less effective against more common forms of cancer such as lung, colon and breast. The area of immunotherapy remains a highly promising one, however, and much encouraging work continues to be done," says Dr. Laszlo.

CANKER SORES AND COLD SORES

Sometimes all it takes is anxiety over a hot date or a bite into a spicy meatball to spark a mouthful of woes. Just ask anybody who suffers from cold sores (also known as fever blisters) or canker sores.

"There are so many triggers for cold and canker sores that you can't count them all," says Steven Vincent, D.D.S., an associate professor in the Department of Oral Pathology, Radiology and Medicine at the University of Iowa College of Dentistry in Iowa City.

Although both cold sores and canker sores attack the mouth, and *occasionally* may be triggered by the same things, they are actually quite different.

KNOWING ONE FROM THE OTHER

Cold sores occasionally form on the inside of the mouth (and occasionally on the nostrils, fingers and even eyelids), but their favorite place to pop up is on the lips. A cold sore actually begins as several small blisters that swell up and form one large blister. That blister eventually ruptures, forming an ulcer. An unsightly yellow crust forms and finally heals in seven to ten days, without scarring. Cold sores affect about one-third of all Americans.

Unlike canker sores, cold sores have a known direct cause—the herpes simplex (almost always type 1) virus. Don't let that "herpes" stuff scare you. "When people hear of herpes, they automatically think of genital herpes (type 2), but this is a much different and separate phenomenon," says Brad Rodu, D.D.S., associate professor in the School of Dentistry at the University of Alabama in Birmingham.

A canker sore is a pinhead- to pea-size white or yellowish ulcer that forms on the tongue or inside the cheek or lip. The medical term for cankers is *aphthous ulcers,* which means "fire sores," an apt phrase considering how painful they are. Canker sores are probably just about as common as cold sores, but they appear to be somewhat hereditary.

A canker sore usually lasts a week or two and can make eating, drinking and even talking feel as if a missile just exploded in your mouth. Most people get only an occasional canker, but some severely afflicted individuals may have clusters of them forming all the time.

COOLING A COLD SORE

The virus that causes cold sores is so common that 90 percent of Americans have been exposed to it by age five. The virus lies dormant, often for years, in a nerve until a triggering factor such as stress, cold winds or exposure to sunlight activates it. Some other triggers include fatigue, fever, upset stomach and menstruation. Many sufferers get warning signals such as tingling, itching or burning on the lips 36 to 48 hours before a cold sore appears. Unfortunately, at that stage there is little that can be done to stop it. However, there are things you can do to prevent cold sores in the first place or to help soothe the pain once they erupt.

Wear a ski mask in cold weather. The rush of cold wind is notorious for bringing out cold sores.

Always wear a sunscreen. Not only will you protect your skin from damaging ultraviolet rays that can cause skin cancer, you'll also reduce your chances of developing cold sores. Pay special attention to the lips. Wear lip sunscreen and a broad-brimmed hat whenever venturing out into the sun.

Keep stress in check. Excessive worrying seems to bring out the worst in cold sores. "I see a lot of them among students before final exams," says Dr. Vincent (for tips on combating stress, see "Stress" on page 472).

Consider L-lysine. Some people say this over-the-counter amino acid supplement has helped them to fend off or treat cold sores. "It may simply be a psychological effect," Dr. Vincent says, "but some people swear by it." Those cold sore sufferers who have reported success generally take daily doses ranging anywhere from 300 to 3,000 milligrams. Of course, you shouldn't take this or any other supplement without the advice and consent of your doctor.

Use moisturizing ointments. Petroleum jelly or other moisturizing ointments can help prevent cracking (which would make the blister look and feel worse). Analgesic solutions will reduce the pain, but avoid using products that contain cauterizing agents or astringents such as silver nitrate or tannic acid that can burn the skin, says Dr. Vincent.

Avoid squeezing or picking at a cold sore. It can become infected. If you notice yellow pus around the sore, see your doctor or dentist.

In addition to what you can do on your own, your doctor may also be able to help battle your cold sores with a prescription drug called acyclovir.

It comes in either ointment or pill form and is most helpful when applied soon after the onset of symptoms. "Acyclovir prevents the replication of the virus and helps prevent tissue damage. For some, it may diminish symptoms as well as the duration of the recurrence," Dr. Vincent says. "In other words, if you use acyclovir, you may only develop one or two small blisters that last a few days instead of a crusted ulcer that lasts two weeks."

TAMING THE WILD CANKER

As with cold sores, there are a number of ways to both prevent and treat canker sores.

Keep calm. Stress is the one factor that seems to trigger both canker sores *and* cold sores. In the case of canker sores, however, doctors aren't certain whether it's the stress itself or the biting of our lips and cheeks that accompanies stress. No matter. Staying relaxed is advised.

Watch what you eat. Some people find that the onset of canker sores is related to the foods they eat. High on the hit list are cherries, plums, pineapple, tomato products, nuts, chocolate and other sweet, spicy or acidic foods. "A lot of patients also say bananas give them trouble, and I can't quite figure that out, because bananas seem pretty bland," Dr. Vincent says.

Try an elimination diet. That's probably the best way to determine which foods are causing sore points in your mouth, says Sol Silverman, Jr., D.D.S., professor and chairman of the Division of Oral Medicine at the University of California, San Francisco. Start by slashing all of the foods listed above from your diet. Then reincorporate each at regular intervals. For example, if your canker sores generally show up every four weeks, wait a month before adding the first food back into your diet. If that doesn't create problems, then move to the next food the following month. Notice when the sores develop, and you might be able to isolate your problem causer.

Give yogurt a try. "I've had patients who've told me that if they eat yogurt once a day or once every other day, they don't get canker sores," Dr. Vincent says. "Of course, that's all anecdotal, and there isn't any firm clinical research to support that." But it can't hurt to give it a try.

Eat foods rich in folate, iron and B vitamins. Several studies have found that about 15 percent of people who get canker sores are deficient in these nutrients. If you are deficient, consuming plenty of foods containing these nutrients or taking supplements in moderation may help eradicate the sores. Check with your doctor if you suspect a deficiency.

Rinse your mouth. A solution made by mixing 1 teaspoon of salt in 1 pint of water may help soothe cankers and relieve their irritation. Use as needed.

Be patient. "The best thing to remember is that in seven to ten days, these things are going to go away," says James Stankiewicz, M.D., vice chairman of the Head and Neck Surgery Department at Loyola University Medical Center in Maywood, Illinois.

In case you've tried all of the above and still find your canker sores hard to live with, see your doctor or dentist. He may prescribe a steroid rinse to ease your discomfort. "We find it's very effective for the vast majority of people we see who have canker sores," Dr. Vincent says. "We advise them to rinse their mouth with it four times a day when they have an active sore."

HEALING FROM WITHIN

You've tried *everything,* and nothing, absolutely nothing, has helped rid you of your mouth sores. Perhaps you're trying too hard. Preventing and healing your cold sores or canker sores may be as simple as using some positive thinking and a bit of imagination.

Visualization techniques can be powerful tools in combating cold and canker sores, says Dennis Gersten, M.D., a San Diego psychiatrist who specializes in the use of mental imagery. Such techniques may work by boosting the power of your immune system and increasing local blood circulation, he says.

In one study of seven people who suffered from chronic canker sores, researchers at Pennsylvania State University and Case Western Reserve University found that visualization may indeed help. After several weeks of practicing visualizations twice daily, all seven people reported fewer days with sores—and six experienced a decrease in the number of sores.

If you want to give visualization a try, Dr. Gersten suggests, practice this three-step process twice a day.

1. Relax your body. Lie down, close your eyes and breathe slowly. Imagine you're a feather in the air, floating softly and slowly downward. By the time you reach the ground, which should take about 1 minute, you should be totally relaxed.
2. Mentally repeat one uplifting word or phrase of two or more syllables. Continue chanting your "mantra" for 4 to 5 minutes.
3. With your eyes still closed, imagine—visualize—a light shining on your sores. For the next 5 minutes, see the light penetrate the sores, and see it begin to heal them from the bottom up (that's how they naturally heal). The technique can be used both to heal sores you currently have and to prevent future sores from erupting, he says.

CARPAL TUNNEL SYNDROME

Karen, a typist, gets shooting pains in her hands. Bruce, a carpenter, wakes at midnight with tingling fingers. Skip, a former butcher, retired early when his right hand went numb.

Karen, Bruce and Skip have one thing in common: carpal tunnel syndrome. Caused by doing the same thing—typing, sawing, cutting meat—over and over again, carpal tunnel syndrome can cause numbness, prickling or burning sensations in the hand, thumb and fingers. And it's on the rise, says Jeffrey N. Katz, M.D., a rheumatologist (a specialist in bones, muscles and ligaments) at Boston's Brigham and Women's Hospital and an assistant professor of medicine at Harvard Medical School. In today's high-speed workplace, it's common for people to repeat the same motions thousands of times an hour. Bit by bit, their hands and wrists show the strain.

NERVOUS BREAKDOWNS

Let's take a look at the wrist, the source of carpal tunnel syndrome. First feel the bony back of your hand where it meets the wrist—those are the carpal bones. Turn your hand over and bend it upward—beneath those creases is the carpal ligament. Now between the carpal bones and the carpal ligament is a passageway called the carpal *tunnel*. And inside this tunnel is the median nerve, which transmits sensations through the hand, thumb and fingers.

Normally this nerve is well protected. But in today's fast-paced world of computers and assembly lines, the wrist often does more than it was designed for. "You can outpace the ability of your joints and ligaments to produce sufficient lubricating fluid," says Steven J. Barrer, M.D., a neurosurgeon and carpal tunnel expert in Abington, Pennsylvania. "People who do frequent rapid hand motions with no rest are working without oil, so to speak."

Over time, this can cause tissues inside the wrist to become inflamed and swollen. As they swell, they begin to press on the sensitive median nerve. This is what causes pain, numbness and other symptoms of carpal tunnel syndrome.

TOO MUCH, TOO LONG

You wouldn't think that tapping a keyboard could cause serious injury. But a fast typist makes thousands of keystrokes an hour, each of which sends slight jolts into the fingers and wrists. Multiply each jolt several million times, and you can see how each letter you strike turns into a *pound sign.*

"Light" factory work can also take a heavier toll than you might think. "I've seen people on assembly lines do the same motions for their entire 8-hour shift," says Janna Jacobs, a physical therapist and president of the Hand Rehabilitation Section of the American Physical Therapy Association.

Working at home also can cause carpal tunnel pain. Painting—a row of apartments or a masterpiece on canvas—can cause trouble. So can knitting, crocheting or playing a musical instrument. "For a lot of people, it's what they do at home plus what they do on the job that causes problems," says Jacobs.

There are some underlying physical conditions—arthritis is one, pregnancy is another—that can cause carpal tunnel syndrome, Dr. Katz adds.

Since women (even nonpregnant women) get carpal tunnel syndrome two to five times more often than men, doctors suspect that changing levels in women's hormones may play a role.

HANDY ADVICE

For people who do work with their hands, reducing the time spent on repetitive tasks is the best way to prevent trouble later. Varying your routine can also help. But there's more.

Warm up. Athletes know that starting work with cold muscles is inviting trouble. The same is true for keyboard and assembly-line athletes. By stretching before you start to work, Jacobs says, you can reduce wrist strain and the potential for carpal tunnel syndrome.

Here's one stretch: First clench your fist. Then fan out the fingers as far as they'll go. Repeat five times. Or lean forward and gently press your hands on a tabletop, stretching the fingers and wrists. Hold for 5 seconds, then repeat.

Adjust your keyboard. Typing a letter is easy. Typing dozens of letters, from A to Z, is hard work. To reduce the strain, good positioning can help, Jacobs says. With your upper arms by your side, your elbows at 90 degrees and your forearms level, the keyboard should be slightly higher than your hands. This allows your fingers to roam without putting crimps in your wrists. Also, striking the keys gently can help reduce the strain.

Keep your wrists straight. Whether you're a typist, mechanic or home hobbyist, flexing your wrists up or down can put unwanted pressure on the carpal tunnel, Dr. Katz says. When you work, try to keep your wrists in a straight line with the forearms.

Don a pair of gloves. This can be particularly helpful if your job requires you to pick up slippery objects—boning knives, for example—which require a strong grasp. By adding friction, gloves reduce the strain, Jacobs says. They also reduce vibration, another potential cause of carpal tunnel symptoms.

Take frequent breaks. Your hands need recovery time, Jacobs says. Try to allow a 5-minute break at least once an hour. You don't have to stop working. Just do something different. For example, stop typing and return a phone call. Clean out your desk. Read the rest of this chapter. *Then* return to work.

STOP THE PAIN

You may have had coaches in high school who told you to "work through the pain." That's terrible advice, particularly for carpal tunnel syndrome. Continued pressure on the nerve can only cause continued pain—and perhaps long-term damage, Dr. Barrer warns. If you have signs of carpal tunnel syndrome, you should see a doctor right away.

Still, your doctor may suggest treatments you can do at home. For example:

Put it to bed. Resting your hands and wrists can be the best medicine for carpal tunnel syndrome, says Dr. Katz. You don't have to rest them entirely, though. Just stop the motions that caused the damage. As the injured tissues heal, the pain will often disappear.

Put it on ice. This can help reduce swelling and pressure on the tender nerve, says Dr. Barrer. Don't put ice directly on the wrist, however. Wrap it in a towel or washcloth first, then apply it for a half hour, several times a day.

Add some heat. "If there's no inflammation but your wrist is stiff, heat is very effective," Dr. Barrer says.

MEDICAL RELIEF

Many people with carpal tunnel syndrome have such mild symptoms—occasional pain, a twinge, a moment's numbness—that they never need treatment. But for others the pain can be relentless. Medical treatment can help.

The first thing your doctor may try is giving you a splint to wear for a week or two. By keeping the wrist straight and immobile, splints are "dramatically effective" for relieving carpal tunnel syndrome, says Dr. Katz.

For short-term relief, your doctor may also recommend an injection of steroids, powerful drugs that quickly reduce inflammation, says Dr. Katz. Since steroids don't affect the underlying problem, however, they often provide only temporary relief of symptoms.

Among older women, carpal tunnel syndrome has been linked to changing hormones. Hormone replacement therapy may help. In a British study, 42 postmenopausal women with muscle-skeletal problems (including carpal tunnel syndrome) were given hormone replacements. After six months, the women had "improved significantly"—possibly, the researchers suggest, because the hormones blocked the reduction in forearm fat that generally occurs after menopause. Protecting this extra "cushioning" may have helped save their wrists from injury.

For serious cases, surgery can help. In a relatively simple, outpatient procedure, the carpal ligament—the one pressing against the nerve—is cut. This essentially raises the "roof" over the carpal tunnel, giving the nerve extra room.

There are many ligaments in your hand, so cutting one isn't likely to change the ways your hand functions. Of course, it may be a few weeks before you feel entirely recovered from the surgery. For many people, the operation works well, adds Dr. Katz. "If you had to divide the world of surgery into lousy, mediocre and good operations, this would be a good operation."

CELIAC DISEASE

W hat comes to mind when you think about bread? Perhaps you think of crusty French bread, or chewy Jewish rye, or the plump, fragrant loaves Mom baked fresh on Saturday mornings. Most of us eat bread or its brethren—muffins, pancakes or croissants—nearly every day. No wonder it's long been considered the "staff of life"!

If you have celiac disease, however, the staff of life—or more precisely, the gluten found in common grains—becomes the wrath of life. You can eat a lot or a little, two meals or ten, but your gluten-damaged intestines simply can't extract the nutrients they need. Here's why.

HUNGER AMIDST PLENTY

Your small intestine is packed with millions of threadlike projections called villi that absorb nutrients from digested foods. These nutrients then travel through your intestine, into your bloodstream and on to hungry cells throughout your body. But if you have celiac disease (also referred to as sprue), gluten, a protein found in wheat, rye, oats, barley and other grains, actually flattens the villi, which prevents nutrients from getting in, explains Steven R. Peikin, M.D., author of *Gastrointestinal Health* and an associate professor of medicine and pharmacology at the Medical College of Philadelphia's Thomas Jefferson University Hospital.

"If celiac disease occurs before puberty, growth failure is very common," Dr. Peikin says. "It can cause severe bone disease, because you're not absorbing calcium from your diet. Many people experience severe malnutrition. Left untreated, it can lead to severe sickness and even death."

Doctors aren't sure what causes celiac disease, which is characterized by severe intestinal distress. Recurrent diarrhea, stomach cramps and unpleasant bowel movements are common symptoms. They speculate that a virus or bacterium may make the intestine particularly sensitive to gluten. It also seems to be an immunological disease—that is, something about the gluten encourages the body, rather stupidly, to attack itself. In addition, the disease is believed to be hereditary: Doctors call some regions of Ireland, generously populated with afflicted families, the "sprue belt."

There isn't a cure for celiac disease, but staying away from gluten is the next best thing, Dr. Peikin says. In fact, people who eliminate this pestiferous protein from their diet can be symptom-free in just a few weeks.

Bootin' Gluten

If gluten appeared only in bread, it wouldn't be so tough to avoid. But gluten can be found in just about anything. It can hide in soups and condiments, lunch meats and cheese spreads, soy sauce and ice cream. "You have to be very fastidious and careful, because gluten is in all kinds

---

PROFILE IN HEALING

LEON ROTTMANN: BREAKING AWAY FROM BREAD

At one time, Leon H. Rottmann never hesitated before packing in a pizza or gnawing on a thick slice of wholesome wheat bread. But in his early fifties, Leon developed celiac disease—the "malabsorption syndrome." Caused by the gluten found in wheat, rye and other grains, the disease steadily damaged Leon's small intestine, preventing nutrients from filtering through his body. He got plenty to eat, but he was starving to death.

"I had bone aches and muscle pains, and I was tired all the time," says Leon, a professor of human development and the family at the University of Nebraska at Lincoln. "I went from 185 pounds down to 134. I starting having uncontrollable diarrhea three or four times a day. I had days when I had diarrhea 20 to 25 times. I got so weak that I wasn't sure I could drive to the hospital."

Leon did make it to the hospital, and he stayed 16 days. When he was discharged, his orders were clear: no more foods containing gluten. No small task, since gluten is found in breads and pastries, sauces and spices, even in medicines. And it doesn't take much to make him sick. "If I go into a bakery and wheat flour is in the air, I'll get sick," says Leon, whose experience has led him to his volunteer

---

of things," Dr. Peikin says. "You have to be a detective if you're going to avoid it."

Read the label. If it comes in a bag, can, tube or bottle, assume the worst, advise officials at the Omaha headquarters of the Celiac-Sprue Association of the United States of America, Inc. Read all product labels—and don't assume "gluten" will jump off the page in capital letters and neon lights. Ingredients that may contain gluten include malt, bran, semolina or hydrolyzed vegetable protein (HVP). Instant coffees can contain gluten. So do beers, bourbons and whiskey blends. Even white vinegar can be a problem.

Get rid of grains. Rice and corn contain no offending glutens and are the only grains you should consider safe, Dr. Peikin says. You should give all other grains the heave-ho. But before you celebrate your new diet with a panful of corn pone, peruse the package: Some commercially packaged cornmeal actually contains wheat flour.

Take a culinary cruise. Many Asian foods are wheat-free, so you

---

job as executive director of the Celiac-Sprue Association of the United States of America, Inc.

But he doesn't dwell on his culinary misfortunes. Instead, he concentrates on the future—on the new, gluten-free recipes he wants to try, on the healthy twists he plans to put on his old favorites. Pizza, for example—he wasn't about to give it up. "I have a pizza pan at home, and I make a rice flour and potato starch crust," he says. "I take that to a neighborhood pizza place, and they put the toppings on and bake it for me."

Leon goes out to dinner, too. Sometimes he will call ahead to ask what, *exactly*, goes into different foods on the menu. He always asks lots of questions. Is gluten in the margarine? Is gluten in the spices? Is gluten in the salad dressing? "At the beginning I was self-conscious, but this is something I have to do," Leon explains. "Otherwise, I'll be ill for days."

Some people never get used to their gluten-free diets, Leon says. "They see it in the negative sense, as 'can't do, can't have,' and that's a real problem. But there are hundreds of fruits, vegetables and fresh meats I can eat. I have an excellent recipe for pancakes and a reasonably good one for cinnamon rolls. It's really a very good, very healthy diet."

can tempt your taste buds with exotic stir-fries or curries. Of course, all fresh meats and vegetables are gluten-free, as are fish, rice cakes and garden-fresh salads.

Take your tastes on the town. Dining out may be a little tricky if you have celiac disease, but it needn't be out of the question. Many restaurants routinely take requests—and questions—from diners with celiac disease who are concerned about having a "safe" meal. To play it even safer, you can always take your own condiments—salad dressing, for example.

WHEN TEMPTATION KNOCKS

After a few months on a gluten-free diet, you should be feeling pretty good, and you may be tempted to cheat just a little bit. After all, you ask yourself, how much harm can a teeny, tiny crust of bread do? Plenty, Dr. Peikin says. Even if you don't get sick immediately, your insides won't forget the insult. Sooner or later they will retaliate, and your symptoms will come right back.

"Most people know what will happen to them if they do cheat, so they tend to be pretty careful," Dr. Peikin says. "But you can have some very good meals once you know what you're doing. You don't have to have a crummy life just because you have celiac disease."

CERVICAL DYSPLASIA

The last word any woman wants to hear following a Pap smear is "abnormal." It is not, however, a reason for panic. "Abnormal" findings are extremely common and are usually due to easy-to-treat conditions such as inflammation, an infection or cervical erosion. It's also possible to learn that you have what doctors call cervical dysplasia.

This condition often causes no symptoms—it's simply the growth of abnormal cells on the cervix. (The cervix, located deep within the vagina, is the opening to the uterus.) But because some kinds of cervical dysplasia set the stage for the development of cervical cancer, doctors often treat cervical dysplasia aggressively, removing the cells in moderate or severe cases and, in mild cases, either removing cells or monitoring them closely with frequent Pap smears. (The cells may revert to normal or become increasingly abnormal.)

PROTECTING YOURSELF

Unlike heart disease or lung cancer, cervical cancer—and its precursor, cervical dysplasia—isn't generally thought of as a "lifestyle" disease. But population studies do link an increased risk for cervical cancer with some factors that *are* within your control. Following these tips will help you reduce your risk.

Get regular Pap smears. "The biggest risk factor for invasive cervical cancer is infrequent Pap smears," says Ruth Peters, Sc.D., a professor of preventive medicine at the University of Southern California School of Medicine in Los Angeles.

Most experts recommend that you begin getting Pap smears as soon as you become sexually active. After you've had *three* consecutive annual Pap smears that show all is normal, you shouldn't need another for three more years. If the test shows that something cancerous may be brewing, more frequent testing is highly advisable, says Dr. Peters.

One study by researchers at the University of Washington found that women who hadn't had a Pap test in ten years or more had *12 times* the cancer risk of women who got checked more regularly.

Make it monogamous. The more sexual partners you've had, the higher your risk for cervical cancer. And if you're faithful but he's been sleeping around, your risks also shoot up. Why? Chances are you, through your mate, have been exposed to a virus associated with cervical cancer. "Strains of human papillomavirus (HPV) have been found in more than 90 percent of cervical cancer tissue samples," says Ralph Richart, M.D., director of the Division of Gynecological Pathology and Cytology at Columbia Presbyterian Medical Center in New York City.

Wait till you're twentysomething. Because it may expose cervical cells to the sexually transmitted factor (perhaps HPV) at a time when they are particularly vulnerable, sex at an early age ups your risk for developing cervical cancer later, Dr. Peters says. "In one recent study, one partner before age 20 tripled a woman's risk, and three or more sexual partners before age 20 increased the risk tenfold," she says.

Use barrier methods of birth control. Condoms and diaphragms protect the cervix from contact with lots of potential irritants, including the HPV virus. In her study, Dr. Peters also found contraceptive creams, jellies and foams reduced cancer risks. Why? "They kill sperm, and they probably also kill whatever else might be transmitted," she says.

Douche with discretion. Don't douche unless your doctor tells you to. There is a misperception among many women that regular douching keeps you fresh and clean. Instead, it seems to reduce the body's natural ability to fight off disease. "In one recent study, douching five or more times a month tripled the risk of cervical cancer," says Dr. Peters.

Ditch your butts, and his, too. Studies show that smoking triples your risk for cervical cancer, Dr. Peters says. "Nicotine and other chemicals from cigarette smoke are concentrated in the cervical fluid," she says. Those same toxins also end up in a man's semen.

One study showed that women exposed to passive cigarette smoke for 3 or more hours a day had a threefold increase in cervical cancer.

Eat better. Numerous population studies have linked the development of cervical cancer with poor nutrition. Adequate intake of vitamins E and C, beta-carotene and folate seems protective.

GET PROPER TREATMENT

What do you need to know if you are told you have cervical dysplasia? In a sense, you should be delighted that your doctor has found these abnormal cells. Early treatment can *prevent* them from turning into cancer.

Next you should be aware that your diagnosis should not be based on a Pap smear alone. "A Pap smear is a screening test, not a method of diagnosis," says Robert Kurman, M.D., a professor and director of gynecologic pathology at Johns Hopkins Hospital in Baltimore.

An abnormal Pap smear indicating dysplasia should be followed by a biopsy of the cervix done with a colposcope, a viewing instrument that provides a magnified view of the cervix and allows the doctor to see any actual lesions, Dr. Kurman says. The biopsy removes small bits of tissue that are examined under a microscope. At the same time, the doctor may also scrape cells from the opening to the uterus, a procedure called endocervical curettage. Based on the examination of these two tissue samples, the doctor will decide how much cervical tissue needs to be removed and how it should be removed.

The tissue is most often removed by freezing (cryosurgery) or carbon dioxide laser surgery, both simple outpatient procedures. If the abnormal cells have invaded underlying tissue, a more radical surgical procedure, or radiation therapy, may be required.

A newer technique that uses a thin, electrically charged wire loop to scoop out areas of abnormal cells may be better than either cryosurgery or laser surgery, though, Dr. Richart says. "The procedure is easy to teach and learn," he says. "It requires less expensive equipment than other methods of removal, allows biopsy and treatment to occur at the same time, which saves patients an additional office visit, and gives a complete tissue sample for examination, which will do away with missed diagnosis of invasive cancer."

CHILDHOOD
INFECTIOUS DISEASES

One hundred years ago, a band of ruthless desperados was ravaging the cradles of America. With names such as Measles, Diphtheria and Whooping Cough (alias the Pertussis Kid), the Infectious Disease Gang killed *one-fifth* of all infants before their first birthday. Another gang member named Polio crippled countless more.

But the sun long ago started setting on the Infectious Disease Gang. Our nation's modern tots are healthier than ever—and the dreaded diseases of yesteryear are still running scared from the long arm of modern medicine.

The arm holds not a gun but a needle and syringe. Modern immunizations shield today's tots not only from the four desperados above but also from tetanus, mumps, rubella (German measles) and *Hemophilus influenzae* (the most common bacteria that cause meningitis). In fact, "probably the only common childhood disease that we *don't* have a handle on at the moment is chicken pox," says George Nankervis, M.D., Ph.D., chairman of pediatrics at Children's Hospital Medical Center of Akron, Ohio, and a member of the Committee on Infectious Diseases of the American Academy of Pediatrics.

That's not to say that kids today never catch anything more than chicken pox. Little people, just like big people, still get colds and common flu. We can't stop that. But *far* too many children suffer from the wholly preventable kinds of diseases. For instance, in 1990, the federal Centers for Disease Control in Atlanta received reports of nearly 28,000 cases of measles.

IMMUNIZATIONS: SMALL RISK, BIG RETURN

Why do some kids still fall prey to the likes of measles, mumps and pertussis? The answer is simple. They slip through the cracks of the system and don't get the vaccinations they need, says Dr. Nankervis.

Even more than they hate vegetables, baths, and Aunt Eva's loud pecks on the cheek, kids *hate* shots. Given a choice, they'd never get them. But childhood immunizations protect against eight very serious diseases—so if ever there was a case for parental persuasion, this is it.

Unfortunately, some *parents* need a little persuasion of their own, says Howard Lederman, M.D., Ph.D., associate professor of pediatrics and co-

THE PERFECT PROTECTION SCHEDULE

If only every disease were as easy to prevent as most childhood infectious diseases! But despite the ease of immunization, and despite the high risks of disease, experts say that approximately one-fourth of all American preschoolers—the most susceptible kids of all—do not get fully immunized. They do get their vaccinations when they report for their first day of school (it's the law), but by then it may be too late to prevent disease.

As a parent, your mission is to see that your child does get complete protection—early on. As you can see from the following schedule, recommended by the American Academy of Pediatrics, your toddler's first vaccination should come at two months. Notice that there are two groups of diseases for which combination shots are offered. The *DPT* vaccination protects against diphtheria, pertussis and tetanus. The *MMR* is for measles, mumps and rubella.

AGE	DPT	(oral) POLIO	MMR	HEMOPHILUS INFLUENZAE	TETANUS/ DIPHTHERIA	HEPATITIS B
At birth						X
2 months	X	X		X		X
4 months	X	X		X		
6 months	X			*		X
12–15 months				*		
15 months			X	*		
15–18 months	X	X				
4–6 years	X	X				
11–12 years			X			
14–16 years					X	

Note: There are two different vaccines for *Hemophilus influenzae.* Those injections indicated by an asterisk (*) are optional, depending on which vaccine your child is started on.

director of the Immunodeficiency Clinic at Johns Hopkins University School of Medicine and Johns Hopkins Hospital in Baltimore. Unfounded fears sometimes drive parents—along with their children—away from doctors' offices, he says. Most prevalent, nasty rumors of problems associated with the combined diphtheria/pertussis/tetanus (DPT) vaccine have resulted in too many kids running around unprotected.

Some years ago a group of British doctors alleged that DPT vaccinations had caused several children to suffer from permanent side effects as serious as cerebral palsy and mental retardation. Their report received much television coverage on this side of the Atlantic, which resulted in a notable drop in the number of kids getting immunized and a notable *rise* in the number of kids catching pertussis.

"Some kids will get high fever or severe irritability for a day or two after receiving a DPT shot, but it is *not* associated with any long-term neurological problems," says Dr. Lederman. A study published in the prestigious *Journal of the American Medical Association* concurs. Nearly 40,000 kids from Tennessee were given over 100,000 DPT immunizations over their first three years of life. Researchers carefully tracked the children—and *not one* developed serious complications.

In the case of polio immunizations, the numbers aren't so crisp. There have been cases of polio immunizations actually *causing* polio (most of them not to the child immunized but to a close contact). The numbers of those infected, however, are extremely small: roughly one infection for every *five million* immunizations. "New vaccines that have been developed recently appear to be just as effective but without even this tiny risk," says Dr. Lederman.

In the case of both polio and DPT—and with all other immunizations, whose side effects usually involve little more than minor swelling and redness—the trade-off between risk versus return is quite clear, says Dr. Lederman. Immunizations save children from death and disability.

TO BAG A CHICKEN

But immunization won't spare kids from chicken pox. In the world of childhood diseases, chicken pox (also known as varicella) is the wild renegade. "It is such an infectious disease that there's not much you can do to protect your child," says Dr. Nankervis. Approximately 3.5 million Americans catch the disease each year, and sooner or later, the chances that your child will be among them are about as likely as tomorrow's sunrise.

But just because you can't prevent the disease itself may not mean that you can't prevent the worst of it!

One of the most exciting studies ever to hit the world of chicken pox appeared in a 1990 issue of the well-respected *Journal of Pediatrics*. More than 100 kids with chicken pox were experimentally treated with a drug called acyclovir (most commonly given for herpes). The children who took the pills saw their fever subside in half the usual time (one day as opposed to two), their skin lesions healed faster (in two days as opposed to three), *and* they had fewer skin eruptions (an average of 336 as opposed to the normal average of, yuck, 500).

No matter how impressive the results, doctors, being the conservative bunch they are, generally like to see research results repeated before they begin to prescribe a particular drug. "Additionally, these results do not imply that all children with chicken pox should receive acyclovir," says Christian C. Patrick, M.D., Ph.D., physician and associate member at St. Jude Children's Research Hospital in Memphis. It's something to discuss with your pediatrician.

TREATMENT BREAKTHROUGH

ONE SHOT CONQUERS ALL

As we gaze into our crystal ball, several future developments in childhood diseases seem virtually certain. Perhaps most imminent, a vaccine for the all-too-common chicken pox may be just around the corner, says George Nankervis, M.D., Ph.D., of the American Academy of Pediatrics. How far in the future? "We have an experimental vaccine right now. I'd say we'll see it licensed real soon," he says.

Another coming attraction in the world of childhood diseases—one that would be super news to toddlers everywhere—may be the development of a single vaccine to replace the many currently given. "I think that will be a while off, but we are working on combining them," says Dr. Nankervis. He adds that kids today too often come out of their doctors' offices "looking like pincushions."

The ultimate goal, of course, would be to wipe out all childhood diseases. After all, one scourge, smallpox, was immunized into oblivion. Measles may be next in line. And other diseases currently being immunized against may eventually follow, says Christian C. Patrick, M.D., Ph.D., of St. Jude Children's Research Hospital in Memphis.

But will we ever vanquish *all* childhood diseases? It's not likely. "Once you think you have all your bases covered, new players come onto the field," says Dr. Patrick. "I think we're always going to find new viruses, new protozoans and new bacteria to keep us busy."

CHRONIC FATIGUE SYNDROME

When Nannette Piscitelli's "flu" lasted almost two weeks during January 1986, she thought she was just run-down. Finally feeling a little better, she went back to her job as a planner at a Fortune 500 company. Then in April, besides feeling overtired, she started getting headaches, lost her train of thought often and had trouble walking. A brain scan found nothing wrong.

In August, a blood test revealed that she had high amounts of certain antibodies (proteins that fight foreign substances) in her blood. By then she was working only half days because of her constant fatigue and pain. The next month, she began having massive migraine headaches. "After a few more months, I didn't feel as much pain or weakness, but I was exhausted," says Nannette. "I no longer was productive in my job. So I stopped."

Nannette's strange malady has been called the "yuppie flu," "Raggedy Ann syndrome" and bunk—but it's for real. It's chronic fatigue syndrome (CFS), an illness of continual dog-tiredness, achy muscles, fever, drowsiness and the blahs lasting months, even years. And tens of thousands of Americans may have it.

Although it seems to be more common among women, anyone can be affected—from 30 to 40 percent of CFS victims are men, and others with the syndrome include children under age ten, teenagers and men and women in their fifties and sixties. The disease strikes people in all socioeconomic groups, races and walks of life, from all over the world.

But although scientists don't yet know exactly what causes CFS, there's new hope for dealing with it. Finally, after a lot of confusion about what CFS really is and even if it actually exists, medical experts are pinning it down and learning more about how to curb it. And they've put out the good word: CFS is not a fatal disease, and most people who suffer from it get better when they learn how to fight it.

TELLTALE SIGNS

About one in five people who walk into a doctor's office complains that fatigue is disrupting his or her life. Yet only 3 to 5 percent fit the criteria for CFS devised by more than a dozen experts, along with the Centers for Disease Control (CDC) in Atlanta.

According to these criteria, people who truly have CFS are those who suffer a debilitating fatigue (or easy fatigability) that has lasted at least six months. They also must have ruled out (with their doctor's help) any other physical or psychiatric diseases that may mimic CFS symptoms, like acute nonviral infections, depression, hormonal disorders, drug abuse or exposure to toxic agents. Then they must have at least 8 of the following 11 symptoms recurring or persisting for six months or more: chills or mild fever; a sore throat; painful or swollen lymph glands; unexplained general muscle weakness; muscle discomfort; fatigue for at least 24 hours after previously tolerated exercise; a headache unlike any previous pain; joint pain without joint swelling or redness; complaints of forgetfulness, excessive irritability, confusion, inability to concentrate or depression; disturbed sleep; and quick onset of symptoms within a few hours or days.

Such symptoms are common to a variety of diseases, and chronic fatigue alone does not a CFS diagnosis make. So it's important to meet fully the CDC's criteria before your doctor can declare you a bona fide CFS victim. After all, some of us, because of our lifestyle, *should* be tired. A mother of three who gets only 4 hours' sleep each night is bound to be physically exhausted. Psychological stresses can also make you tired.

Besides having specific criteria for diagnosing CFS, scientists also know that many CFS sufferers have common traits. Some people with CFS often have several abnormal immune system responses. Some, for example, have high levels of antibodies in their blood, normally a sign of the presence of bacterial or viral agents. CFS sufferers say that their fatigue started abruptly when they had a specific infection, such as the flu. They may even be able to name the exact day they took sick. The syndrome often begins during a stressful time, such as during a divorce, career change or a death in the family. Also, many CFS people say they're depressed, but it isn't clear whether the depression caused CFS or developed later, when "patients are sick and tired of being tired," says Stephen Straus, M.D., chief of medical virology at the National Institute of Allergy and Infectious Diseases.

CFS sufferers also are more likely to have allergies, and their immune systems may not produce the normal amount of chemicals that regulate the body's responses to disease.

GETTING A DIAGNOSIS

If you believe you meet the CDC's criteria for chronic fatigue syndrome, you should be tested and have an adequate workup. Your family physician is probably the best place to start the investigation. With some simple tests, your doctor should be able to rule out other illnesses that

---

TRUE CURES AND FALSE HOPES

To help those with chronic fatigue syndrome (CFS), doctors have tried various drugs to help boost the immune system or to attack specific viruses. It's unclear, though, whether these medications can really help, because they haven't been tested. One drug that was tested, an antiviral called acyclovir, was found ineffective.

But one type of drug—tricyclic antidepressants—appears, theoretically, to be designed specifically for this syndrome. "Depressive symptoms are part of the illness, but elevating depression is not the only reason to use antidepressants," says James F. Jones, M.D., of the National Jewish Center for Immunology and Respiratory Medicine in Denver. "Tricyclic antidepressants have a number of pharmacological activities. They are potent antihistamines, which may help ameliorate allergies. They also are sedating, which can help patients get a good night's sleep. And they have anti-inflammatory effects."

Dr. Jones has been able to relieve the symptoms of 70 percent of his CFS patients using one-tenth the dose of antidepressant generally prescribed to treat depression. He points out that antidepressants have not been evaluated in controlled trials of CFS patients.

Whatever treatment you try, CFS experts recommend that you beware of unproven therapies promoted as sure cures. "Be wary of so-called chronic fatigue syndrome specialists who suggest you fly across the country to see them," says John Renner, M.D., of the University of Missouri. "They are likely to put you on a bizarre treatment." The list of unsubstantiated therapies promoted as effective includes injections of hydrogen peroxide, homeopathic remedies, high colonics and large doses of vitamin C or other food supplements.

"Until a cure is found, focus on safe, best-bet treatments," Dr. Renner says. "And remember that most people with CFS do learn to cope with it, and they usually get better."

---

may look like CFS. Such tests include autoimmune disease tests, a complete blood count, endocrine disease studies, liver and metabolic tests, a kidney screen and a urinalysis.

Most people with CFS end up seeing several specialists to exclude other causes of the flulike symptoms. Nannette, for example, saw a rheumatologist, an orthopedist, a neurologist and a psychiatrist before her family physician felt confident enough to make the diagnosis of chronic fatigue syndrome. University medical centers usually can provide all the consultants necessary to diagnose the syndrome.

Because it's not a simple disease to identify, some doctors are over-diagnosing the illness, leading patients who have not had appropriate workups to believe they have the syndrome. And some doctors who don't know exactly what CFS is are underdiagnosing it.

"Only about 50 percent of the people told that they have chronic fatigue syndrome actually have it according to the CDC criteria," says John Renner, M.D., president of the Consumer Health Information Research Institute in Kansas City, Missouri. He's seen the medical records of hundreds of patients diagnosed with the syndrome. "This is a complicated illness," he says. "First and foremost, it is something that takes a sophisticated medical workup, which includes immune studies (like blood work that looks at antibodies) and all the tests necessary to rule out other diseases. You want someone who understands the sciences of infectious diseases and immunology. If there's any doubt in your primary physician's mind, don't hesitate to consult an immunologist. And you probably will want to get a second opinion."

IT'S NOT ALL IN YOUR HEAD

One myth that CFS experts are trying to dispel is that the illness is all psychological. It's true that most people with CFS become depressed during their illness. But then so do most people with chronic illnesses. The question is whether they have a history of depression before the flulike symptoms appear.

When doctors treat fatigue as just a trivial psychological problem, they do CFS sufferers a disservice. The kind of fatigue they feel is serious and unrelenting. "I can drive to the grocery store and fill a lightweight plastic bag with food, and that's it for the day," Nannette says. "The quality of my life has been reduced tremendously. I can get people to buy groceries for me and to do my housework. But I can't get someone to help me concentrate or think clearly."

Many illnesses—including multiple sclerosis, Legionnaires' disease, lupus and AIDS—have gone through stages of skepticism only to become fully recognized. "Rather than saying that chronic fatigue syndrome is all in the patient's head, the skeptics need to listen to their patients more intently. The patients know their bodies and their emotions," says Orvalene Prewitt, a cofounder of the National Chronic Fatigue Syndrome Association, in Kansas City, Missouri. "We need to pursue all avenues to find an answer for this baffling flulike illness. Both the public and doctors need to know that there are people out there who really are sick."

TREATMENT BREAKTHROUGH

ZOOMING IN ON A CAUSE

In 1949, doctors in Iceland reported a strange rash of complaints about chronic fatigue among their patients. Similarly mysterious outbreaks occurred in and around Punta Gorda, Florida, in 1956 and again in Lake Tahoe, California, in 1984.

Over the years, doctors have come up with unproven and dubious explanations for the malaise: iron-poor blood (anemia), low blood sugar (hypoglycemia), environmental allergy (20th-century disease) and systemic yeast infection (candidiasis). Today, doctors call it chronic fatigue syndrome (CFS), and they admit the cause is unknown.

At one time, scientists considered Epstein-Barr virus (EBV) as a possible cause of CFS, since many—but not all—CFS sufferers have EBV in their blood. New evidence, however, indicates that EBV alone doesn't appear to be the culprit. Some doctors believe that CFS and fibromyalgia, a disorder also associated with fatigue, may actually be the same condition in many cases. But no one is sure.

To study CFS and to try to zero in on what's really behind it, the Centers for Disease Control (CDC) has asked over 400 doctors in Atlanta, Grand Rapids, Reno and Wichita to gather detailed information about the onset of CFS, what symptoms they see and the course of the illness. "We are looking at everything—including pesticides, fertilizers, varnishes, paints, household construction and insect bites," says Walter J. Gunn, Ph.D., former principal investigator of the CFS surveillance system at the CDC. "It's a fishing expedition—to see if there's a common thing that all these people share." So far, the most recent evidence indicates a strong possibility that the common link may be a virus, says Dr. Gunn.

Although it's impossible to say when scientists will find a definite answer, a major breakthrough may be right around the corner. "There are many credible researchers working on CFS," says Dr. Gunn. "I'd be very surprised if we don't know the cause by the year 2000."

FIGHTING BACK

There's no proven cure for CFS yet, but there are treatments that can often help reduce the symptoms. And there's plenty of ongoing research to test new therapies. In part because of the symptomatic treatments, those who meet the CDC criteria usually do not get progressively worse, and many have gradually improved over time.

Most experts say that your best bet for treating symptoms is to:

Take time out. Get adequate amounts of rest. Measured doses of taking it easy do alleviate some symptoms.

Eat right. CFS is not associated with vitamin or mineral deficiencies, but eating meals with adequate amounts of nutrients (including calories) does make a difference in how some CFS sufferers feel. Some report feeling better when the diet is low in sugar and fat.

Push yourself to do something active. Do a small amount of exercise every day, even if it's just stretching. Chronic overexertion tends to worsen symptoms and may prolong the course of the disease. But most experts do not believe people will get better faster if they stay in bed. That can be psychologically and physically devastating.

Ration your limited energy. "Every day, I think of energy credits," says Nannette. "The first credits I use are always for myself—I wash my hair, paint my nails. Then I balance out the rest over the day."

Don't tough it out. If your joints are in a lot of pain, talk to your doctor about pain medication.

Air your feelings. Get help on how to deal emotionally with the disease. You can seek counseling or get support from CFS patient groups. "I went to a support group and found others like myself," says Nannette. "I also saw I needed some help on how to adjust to being chronically ill. After I had stopped working, I didn't call my friends to chat or get involved in any activities. Now I've become the leader of the support group. Helping others helps me feel good."

Those patients who can maintain a positive attitude seem to cope the best. "I focus on living a balanced life and increasing my stamina," says Nannette. "Now I really appreciate the company of others. I'm not waiting to catch up with life. I do things in moderation, but I don't miss out on too much."

If you would like to find a support group in your area or need more information about CFS, contact the National Chronic Fatigue Syndrome Association at 3521 Broadway, Suite 222, Kansas City, MO 64111. Please include a self-addressed, stamped envelope with your request for information.

COLDS

10 –9–8–7–6–5–4–3–2–1 . . . "Ah-choo!"

That's the way it went back on February 27, 1969, the eve of the scheduled launch of spaceflight Apollo 9. One small sneeze by man became one giant snafu for mankind, as the liftoff had to be scrubbed when all three astronauts came down with colds. The postponement cost U.S. taxpayers an estimated half-million dollars. And what irony! Despite being able to rocket ourselves deep into outer space, we haven't yet been able to get off the ground against a group of germs as close as the stuffy nose on our face.

"It certainly hasn't been for lack of trying, however," says Frederick Ruben, M.D., head of the Infectious Disease Unit at Montefiore Hospital in Pittsburgh and professor of medicine at the University of Pittsburgh School of Medicine. "Probably no other illness has received as much attention as the common cold."

More than a few cold sufferers throughout the ages might vouch for that: We've been bewitched, bothered and bewildered not just by colds but by *cold remedies* ever since the first prehistoric sniffle. From the custom of "kissing the hairy muzzle of a mouse" popular during Roman times to the practice of applying throat wraps made of salted herring during the Middle Ages, our efforts against the cold have ranged from the risky to the ridiculous. As recently as the early 1900s, cold remedies were spiked with so much alcohol or narcotics that you really didn't *care* if you had a cold. And surveys of late tell us there are still some of us eating raw peanuts and chugging hot beer in hopes of relieving our sniffly heads.

TREATING THOSE "KILLER T-CELLS" RIGHT

What *does* one do against this age-old and seemingly invincible foe? Do we simply keep our tissue boxes full and *accept* that we'll get our national adult average of four colds a year?

No. Medical science may not be rocketing forward against the more than 200 viruses known to cause colds, but that doesn't mean there isn't a lot *you* can do. Perhaps the most positive thing to come of research in recent years is an increased understanding of how the human immune system might be encouraged to do a better job of fighting colds on its own, without the help of some miracle cure from a test tube and certainly without having to romance any mice.

"We've only recently begun to realize just how fantastically intricate the immune system is and how its optimal efficiency may be more dependent on environmental and lifestyle factors than previously thought," says Varro E. Tyler, Ph.D., professor of pharmacognosy (the medical uses of plants) at Purdue University. "Better immunity through better living might sound simplistic and a little trite, but it represents the state of the art in what we know."

But what constitutes "better living" for things as remote and impersonal as lymphocytes, neutrophils, immunoglobulins and killer T-cells—the nuts and bolts of your immune system? Nothing terribly elaborate, really—things as basic as adequate exercise, stress control, sound nutrition and maintaining a positive attitude.

WALKING AWAY FROM COLDS

You know that exercise is good for your heart, and it can do wonders for firming flabby thighs, but did you know that moderate exercise can stifle a sniffle? So says David C. Nieman, D.H.Sc. (doctor of health science), director of the Department of Health, Leisure and Exercise Science at Appalachian State University in Boon, North Carolina. Dr. Nieman investigated the effects of a 15-week, five-day-a-week walking program on the immune systems of 36 women, half of whom walked for 45 minutes a day at a brisk but comfortable pace. Compared with the 18 women of similar age who did *not* walk, the walkers walked away with some remarkable results.

"Natural killer T-cell activity at one point was up by 60 percent in the walkers," says Dr. Nieman, "and we also saw a marked increase in the activity of immunoglobulins in the exercise group." More important, however, were the real-life results of these increases. "What we found is that the exercise group got colds that lasted only half as long as colds among the sedentary group—3½ days compared to 7—and were less severe," says Dr. Nieman.

Take a step in the right direction. "Exercise seems to keep the immune system in shape," Dr. Nieman says of his results. "We don't know precisely how or why yet, but increased circulation, beneficial hormonal changes and stress reduction all could play a role." Whatever the reasons, walking's benefits are clear. Walking is also fun and (as long as you watch for cars!) about as safe an exercise as you'll find. So step to it!

But don't push, says Dr. Nieman. Studies of marathon runners following the completion of their 26.2-mile jaunts show that exceptionally exhaustive exercise can *reduce* immune function. "So don't think that more is necessarily better with exercise," Dr. Nieman says. "Keep it comfortable and keep it consistent. Moderation seems to be the key."

DECONSTRESSANT THERAPY

And while you're exercising moderation out on the old fitness trail, you might also think about moderating your levels of stress. That's the implication of a study from Carnegie Mellon University in Pittsburgh and

YOUR BEST COLD REMEDY

Not all colds are alike, and not all cold *remedies* are alike either. Use this table to help match your symptoms with the best medication.

SYMPTOM	TYPE OF DRUG	ACTIVE INGREDIENT	BRAND NAME
Congestion, runny nose	Spray or drop decongestant	Phenylephrine	Dristan, Neo-Synephrine, Sinex
		Oxyetazoline	Afrin, Dristan Long-Lasting Nasal Spray, Duration
	Oral decongestant	Xylometazoline Pseudoephedrine	Neo-Synephrine II Actifed, Contac Sinus Tablets, Sudafed
Cough	Cough suppressant	Dextromethorphan	Benylin DM, Delsym, Triaminic DM, Pertussin ES, PediaCare Liquid, St. Joseph Cough Suppressant for Children, Hold 4-Hour Cough Suppressant
		Codeine	Cheracol, Ryna-CX, Naldecon CX, Novahistine DH

two prestigious research institutes in England. The connection between psychological stress and susceptibility to colds has been under investigation for some time, but never with results as convincing as these. Even after all other relevant variables were taken into consideration—age, general health, diet, exercise, smoking and patterns of sleep—people reporting the highest levels of stress were twice as likely to be infected by cold viruses as people reporting the lowest levels.

Stress, of course, can mean a lot of different things to a lot of different people, but it was defined for the purposes of this study as "a general feeling of being overwhelmed," whether by one's job, domestic responsi-

SYMPTOM	TYPE OF DRUG	ACTIVE INGREDIENT	BRAND NAME
	Medicated lozenges	Diphenhydramine Menthol	Benylin N'ICE Sugarless Cough Lozenges
	Expectorant	Guaifenesin	Comtrex Cough Formula, Hytuss, Dorcol Children's Cough Syrup, Nortussin, Robitussin
Headache, muscle aches and fever	Pain reliever	Aspirin	Bayer, Bufferin, Norwich, St. Joseph Aspirin (for adults)
		Acetaminophen Ibuprofen	Datril, Tylenol Advil, Nuprin
Sore throat	Medicated lozenges and spray	Phenol compounds Benzocaine	Chloraseptic Sore Throat Spray Vicks Throat Lozenges
		Hexylresorcinol Menthol	Sucrets N'ICE Sugarless Cough Lozenges

bilities or the unpredictability of life itself, according to the study's lead author, Sheldon Cohen, Ph.D., of Carnegie Mellon. Anger and hostility were also predominant in those reporting high levels of stress.

Why should stress so affect the immune system? "Probably it's hormonal," Dr. Cohen says. "We know that stress can affect the body's delicate hormonal balances in a variety of ways and that these changes can in turn produce changes in immune function. More work needs to be done in this area before these changes can be identified in greater detail, but we have little doubt they occur."

Take control of your life. Does the stress/cold connection suggest you should be popping tranquilizers to escape the sniffles? Not necessarily, says Ronald Podell, M.D., a psychotherapist and director of the Center for Mood Disorders in Los Angeles. But it *does* mean trying to get a better hold on your life. "It's feeling out of control, feeling powerless that's at the real heart of stress," Dr. Podell says. "This in turn produces the anger, hostility and frustration that appear to weaken the immune system. Many of us need to be more accepting and also more realistic. The sooner we stop fighting battles that can't be won, the better off we'll be," says Dr. Podell.

EATING FOR IMMUNE POWER

"Research leaves little doubt that a good diet and a good immune system go hand in hand, but it's a relationship that needs to exist on a day-to-day basis—not just opportunistically once a cold has been caught," says Charles Kimmelman, M.D., professor of otolaryngology at New York Medical College in New York City. With the *possible* exception of large doses of vitamin C, "anything consumed after a cold has hit is basically a case of too little, too late," says Dr. Kimmelman.

Eat well, not wackily. Of principal importance in maintaining a strong immune system appear to be vitamins A and C, "but a deficiency in any nutrient can upset the apple cart," Dr. Kimmelman points out. The best diet for your immune system is one such as those recommended by the American Heart Association or the American Cancer Society. That is, you want a diet low in fat, rich in fiber, varied and well balanced. To make sure you get lots of C and A and other vitamins, you should eat lots of fresh fruits, vegetables and whole grains as well as protein sources such as legumes, lean meats and dairy products.

Don't stuff or starve. As for the age-old question of whether to feed a cold or starve it, the recommendation now is to let your appetite be your guide. "If you feel like eating, eat," says Dr. Kimmelman. "And if you don't, don't. Follow this advice for one or two days. If your appetite hasn't returned after that, see your doctor. Something more than a cold could be going on."

DRUGS, DRUGS EVERYWHERE

We may no longer be wearing necklaces of salted fish, kissing hairy mice or getting blitzed on cold "cocktails" capable of curling the lip of even Dean Martin, but our modern-day cold remedies still are by no means perfect.

Beware of medicinal "shotguns." "Many cold remedies simply try to do too much," says Dr. Kimmelman. "They contain ingredients for treating more symptoms than most colds actually present. It's better to target each cold symptom individually with a product designed to treat that symptom and that symptom only. Not only is this likely to bring more effective relief, it reduces the likelihood of unwanted side effects."

If you have just a stuffy nose and sore throat, for example, how much sense does it make to take a product designed to relieve a headache, muscle aches and cough as well? Not much, so with that in mind, check over the table in "Your Best Cold Remedy" on page 118. "Your goal in medicating a cold should be to be as specific as possible," Dr. Kimmelman says, "Take only what you need and only for as long as you need it."

Avoid the "rebound effect." This warning applies to the use of decongesting nasal sprays especially, Dr. Kimmelman says. Used for too long, they can cause a rebound effect, worsening the very congestion they're designed to relieve and prolonging any infection you may have. Limit your use of such sprays to no longer than three days.

OLD STANDBYS THAT STILL STAND

Oddly, perhaps the most problematic "side effect" of today's pharmaceutical cold remedies is that they can sometimes work too well, says John Stringfield, M.D., a physician in family practice in Waynesville, North Carolina. "People suddenly feel well enough to get back into the world, which not only increases their chances of spreading their infection to others but causes them to avoid the rest they may need to help them recuperate naturally."

That being the case, here are some "low-tech" remedies that can help you feel better, but not falsely so. "They work more in harmony with the healing processes the body is trying to undergo," Dr. Stringfield says.

Give in to the urge to rest. "Probably the biggest mistake people make when hit with a cold is to fight it," Dr. Stringfield says. "They insist upon going about their jobs and domestic responsibilities, which not only compromises the body's cold-fighting efforts but also helps spread the infection. Taking time off at the onset of a cold can be time well spent by helping to shorten its duration."

Drink—and breathe—sufficient fluids. Consuming adequate fluids—at least six to eight glasses a day—is important, because the body needs extra water to help flush itself of the cellular "waste" created by its antiviral efforts. *Inhaling* moist air is also important for preventing nasal and throat passages from becoming dry and cracked and more vulnerable to viral attack. "Keeping your home humidified can be both a cold soother and a cold preventer," Dr. Stringfield says.

You can keep your house humid by leaving bathroom doors open when taking showers, keeping a lot of plants around (they add moisture to the air naturally), putting open pots of water on wood stoves or rear radiators or using a room humidifier with a good filtering system. "It's important to keep humidifiers clean by changing their water and their filters often. You don't want mold developing, because that can present its own type of respiratory ills," Dr. Stringfield says.

Spritz a stuffy nose with saltwater. A spritz or two of saltwater can do nearly as well as a high-powered nose spray—without any rebound effect, says Dr. Stringfield. Simply mix about 1 teaspoon of salt in 8 ounces of water, suck the solution into a nasal aspirator and give a quick spray. Breathe in as you do and hold your head back. Spit the water out after you've made the application and then give your nose a good, but gentle, blow.

Wash your hands often. Cold viruses can survive on doorknobs, handrails, money—you name it—for as long as several hours, so frequent hand washing during the cold season is "paramount," Dr. Stringfield says. This holds true, moreover, for cold sufferers and would-be victims alike. "Not many people realize it, but just because they have a cold doesn't mean they can't catch another on top of it. There are over 200 viruses known to cause colds, so it's very possible to catch a second even before you've gotten over your first."

Keep your sneezes to yourself. Studies show that a robust sneeze can launch virus-laden droplets 12 feet or more—and at speeds of 200 miles per hour—so treat your sneezes with respect. Sneeze into a paper tissue (better than cloth hankies, which can become veritable viral warehouses) and dispose of it properly. "Never block a sneeze, however, because this can risk forcing viral infection into the ears," Dr. Stringfield says. "If you find yourself needing to sneeze unexpectedly, block it with your hands, then head for the nearest bathroom for a *real* good scrub."

Take some C and see. Is it worth taking vitamin C to combat a cold?

IF YOU CAN'T BEAT 'EM, COAT 'EM

You do have to wonder. With vaccines for polio, smallpox, tetanus, measles and mumps—why not colds?

In large part, it's because the culprit is so elusive, says Frederick Ruben, M.D., of the University of Pittsburgh School of Medicine. "There isn't just one virus that causes colds—there are over 200, with new ones still being discovered. This has made finding a vaccine against colds a little like trying to hit an entire flock of birds with just one shot."

Making the hunt for a vaccine even harder is the ability of cold viruses to mutate and become immune to a specific vaccine or antibody over time. "This means that a vaccine that might be effective against a virus or group of viruses today might not be effective several years from now," Dr. Ruben says.

But the news isn't all bad regarding our chances of finding a cure for this fiendish foe. A new approach is under investigation that is looking to render cold viruses inactive by enveloping them in a type of protective coating, says Elliot Dick, Ph.D., a professor of preventive medicine and director of the Respiratory Virus Research Laboratory at the University of Wisconsin.

Cold viruses are characterized by a tiny notch on their surface, which is the key to their ability to latch on to host cells and do their damage, says Dr. Dick. The notch provides an anchoring point for a pronglike projection on the host cell, almost like a keyhole provides the entry point for a key on a door lock. "The protective coating fills this notch in such a way that the host cell's key has no place to fit," says Dr. Dick.

The drug—known as ICAM, which stands for intra-cellular adhesive molecule—is still in experimental stages but "looks very promising," Dr. Dick says.

Also under investigation and looking promising are air-filtration systems aimed at removing cold viruses from the air before they can enter any noses in the first place, Dr. Dick says. "They're similar to currently available devices that remove tobacco smoke from the air, but somewhat more sophisticated. A couple of years' more work still needs to be done before such systems will be ready for public use," Dr. Dick says.

This is controversial. But consider a study done at the University of Wisconsin. Eight men were given 500 milligrams of vitamin C four times daily, while 8 other men were given no C. All 16 men were then locked in a dormitory for a week with other men who had been infected with colds. Results showed not just fewer colds in the C-treated group but also considerably milder colds. The men taking vitamin C experienced only one-third the coughs, one-third the sneezes and one-half the number of nose blows.

Vitamin C is found in many fruits and vegetables. Those with the most include broccoli, brussels sprouts, oranges, strawberries and grapefruit. Short-term supplements of C are generally considered safe in the amount taken by the men in the Wisconsin study (2,000 milligrams a day). This may, however, cause diarrhea.

Know that hot spice can be nice. If a food makes your eyes water and your nose run, it's doing so by causing your mucous membranes to secrete more liquid. And this secretion, says Dr. Tyler, provides a little boost to the body's efforts to rid itself of cold-related viral waste material. So don't be shy with the peppers and other hot seasonings. They can be healthful as well as tasty.

Get on the mend with menthol. A study from British researchers at the University of Wales found that lozenges containing menthol increased people's feelings of airflow through their noses almost immediately. The effect lasted at least 30 minutes, moreover, even though only 10 minutes were required for the lozenge to dissolve.

Don't eschew exercise. In addition to keeping the immune system "in shape" for resisting cold infection in the first place, a little exercise may also help reduce cold symptoms once a cold has hit, says Bryant Stamford, Ph.D., director of the Health Promotion and Wellness Center at the University of Louisville School of Medicine. Wait until the acute symptoms have passed—usually about three days—and go easy, Dr. Stamford says. Do *not* exercise, however, if you are still experiencing chest congestion, aching muscles, a hacking cough or a fever. You could *slow* your recuperation if you do.

CONSTIPATION

G ladys finished her double cheeseburger, slugged down the last 3 inches of cold brunch cola and frowned until her forehead ached. "Well, it's that time again," she muttered to herself as she picked up *TV Today,* trudged to the bathroom and started reading. She read about her favorite show, "Legal Beagles." She read about Warren Beatty and his latest movie. She even read the recipes calling for lime gelatin, marshmallows and candied plums. But after 20 minutes, her frown deepened. "It's been three days, by gosh, and I'm gonna sit here till I go!"

Gladys is always bemoaning her blocked-up bowels. Most mornings, she can't go at all. When she finally does have a bowel movement, it often hurts, and she's rarely pleased with the results. But Gladys is hardly alone in experiencing these uneventful morning—or afternoon or evening—rituals. In fact, doctors say that constipation—the word is derived from the Latin *constipare,* "to crowd together"—is the most common gastrointestinal complaint in the United States.

But sometimes constipation, like beauty, exists only in the eye of the beholder. Even though a majority of Americans believe that daily bowel movements are necessary for good health, this just isn't so, says David R. Rudy, M.D., chief of family medicine at the University of Health Sciences at Chicago Medical School. "Some people have a bowel movement three times a day, while others have one every four days," Dr. Rudy says. "There is a wide variation in 'normal' bowel activity."

But if you have fewer than three bowel movements a week, and the stools are difficult to pass, you really are constipated, doctors say. If your lack of bowel movements is accompanied by a fever or abdominal pain, there could be something seriously wrong—an intestinal tumor, for example, or a malfunctioning thyroid gland. But constipation is rarely caused by disease. More often, we get constipated because of habits we cultivate when we're *not* in the john.

ALTERED TASTES

Until the early 1900s, just about everyone ate their fill of fiber. Meats (which are devoid of fiber) were expensive, and many of the low-fiber foods we live on today hadn't been developed yet. People ate what they could afford: beans, fruit, vegetables and whole-grain breads. The average Westerner probably ate 40 grams of dietary fiber a day. People who eat foods containing lots of dietary fiber have less chance of getting constipated.

But with progress, things changed. Today, Americans eat closer to 11 grams of fiber daily. That helps explain why constipation is now the most frequent complaint heard by gastroenterologists.

"It's getting worse all the time," says Betty Garrity, a registered dietitian and nutritionist at the University of California, San Diego, Medical Center. "People rely more on fast foods, processed foods and convenience foods than on fresh, natural types of foods. If you're not getting fiber—you really need between 25 and 35 grams a day—you're going to get constipated."

For more than ten years, doctors have been telling everyone who will listen—and many more who won't—that dietary fiber is the cure for constipation. People aren't quite catching on, Garrity says. "They're more aware than they used to be, but being aware of what you need to do and actually changing your habits are two different things. In this fast-paced society, we want quick and convenient. That usually means *more* processed food and *less* dietary fiber."

FIGHTING WITH FIBER

Basically, eating a high-fiber diet is like dropping thousands of tiny sponges into your gut, Dr. Rudy explains. The sponges proceed to pull in water, and that makes the stools softer, larger and easier to pass.

A warning: Any time you start eating more fiber, you may notice some rather uncomfortable (not to mention unsociable) consequences. To prevent flatulence, abdominal cramps or diarrhea from taking over, begin increasing your fiber intake slowly, Garrity advises. "Start with some whole-wheat bread in the morning, for example, and maybe a few pieces of fruit. Then you can work up from there."

Bring on the beans. There are legions of legumes, and they're all rich in dietary fiber, Garrity says. A half cup of canned chick-peas, for example, contains more than 6 grams of fiber, and the same amount of canned kidney beans contains a whopping 9 grams—one-third of your total recommended daily fiber intake!

All fruits and vegetables contain fiber, so eat your fill, Garrity advises.

And don't forget the prunes. Not only are they high in fiber, they also contain substances that stimulate the bowel muscles and help get things moving.

Bring on the bran. Any of the brans—oat, wheat, rice and corn bran are all packed with fiber—can help your intestinal engine run on time. Unfortunately, pure bran also has the texture—some would say the taste— of pencil shavings. Taken in large amounts, it can be hard on your gut as

FOOD SOURCES OF FIBER

Dietary fiber, often called roughage or bulk, helps relieve constipation and may also help prevent hemorrhoids, colorectal cancer and diverticular disease.

Experts recommend that we consume approximately 20 to 35 grams of fiber per day—which is just about twice as much as most of us get. The foods on the following list are some of the top sources of fiber.

FOOD	PORTION	DIETARY FIBER (g.)
Pearled barley, cooked	1/2 cup	12.3
Pears, dried	5 halves	11.5
Cowpeas, boiled	1/2 cup	8.3
Corn bran, raw	2 Tbsp.	7.9
Blackberries	1 cup	7.2
Chick-peas, canned	1/2 cup	7.0
Kidney beans, boiled	1/2 cup	6.9
Lima beans, boiled	1/2 cup	6.8
Refried beans, canned	1/2 cup	6.7
Baby lima beans, boiled	1/2 cup	6.6
Black beans, boiled	1/2 cup	6.1
Ralston cereal, cooked	3/4 cup	6.0
Raspberries	1 cup	6.0
Apples, dried	10 rings (app. 2 oz.)	5.6
Whole-wheat spaghetti, cooked	1 cup	5.4
Peaches, dried	5 halves (app. 2 oz.)	5.3
Figs, dried	3 (app. 2 oz.)	5.2
Lentils, boiled	1/2 cup	5.2

well. So try mixing your bran, a few teaspoons at a time, into other foods—for example, meat loaves, casseroles or milk shakes.

Psyllium makes it simple. Found at health food stores and in some over-the-counter laxatives, ground psyllium seeds are a concentrated source of fiber. "Food is really a better way to get your fiber, but if you're not crazy about whole-grain or bran breakfast cereals, then take psyllium," Dr. Rudy says.

FILL UP ON FLUIDS

If you've ever made fresh pasta, you know how important it is to add just the right amount of water to the flour. If the dough gets too dry, the pasta machine will surely jam. If you get too dry, *your* machine will jam.

One reason there are so many plugged-up people in the world is because they're simply too busy to drink enough water. Extra water is particularly important if you've already begun your high-fiber diet, Garrity says. Like a garden topped with sawdust, your insides will need lots of water to stay moist and keep things moving. "If you eat a lot of fiber without drinking lots of water, you run the risk of fecal impaction, and that can be serious," Garrity says. Dr. Rudy concurs.

It's nearly impossible to drink too much water. "You should drink at least six to eight glasses of water a day," she says. While you're at it, go easy on the coffee and caffeinated soft drinks. Caffeine is a diuretic. That means it could actually help deplete the body's water supply.

Of course, you can't appease an intractable bowel merely by stuffing it with fiber and water. There are other habits you may need to change as well.

THE BATHROOM BASICS

Gladys does it all wrong. Not only does she scarf doughnuts by the dozen, her only exercise comes from pressing a heavy thumb on the TV remote control. No wonder she's all plugged up!

Your bowels won't move until you do. Researchers have discovered that constipation occurs most often among people who get the least exercise. This doesn't mean you have to be a track star just to reach the finish line, Dr. Rudy says. Any exercise—riding your bike, walking around the block or working in the garden—can help loosen things up.

Heed the call. Gladys usually ignores it. For example, if she gets the urge during her favorite TV show, she waits for the commercial break before heading down the hall. Of course, by then it's too late. "You should 'listen' to what your body is trying to tell you," Dr. Rudy says. "Generally, you should take advantage of the time right after meals, which is when most people are ready to go."

Give yourself time. If every morning you sleep late, yank on your clothes and dash for the bus, your bowels simply won't have time to cooperate. Try getting up a little earlier. Adding a little quiet time can help you *and* your bowels get off to a better start.

THE BIG GUNS

Even though exercise and fiber diets are natural and easy solutions for constipation, too often people reach for over-the-counter relief. Each year, millions of Americans spend $300 to $400 million for laxatives. While most laxatives will work, some of the more powerful potions can work *too*

COFFEE: MORE THAN AN EYE OPENER

Ever since a handful of patriots dumped British tea into Boston Harbor, coffee has been celebrated as America's number one wake-up call—and the answer to nature's call. Not only does this pungent brew brush off morning cobwebs, some devotees say it warms up the bowels as well.

Researchers agree that coffee's folkloric reputation as a mild purgative isn't entirely unfounded. In one study, British researchers gave volunteers regular coffee, decaf or warm water to drink. They found that people who drank coffee (with or without caffeine) had a significant increase in rectal activity. The water drinkers' bowels, on the other hand, showed no such change.

Does this mean a morning cup of joe really does help waken sleepy bowels? It might, says *Prevention* adviser Manfred Kroger, Ph.D., professor of food science at Pennsylvania State University. Then again, many foods and drinks can have the same effect. "If you eat a pound of onions, that will loosen your bowels," says Dr. Kroger. "So will some beer or some wine. One of my aunts drank a cup of warm water in the morning, because coffee wasn't available. She thought that helped."

No matter what you eat, your body's "gastrocolonic response" automatically kicks in to move things along, explains Dr. Kroger. In fact, doctors often advise people to head for the bathroom soon after they eat, when the response is strongest. Any time you're constipated, Dr. Kroger says, "you want to get something into your stomach to initiate the intestinal contractions."

---

well, giving you unpleasant repercussions. Used too often, laxatives can also weaken the muscles in your intestines—muscles you use every time you have a bowel movement.

Doctors say, however, that *occasional* use of laxatives is safe. And you should be aware that some laxatives are safer for you than others. Here's a rundown of what's available at your drugstore.

BULK-FORMING LAXATIVES. For most people, these should be the laxative of choice, Dr. Rudy says. Like dietary fiber, these work by drawing water into the stool, making it larger, softer and easier to pass. They also help trigger the intestinal contractions that get things started.

STIMULANT LAXATIVES. Drugs such as castor oil and phenolphthalein (Ex-Lax) trigger bowel movements by irritating the intestinal lining. Because these powerful laxatives can produce uncomfortably dramatic bowel movements, they should be avoided or used only as a last resort.

SALINE LAXATIVES. Less powerful than the stimulant laxatives, over-the-counter drugs such as Milk of Magnesia are safe and usually mild, Dr. Rudy says. Since they work by drawing lots of water into the bowel, however, be sure you drink extra water to prevent dehydration.

LUBRICANTS. Drugs such as mineral oil and docusate calcium (Surfak) soften and lubricate hard stools, allowing them to slide right through. But mineral oil can decrease your body's absorption of the fat-soluble vitamins (A, D, E and K), and docusate calcium can be toxic to liver cells. Before using stool softeners, check with your doctor.

If you get enough fiber, water and exercise, you may never need a laxative, Dr. Rudy says. "If all of a sudden you're constipated and you never were constipated before, that could signal a problem," he warns. "Intermittent constipation and diarrhea can also be a warning sign, particularly so if there is also blood in the stool. If that happens, you should see a doctor."

DANDRUFF

I ntelligent and hardworking, Dusty Chalders has a good job, a loving wife and healthy, obedient children. He also has a little problem.

"Hey, Dusty, is it snowing outside?"

"Say, Dusty, did you drop your powder puff?"

"Yo, Dusty, have you been painting today?"

After fielding hundreds of personal comments from a few insensitive "friends," Dusty went to his doctor for help. "Doc, you've got to help me get rid of this dandruff," he pleaded. "I can't even wear my good blue suit."

GETTING A LITTLE FLAKY

Doctors aren't sure why, but sometimes skin cells on the scalp proliferate—form, die and flake off—at an accelerated rate. "Dandruff is skin that comes off as a cohesive chunk," says Guy F. Webster, M.D., Ph.D., an assistant professor of dermatology and director of the Center for Cutaneous Pharmacology at Thomas Jefferson University Hospital in Philadelphia. "It gets worse in the winter, when the air is dry, because each individual flake is less prone to stick to your scalp if it's not moist."

While dandruff can be itchy, and perhaps a little unsightly, the biggest concern you probably will ever have is putting up with its appearance—and perhaps a few jokes. Because dandruff is present in nearly everyone, it's hard to call it a disease.

DERMATITIS BY ANOTHER NAME

The problem with dandruff, however, is that it can be a serious problem cosmetically. Some people get dandruff so badly that it can dump a veritable snowstorm on their shoulders day after day. This type of flaking is called seborrheic dermatitis, a disease characterized by a profusion of flaky, itchy head scales.

In fact, dandruff and seborrheic dermatitis are so much alike—they're even treated alike—that some doctors believe they simply are variations of the same condition. "Some people believe they're part of a spectrum, that the most mild form of scaling disease is dandruff and that if it's a little worse, it becomes seborrheic dermatitis," Dr. Webster says.

But there are differences. Dandruff usually stays at home on the scalp, but seborrheic dermatitis can wander to the eyebrows, outer ears and other parts of the body. It is also accompanied by inflammation and can be quite itchy as well.

Both, however, are a needless embarrassment, says Dr. Webster, because it isn't necessary to bear either of them on your shoulders. Dandruff and seborrheic dermatitis can easily be controlled. All it requires is a little attention to your hair a little more often than you are currently used to.

THE SOAP AND WATER CURE

If you have dandruff, says Dr. Webster, chances are you are not washing your hair often enough. Since dandruff is nothing more than flaking skin, washing it away will get rid of it. How fast the flaking proliferates should determine how often you wash your hair, not whether or not your hair feels dirty. The same goes for seborrheic dermatitis. The more you wash away, the less you have to display.

Every day is best. Some people can wash their hair once a week and still be dandruff-free, Dr. Webster says. People with dandruff problems usually have a problem only because they let it go too long. The notion that shampooing causes dandruff by drying out the scalp is simply not true. Washing your hair—every day, if possible—can be the cure. But you also need to know how to wash it right.

Get the right shampoo. Over-the-counter dandruff shampoos work quite well, Dr. Webster says. The best are those containing selenium sulfide (Selsun blue) or zinc pyrithione (Head & Shoulders), both of which help slow cell growth. You might also try shampoos containing salicylic acid, which can help soften and remove itchy scales.

These shampoos work best if you leave them on for 5 to 10 minutes. Whip up a good head of lather at the beginning of your bath or shower, then thoroughly rinse it out when you're nearly done. Since these shampoos can dry your hair, you might want to use a good conditioner for the crowning touch.

Treat it with tar. Tar-based shampoos not only, well, beat the tar out of dandruff, they pump in extra body as well. You should, however, use these preparations only if you're dark haired, Dr. Webster warns. "If you are very fair haired, tar-based shampoos may turn your hair green."

Oil it up. If you have thick scales on your scalp that create a lot of flaking, try loosening them up by rubbing them with a little warm mineral or olive oil. Let the oil soak in for a few hours, then shampoo as usual.

Finger the fungus. It hasn't been convicted yet, but a fungus called *Pityrosporum ovale* may somehow be involved in triggering dandruff. A cream containing ketoconazole, rubbed into the scalp, can exterminate the fungus and perhaps some of the dandruff as well. For most people, the less expensive antidandruff shampoos will work just as well, Dr. Webster says.

Get used to it. Even though you can control a flaky scalp, it's impossible to eliminate it. Don't even try, Dr. Webster says. "No good is served by stirring up the scalp to see if you can get the last scale off," he says. "You can always stir up another scale."

DEPRESSION

Depression comes in several varieties. There's the Monday morning variety, when you wake up realizing you have to face yet another week at your law firm—Boyd, Dewey, Cheatham and Howe. There's the midweek variety, when you notice your laundry basket is sending cascades of socks and underwear over its sunken edges. And there's the midwinter variety, when the Ice Age descends like your neighbor's slide shows of his trip to Lake Woissamee. Then there's the real big, serious kind of depression, which saps all your vitality, digs a hole of misery, tosses you in, throws the dirt in after you and packs it all down with a steamroller.

It's the nature of depression, no matter how big or small, to hide hope under a black cloud. But there is actually every reason for hope, says psychiatrist Michael Gitlin, M.D., associate clinical professor of psychiatry and biobehavioral sciences at the Neuropsychiatric Institute and Hospital of the University of California, Los Angeles. "Depression is more treatable now than it has ever been," he says.

BEATING BACK THE BLUES

Unless your funk is really lasting and bad, you should be able to pull out of it all by yourself. (To help tell the difference between a minor funk and a really bad depression that warrants serious attention, see "When It's Time to Seek Professional Help" on the opposite page.) Here are ways to get a handle on the run-of-the-mill blues.

Get busy. Wintertime especially is tough, because it cuts down on the time you spend outside, going to visit friends, going out to dinner or the movies, going shopping and exercising outdoors. But sometimes to break out of a funk you have to make that extra effort to get involved in life, says psychologist William Leber, Ph.D., associate professor of psychiatry and behavioral sciences at the University of Oklahoma Medical

School and director of clinical neuropsychology at the Veterans Administration Medical Center in Oklahoma City. "Revving up the body to a higher speed tends to have a counteractive effect on depression," he says.

But how can you drag yourself out of bed to exercise and socialize when all you want to do is lie under the covers and pout, watch TV and eat cookies? "It's hard, but you can do it," Dr. Leber says. "You get up and go to work, don't you? Well, when you come home, add exercising and socializing on to the end of your day, before you let yourself get close to your bed. Or you might get up earlier and exercise or play before you go to work," he says.

Talk it out. But not to the point where people hide when they see you coming. "It's good to talk to people who are close to you," Dr. Leber

---

WHEN IT'S TIME TO SEEK PROFESSIONAL HELP

Clinical depression—the serious kind that deserves professional care—is more than a negative outlook on life. Experts at the National Institute for Mental Health say that if you have at least four of the following symptoms most of every day for at least two weeks, you probably have clinical depression.

- Problems with eating—you don't feel like eating and you start losing weight, or you start eating more than usual and packing on the pounds.
- Problems with sleeping—you can't sleep, or all you do is sleep.
- You slump through the day as if you're Jacob Marley dragging his chains around Ebenezer Scrooge's bedroom. Or you're so hyper that you're up all night polishing the silver and scrubbing the floor.
- Your sex drive doesn't shift out of low gear.
- You tell yourself that you're worthless, punish yourself for things you think you said or did and blame yourself for everything that goes wrong.
- You can't concentrate on what you're doing; you can't even decide what to have for dinner. You feel as if you can't figure out the simplest matters.
- You keep having thoughts and images of killing yourself or wishing you were dead, or you actually try to commit suicide.

Notice that you don't necessarily have to feel overtly sad to be clinically depressed—changes in basic drives such as eating, sleeping, energy and sex may be the only signs you have.

says, "but it's not good to dump on everybody you come in contact with." It's best to ask permission before unloading: "Hey, John, I've been feeling down lately—mind if I talk to you about it?"

Change your routine. It's a way to psychologically bring sunshine into your life, Dr. Leber says. "It could be something as simple as going out for lunch more often instead of eating at your desk or at home."

Change your thoughts. Instead of dwelling on the way things "should" be, make an effort to be more flexible, says Dr. Leber. Think positively about how you can adapt to reality and even try to change it. For example, if it has rained all week and you're furious because you can't spend time outside, reconsider reality. Actually you *can* go outside and enjoy yourself. Get into your raincoat and rubber boots, open that umbrella and go jump in puddles!

Stay booze-free. Alcohol is one of the most powerful depressants known. The more you drink, the more you risk making your blues worse.

A DEEPER SHADE OF BLUE

For depressions that go deeper than the Monday morning blahs, professional help may be in order.

This deeper kind of depression, known as clinical depression, hits many people sometime during their lives. At any one time, 2.5 million Americans have clinical depression. For some reason, the number seems to be rising every year—although this may be due to better recognition and reporting of the problem.

"The hot thing in psychotherapy these days is brief therapy," says Dr. Leber. Problem solving in four to six months is the goal of many of the newer forms of therapy. "They focus on immediate problems as opposed to life history, and the therapist is both active and interventionist," says Dr. Leber.

Cognitive therapy is probably the most popular of the new styles, Dr. Leber says. "It helps you examine your thought patterns and how those patterns keep your depression going. The therapist helps you discover some fallacy in the way you see yourself and the world," he says.

Another major form of brief therapy is interpersonal therapy. "It focuses on the relationships in your life, and it uses relationships to help you gain insights into why you're depressed," says Dr. Leber. Interpersonal therapy also examines the transitions a person goes through from one stage of life to another—marriage, giving birth, divorce, changing jobs, retirement, death.

Traditional psychoanalysis is still an avenue for some. "After you've dealt with your immediate problems and you're feeling better, you may want to go into a longer-term therapy that deals with your major life issues,"

PSYCHOTHERAPY ENTERS THE COMPUTER AGE

Morton doesn't look like any therapist you've ever seen, but someday you may come to Morton seeking help for depression. Morton is a computer program.

Some human therapists are unhappy about Morton. "At meetings they glare at me," says Morton's designer, Paulette M. Selmi, Ph.D., a psychologist in private practice and director of psychology at Desert Vista Hospital in Mesa, Arizona. Why the glares from other psychologists? "They think I'm looking to put them out of business," she says.

Morton gained notoriety among therapists when it made print in the *American Journal of Psychiatry*. A study by Dr. Selmi looked at 36 people who were feeling down. Some were given six therapy sessions with a flesh-and-bones therapist. Others were treated to an equal number of sessions with metal-and-microchips Morton. Both Morton and its human counterpart used a style of therapy called cognitive-behavioral, known to be effective in beating the blues.

How does Morton work? During your first session, it might flash on the screen something like "Hello, Jane, my name is Morton. I hear you've been feeling depressed lately. Is that true?" Every question is followed by several possible responses. You answer by pushing the right choice on the keyboard. "Well, how long have you been depressed?" asks Morton. "Was there anything particular going on in your life at that time?"

"Some people can relate to the computer as if it were a person," says Dr. Selmi. "They have a feeling that Morton is 'real.' There's a sense that the computer has really listened to them," she says.

How good a therapist is this hunk of hardware that appears to "listen"? In this one study, Morton proved "as effective in the treatment of mild to moderately depressed outpatients as a therapist," concluded Dr. Selmi and her associates. But Dr. Selmi asserts that she is *not* looking to put therapists out on the street. Despite Morton's class performance, "I don't see the computer as a replacement for human beings. I see it as a tool that may assist the therapist and reduce costs for the patient," says Dr. Selmi.

For now, computer programs are still experimental. But Dr. Selmi calculates that by the start of the 21st century, many therapists may be using computers to help with patients' depressions.

says Dr. Leber. "It depends on you; some people are better off with one kind of therapy over another," he says.

MEDICATIONS TO THE RESCUE

The more severe your depression, the more likely it is that medication is warranted, says Dr. Gitlin. The so-called tricyclic antidepressants— imipramine, amitriptyline, nortriptyline—have fewer side effects than the monoamine oxidase (MAO) inhibitors—pargyline, phenelzine, isocarbox-azid. But newer drugs such as bupropion (Wellbutrim) and fluoxetine (Prozac) have the least side effects of all.

Prozac quickly became America's favorite choice after its introduction in 1987. Its popularity, says Dr. Gitlin, was due to a resounding success rate and apparent safety. But several years later, the drug became embroiled in controversy, where it remains today. Some people have reported reacting badly to Prozac, even to the point of attempting suicide. Yet suicidal thoughts are often a part of depression, so it's hard to tell if the drug actually causes them, Dr. Gitlin says. If it does, this occurs in only a very small percentage of the people who take it. "Prozac has probably saved a lot of lives," he says, "and more people can tolerate it than other antidepressants."

The argument over Prozac clearly illustrates why you and your doctor have to discuss your symptoms and your drug reactions thoroughly— what works for someone else may not work for you.

DERMATITIS AND ECZEMA

The worst part isn't the dryness, the itching or the painful sores. It isn't even the blizzard of skin flakes that can follow you like a winter storm. "The worst thing is always feeling different because your skin doesn't look like everyone else's," says Irene Crosby, a board member of the Portland-based Eczema Association for Science and Education. "I've had people refuse to sit next to me on buses or let me try clothes on."

Now in her fifties, Irene has been having outbreaks of atopic dermatitis, also called eczema, since she was a baby. "You always have to be aware of it, plan your day around it," she says. "You start thinking of your skin as a separate entity. You ask yourself, 'Today, can I garden? No, my hands won't let me do it.' Your skin is the largest organ of the body, and you become very aware of it," she adds.

MORE THAN SKIN DEEP

As you can tell from the *-itis* in *dermatitis,* this dry, crackly condition is an inflammation of the skin—an inflammation that for some people lasts a lifetime. Irene's hands, for example, have been itchy, scaly and sore for 35 years.

"Eczema often causes a very intense itch reaction, so the person is always rubbing and scratching," says Bruce Bart, M.D., a clinical professor and chief of dermatology at Hennepin County Medical Center in Minneapolis. Irene agrees. "People say you should just stop scratching, but you can't do it. My mother used to tie mittens on my hands, and I would still find ways to scratch."

Doctors are also scratching—for more information about this mysterious, uncomfortable skin disease. They do know eczema runs in families, and sufferers can never be sure when the next outbreak will occur or which part of the body will be affected, Dr. Bart says. They don't even know what to watch out for. Dry air often causes problems. So does stress, costume jewelry, cold air or rough fabrics. "Just walking through a room can start you itching," Irene says.

There is no cure for atopic dermatitis, Dr. Bart says, but there are things you can do to prevent flare-ups from getting under your skin.

DITCH THE ITCH

Sometimes that's as easy as steering clear of things you're sensitive to. If you react only to wool sweaters, for example, wear cotton instead. But eczema rarely is so predictable. To keep it at bay:

Stay calm. Doctors aren't sure if stress causes eczema or if people with eczema just naturally are a little tense. In either case, avoiding stress does seem to reduce flare-ups, Dr. Bart says. (For tips on how to control stress, see "Stress" on page 472).

Catch some rays. Sunshine—or the ultraviolet light from sun-lamps—can often prevent eczema, he says. Of course, too much sun can be as troublesome as too little. Ask your doctor to recommend safe exposure times and an appropriate sunscreen.

Keep cool. Anything that makes you sweat—hot rooms, heavy blankets, even hot baths—can turn up the pitch on your itch. Turn it back down with light blankets, cool water and cool, comfortable temperatures.

Add some vapor. People often have eczema outbreaks in the winter because central heating robs skin-protecting moisture from the air. You can replace moisture simply by turning on the humidifier, Dr. Bart suggests.

Since eczema is so unpredictable, these precautions may not always help. You still can get the upper hand, however, by giving your skin some timely, much-needed attention.

SOOTHING YOUR SKIN

Skin with eczema is extremely dry skin, Dr. Bart says. Like a sponge without water, it becomes rough, crusty, inflexible. To be smooth again, it needs moisture—lots of it.

Take a bath. Or two or three. Your crusty sponge of a skin simply can't soak up too much moisture, Dr. Bart says. Just make sure the water is cool, he adds. Hot water increases blood flow to the skin and makes it itch more. Cool water, by contrast, reduces blood flow, cools the itch and adds some much-needed lubrication to your dry, crackly hide.

To make your bathwater even more soothing, stir in some colloidal oatmeal—oatmeal ground so fine it stays suspended in the water while you bathe. Look for Aveeno brand in your local pharmacy.

Take a whirl in the whirlpool. While the water moistens your skin, the whirling action helps remove dried-up, itchy scales.

Seal it in. After your bath, gently pat yourself dry. Then apply a lotion to seal in the moisture. "In dry climates like we have here in Minnesota, especially in the winter, we use fairly heavy emollients, even Vaseline," Dr. Bart says. "If you're in a humid place, a cream or lotion should be enough." You can't apply too much lotion, he adds. Irene says she rubs her hands with petroleum jelly at least 20 times a day, then tucks them into cotton gloves for extra protection. "At night, I sleep with my hands in a light pair of cotton gloves, and I put vinyl exam gloves over that," she says.

Wear a wet dressing. Lay a damp strip of gauze, cotton or linen on the affected skin. As moisture evaporates from the dressing, the itching should evaporate as well. Repeat the cycle every few minutes for 15 to 30 minutes several times a day.

Buy a gentler wardrobe. Tight clothes and abrasive fabrics can be murder on your sensitive skin. Stick with loose-fitting, natural-fiber garments.

Watch what you eat. If you suspect that certain foods—eggs, seafood and dairy products are common culprits—are causing your outbreaks, abstain for a while and see what happens. If your skin clears up, voilà—you've found a solution.

MEDICAL FIRST AID

Since scratching often causes more problems than the disease itself, your first line of defense may mean medication. One effective, if sometimes odoriferous, remedy is coal tar, for years the treatment of choice, Dr. Bart says. Today's coal tar preparations, available at your pharmacy, are less unpleasant than their predecessors, although some can stain your clothes, he warns. Some people use them only at night, so that they can limit the damage to one (preferably old) pair of pajamas.

Less messy are the steroid ointments, which have revolutionized the treatment of eczema, Dr. Bart says. Drugs such as hydrocortisone, available over the counter, quickly quell itching and inflammation. Many people use hydrocortisone every day for years with no side effects. For more serious outbreaks, the stronger steroids, sold by prescription, can help. Unlike low-dose hydrocortisone, however, these can cause side effects—skin atrophy, for example, or suppression of the adrenal glands. They're usually used only for serious flare-ups, Dr. Bart says.

Another treatment is PUVA. The *P* stands for a light-sensitizing drug, psoralen, and the *UVA* refers to ultraviolet light. Basically, the affected skin is exposed to controlled amounts of healing light for several months.

After 20 to 30 sessions, the eczema can be much improved or even eliminated, Dr. Bart says. But PUVA isn't without drawbacks. There's the inconvenience of going to the doctor's office week after week. As time goes
by, PUVA often becomes less effective. Finally, all that concentrated light
can cause premature aging of the skin and boost your risk of skin cancer
and cataracts as well.

Some people turn to antihistamines, Dr. Bart says. Drugs such as
Benadryl and Dimetane help block the action of a chemical in your body
called histamine, which causes all that itching. Antihistamines can also
make you sleepy, which further suppresses the itch, he says.

TOUGHING IT OUT

Not everyone with eczema has a serious problem, Dr. Bart adds. Most
of the time, it causes nothing worse than an itchy elbow or a bit of scale
on the knee—inconveniences easily treated with a bit of hydrocortisone
cream. But for many, as Irene can attest, eczema is an all-consuming
disease. "It can go out of control to the point you have a total head-to-toe
rash," she says. "It's like all your systems just break down."

Occasionally the disease can simply disappear, but most likely, it will
come back. Irene, for example, had one "clear" period that lasted ten years.
Remissions are rare, says Dr. Bart, so don't expect miracles.

It can be tough on the family system, too. "My mother had to deal
with both her husband and me," Irene remembers. "We'd be scratching
away like mad, totally oblivious, and my mother would be saying 'Jimmy,
stop scratching, Irene, stop scratching!'

"It had one added benefit," she adds. "I had my own bedroom, because
my scratching drove my sister nuts."

DIABETES

This isn't to point fingers or anything, but whether you have diabetes or not, you're a sugar junkie. Your body has quite a sweet tooth. Even if you take your coffee black, your tea unsweetened and your oatmeal plain, you need sugar to survive. We're talking not about the white stuff you sprinkle on cereal but about glucose, the simple sugar your body extracts from fruits, vegetables and many other foods. Every single cell of your body uses glucose for fuel. Your red blood cells consume more than 1 ounce every day; your central nervous system gobbles about 5 ounces.

If you're healthy, your body extracts from your diet exactly the right amount of glucose, then stores the rest. But if you have adult-onset (Type II) diabetes, much of the glucose isn't used or stored. Instead, it remains in the blood, where it creates all kinds of problems. Here's what happens.

A SWEET POISON

To picture how your body makes use of sugars, imagine a counter stacked high with glucose—glucose entrées, glucose salads and glucose desserts. Every cell in your body is ready to eat, but where's the waiter? Enter insulin, a hormone produced by your pancreas. Basically insulin makes it possible for glucose to move from your bloodstream (where it accumulates after you eat) into your hungry cells.

People with adult-onset diabetes do produce insulin. But because of an abnormality at the cell level, the insulin cannot work as efficiently as it should. The glucose cannot get into cells in the normal manner, and so it accumulates in the blood. This condition is called hyperglycemia."You may be eating tons of food, but if your body can't use it, you're starving," says Priscilla Hollander, M.D., vice president for adult diabetes and special studies at Park Nicollet Medical Center in Minneapolis.

Your cells don't get enough to eat, so you're often tired and run-down. You probably drink and urinate a lot—your body's futile attempts to eliminate surplus glucose. What's more, glucose at high concentrations can damage nerves, blood vessels and even the arteries leading to your heart. In fact, more than half of those with diabetes will eventually die from heart problems, Dr. Hollander says.

Even though you can't *entirely* prevent this hereditary disease, you can slow its progress—or, occasionally, even reverse it, Dr. Hollander adds.

THE BEST TREATMENT— POUND FOR POUND

Doctors aren't sure why, but as your pounds add up, your insulin efficiency goes down. In fact, at least 80 percent of the people with adult-onset diabetes are overweight. So even though you can't change your genes, you may be able to control the disease or to prevent it from even becoming a problem by keeping your weight in check. Here's how the right diet can help.

Cut the calories. "For many people, the day they cut the calories down is the day they see an effect on their blood sugar. There's an immediate response," says Linda M. Delahanty, a clinical and research dietitian at Massachusetts General Hospital in Boston.

Of course, your blood sugar will quickly rebound if you feast on ice cream to celebrate your successful weight loss. Like diabetes itself, a successful diet is forever. But you don't have to be model-thin to experience long-term benefits. Some people can significantly lower their blood sugar by losing as little as 10 pounds.

Trim the fat. It doesn't take long for high-fat foods to contribute to a high-fat you. Not only will extra weight make your insulin work less efficiently, it can also raise your cholesterol—bad news for people with diabetes, who are already at risk for heart disease. To stay lean, consume less than 30 percent of your calories from fat, the American Diabetes Association advises.

Load up on complex carbohydrates. Now that you're cutting back on fatty foods, your diet should include more grains, potatoes and other complex carbohydrates, says Dr. Hollander. Although these foods are packed with glucose, they won't substantially raise your blood sugar, she adds. Complex carbohydrates slowly release glucose to the body over a long period of time.

Say sayonara to sweets. Pure sugar, on the other hand, can be pure trouble. Unlike complex carbohydrates, pure sugar is dumped into your bloodstream all at once. Your insulin won't have a chance to catch up.

If you must have a sweet, be sure you are eating one that is not made up mainly of sugar but that has other things in it as well. Proteins, fats and complex carbohydrates will aid in slowing your body's absorption of the sugar. In other words, you're going to be better off with a slice of cake or a bowl of ice milk than with a handful of jelly beans or a tangle of cotton candy.

Nosh between meals. If you eat a lot at one sitting, your body will be hard-pressed to meet the increased demand for insulin. To prevent sudden rises in glucose levels in the blood, "distribute your food throughout the day, so that any one meal isn't so large that it overwhelms the pancreas," Delahanty suggests.

Fill up on fiber. Beans, oat bran and other high-fiber foods not only will help lower your cholesterol but also will put the brakes on glucose as it enters your bloodstream. That may lower your need for insulin.

WORK IT OUT

If the fitness craze has left you cold, here are three good reasons to get warmed up: Diet plus exercise equals weight loss—and, more important, lower blood sugar levels. Regular exercise can lower blood pressure, cholesterol and your risk for heart disease. Finally, exercise can help make your insulin work more efficiently, says John Ivy, Ph.D., a professor of kinesiology at the University of Texas at Austin and director of the school's Exercise Science Laboratories. "Exercise may help by increasing the number of insulin receptors in the body, as well as the number of glucose transporters," Dr. Ivy explains. His suggestions:

Put on your walking shoes. "People can benefit greatly just by doing some good, brisk walking," Dr. Ivy says. Unfortunately, many people with diabetes also have diabetic neuropathy, a nervous system disorder that causes pain, tingling or numbness in the feet and legs. If walking makes you uncomfortable, don't despair, Dr. Ivy says. You have some choices.

Get the upper hand. How? By working your upper body. Exercises such as rowing, pull-ups or lifting weights can keep you in tip-top shape without straining your feet and legs.

Push the pedals. Bicycling is an excellent way to work your legs without overworking your feet, Dr. Ivy says.

Take the plunge. Swimming exercises just about every muscle in your body without putting pressure on your joints or limbs. If you can't swim, *walk* through the water, Dr. Ivy suggests.

Do it daily. You don't have to join a health club to stay in shape, Dr. Ivy insists. The trick is looking for opportunities. For example, get off that tractor and push a push mower instead. Take the steps instead of the elevator. Walk, don't drive, to the corner store. "One of the major reasons we have adult-onset diabetes is obesity," Dr. Ivy says. "Some people have a predisposition for diabetes, but it can be prevented—and often even reversed—if people eat properly and exercise."

TREATMENT BREAKTHROUGH

DELIVERING A CURE

It is difficult for doctors to control with precision the complex interactions between insulin and blood sugar. In fact, it's virtually impossible to duplicate with drugs your body's ideal chemical balance, says Richard A. Guthrie, M.D., professor of pediatrics at the University of Kansas School of Medicine and president of the Mid-America Diabetes Association.

Researchers are beginning to investigate new technologies—cell transplants, state-of-the-art monitors and in-the-body sensors—that someday may help your body help itself.

For example, scientists now are developing machines that will analyze blood sugar levels right through the skin, which will allow you to keep a sharp eye on what's going on inside. Better yet, you don't have to prick your finger for a drop of blood!

Researchers also are working on implantable sensors. "They will sense what your blood sugar is and broadcast that to a receiver—a wristwatch, or something like that," Dr. Guthrie says. "You can look down periodically and see what your blood sugar is."

The next step will be what doctors call a closed-loop system—that is, a surgically implanted sensor, pump and reservoir. The sensor would sense changes in blood sugar, then signal the pump to release exactly the right amount of insulin. Essentially this system would be an artificial pancreas, Dr. Guthrie says.

In addition, researchers hope to grow in the laboratory healthy pancreas cells that could be transplanted into misfunctioning organs, Dr. Guthrie says. If the technical difficulties can be overcome, cell transplantation could actually be a cure for diabetes.

As doctors get a better handle on the disease, their attention will turn to prevention. With advances in genetics, they may learn to diagnose—and treat—diabetes long before it becomes a problem. By the year 2002, says Dr. Guthrie, "we will probably screen the cord blood of all newborn infants for it, just like we screen them now for thyroid dysfunctions," he says.

Times That Try Men's (and Women's) Soles

Diabetic neuropathy can be the most uncomfortable aspect of this generally uncomfortable disease, says Richard A. Guthrie, M.D., coauthor of *The Diabetes Sourcebook* and a professor of pediatrics at the University of Kansas School of Medicine. Caused by the nerve damage resulting from high levels of blood sugar, neuropathy can cause tingling, pain and finally numbness in the feet and legs. "When you lose all sensation, that nerve is dead," Dr. Guthrie says.

To keep your heels on an even keel, try the following.

Peek at your feet. It's not uncommon for people with diabetes to injure their feet without even knowing it. Worse, they're particularly prone to infections. This means that little injuries can turn into big problems: Among diabetics, about 20,000 toes, feet and legs are amputated every year. Stay on the lookout for blisters or cuts, Dr. Guthrie says. If you have a cut that won't heal or a rash that won't go away, call your doctor.

Keep your shoes on. Even if your idea of paradise is walking barefoot through the park on a hot summer day, don't take chances. Protect your feet from sharp objects by wearing shoes whenever you leave the house.

Soap your soles. You don't want to give bacteria opportunities to cause trouble. Clean your feet every day. Keep your toenails trimmed and free of ragged edges. Can't reach your feet? Ask a friend to help. Better yet, get a pedicure. Once you quit giggling, you may be hooked!

Wear soft socks. Socks made from cotton or other absorbent materials not only feel good but also can wick rash-causing moisture away from your tender toes. And while you're putting on those new socks, check your shoes, too. Shoes that don't fit will very likely rub you the wrong way.

When Self-Care Isn't Enough

Just about everyone with adult-onset diabetes will eventually need medication—either synthetic insulin or drugs that make their natural insulin work more efficiently, Dr. Hollander says. "The pancreas is not operating at full steam, and over time it tends to slow down," she explains.

In the early stages of the disease, before your insulin/blood sugar balance becomes dangerously skewed, your doctor may prescribe drugs, taken orally, that will help your pancreas churn out more insulin. Called sulfonylureas, these drugs not only boost your insulin supplies but also increase the number of insulin receptors. This makes the insulin you produce work even more efficiently.

In more advanced cases, people often need regular injections of synthetic insulin to augment their natural supplies, Dr. Hollander says. If you're lucky, your pancreas may recover after a few weeks or months of injections, thus allowing your blood sugar to remain at safe levels without further treatment for a while. More often, however, you will need insulin—sometimes a little, sometimes a lot—for the rest of your life.

Unfortunately, insulin isn't without side effects, Dr. Hollander says. For starters, it may stimulate the appetite in some people—exactly the opposite of what you want! It may also encourage the formation of artery-clogging plaque, which can further increase your risk for heart attacks. Finally, there is the risk of hypoglycemia, a condition in which your supply of glucose, rather than being too high, precipitously falls, sometimes to dangerously low levels. Ask your doctor how to manage this powerful, lifesaving drug.

Researchers currently are investigating a third type of drug, alpha glucosidase inhibitors, that may help slow the passage of glucose from the intestines into the bloodstream, Dr. Hollander says. This would give the insulin more time to prevent your blood sugar from rising to unmanageable levels. But even if alpha glucosidase inhibitors don't pan out, additional drugs for diabetes clearly are needed, she says. "Right now, we only have the oral drugs and insulin. They're very good, but they can't do everything."

DIVERTICULAR DISEASE

Telephone answering machines, VCRs, cruise controls—lots of today's conveniences didn't exist 100 years ago. And neither did diverticular disease. Well, it existed, but it was *very* rare. Today, however, this intestinal disorder is thought to affect as many as 50 percent of older Americans. So what happened to make the disease as common (and sometimes as annoying) as a telephone answering machine?

To really understand the origin of diverticular disease (sometimes called diverticulosis), we have to take a look at the walls of the colon.

INTESTINAL POCKETS

Diverticula are small bulges or pockets that sometimes form in the lining of the "tubular" organs—the esophagus, for example, the stomach or the small intestine. But when doctors talk about diverticular disease, they generally mean colonic diverticula—bulges in the wall of the colon.

The colon usually is smooth and taut. But as it ages, the walls get progressively weaker. Where they're weakest, high intestinal pressures can force small bubbles—diverticula—to bulge outward, explains William Ruderman, M.D., chairman of the Department of Gastroenterology at Cleveland Clinic Florida in Fort Lauderdale. Diverticula range from pin-head-size to quarter-size or larger, although most are considerably smaller than a dime. You can have one diverticulum or hundreds, and the diagnosis is the same: diverticular disease.

Does this mean your colon and its high-mileage bubbles are on the verge of a blowout? Probably not, although it can happen, says Joseph Katz, M.D., a gastroenterologist in private practice in Indianapolis. "Most diverticular disease, unless it bleeds or becomes infected, is silent." In fact, as many as eight out of ten people with diverticular disease never have symptoms. Doctors simply discover it during unrelated medical examinations. "If I didn't tell them they have it, they'd never know," says Dr. Katz.

Unfortunately, diverticular disease isn't always silent. Doctors aren't sure why, but some people have attacks of cramping, constipation and diarrhea. Another more alarming symptom is rectal bleeding, caused by ruptured blood vessels inside the diverticula. More commonly, diverticulosis can progress to diverticulitis, an infection that can be very painful and sometimes quite serious.

Short of surgery, there's no way to eliminate diverticula that already exist in your colon, Dr. Katz says. But you can prevent new ones from forming.

A MANUFACTURED DISEASE

Until the 1900s, people in the United States, Great Britain and other Western countries ate lots of fruits, beans, vegetables and whole-wheat bread. Diverticular disease was rare. Then the Industrial Revolution rattled in. People began to eat more meat, white bread and other processed foods and less dietary fiber. Diverticular disease became quite common.

By contrast, in nonindustrialized parts of the world—most of Africa, for instance—people to this day eat large amounts of dietary fiber. For them, diverticular disease remains a rarity.

The link is this: Dietary fiber makes stools larger, softer and easier to pass. This in turn decreases—or at least distributes—the force exerted by the colon to move the stool along. By decreasing pressure, fiber reduces the risk for blowouts, Dr. Katz explains. "Fiber basically retrains the colon to work the way it's supposed to."

SUPPRESSING THE PRESSURE

You don't need a time machine (or a plane ticket to Africa) to prevent diverticular disease. Here's what you do need.

Fill up on fiber. When you eat foods that contain large amounts of dietary fiber—particularly vegetables and certain types of bran—the fiber particles soak up water in your intestine like so many tiny sponges. The water makes the stools bulkier and softer, and *that's* good for your colon, Dr. Ruderman says.

In a study conducted at three medical centers in Great Britain, researchers placed 21 people with diverticulosis on high-fiber diets. After 12 weeks, the patients reported having regular bowel movements and a decrease in the severity of abdominal pain that accompanied their disease.

Experts recommend you eat 25 to 35 grams of dietary fiber a day. This sounds like a lot, but by the time you've eaten a bowl of bran cereal (6 grams), three dried figs (5.2 grams), a serving of kidney beans (6.9 grams) and an orange or two (5.8 grams each), you're almost there!

Add fiber to fiber. If for some reason you can't get enough fiber from the fruits, vegetables and other foods in your diet, you can supplement it with highly concentrated forms of fiber such as crushed husks of psyllium seeds (found in Metamucil and Hydrocil) or methylcellulose (Citrucel). These are available over the counter at pharmacies, says Dr. Katz.

If you're currently in pain because of a diverticular flare-up, however, you probably should stay *off* the fiber until the symptoms abate, he adds.

Heed the call. Irregular bathroom habits lead to constipation, which, Dr. Katz says, raises pressure in the colon. For most people, the urge to defecate, called the gastrocolonic reflex, is strongest in the morning after breakfast. Give yourself a little extra time before going to work to obey it, he says.

Get a workout. Doctors often tell people that their bowels won't move unless they do. Regular exercise won't cure diverticular disease, but it can improve your overall bowel health. Think of it as preventive maintenance: By keeping your bowels healthy today, they won't fail you tomorrow!

Question certain snacks. Some doctors believe that nuts and seeds, should they lodge inside a diverticulum, can cause inflammation. In fact, there's little evidence in the medical literature to suggest this, Dr. Ruderman says. You might want to ask your doctor for *his* opinion.

WHEN PROBLEMS FLARE

For most people, diverticular disease never causes serious problems. But others aren't so lucky. When a blood vessel inside a diverticulum tears, causing rectal bleeding, it can be terrifying, Dr. Katz says. "It's not going to be a little bit on the toilet paper or a little bit mixed with the stool. When diverticula bleed, they usually bleed profusely." To stop the bleeding, your doctor may try to pinpoint the blood vessel in the colon that has ruptured. Then he can inject drugs to stop it. But people who have one attack of bleeding very frequently have another. Rather than patching you up, your doctor may recommend resection—surgically removing the damaged section of bowel. This will stop the bleeding *and* prevent recurrences—at least from that particular diverticulum.

Some 10 to 20 percent of people with diverticular disease may eventually develop diverticulitis, Dr. Ruderman says. Here's what happens. The bacteria that normally live inside the colon—and inside the diverticula as well—rarely cause problems. You're used to them, and they're used to you. But sometimes they work their way into the colon wall. There they're attacked as enemies, and the resulting infection can cause fever, abdominal cramps, tenderness (particularly in the lower left side of the abdominal area) and diarrhea or constipation. If the infection isn't treated right away, it can spread all the way through the colon wall and into the abdominal cavity. If that happens, the result can be peritonitis, a potentially life-threatening infection, Dr. Katz says.

Fortunately, diverticulitis is easily treated. Antibiotics—given orally or, in more serious cases, intravenously—will quickly squelch most infections. As with diverticular bleeding, however, one attack of diverticulitis is frequently followed by another. Your doctor may recommend surgery to prevent problems in the future.

EAR PAIN

Ears can come in handy. But expose them to a bunch of germs, dunk them in a pool or take them for a ride, and they can dish out a lot of pain.

Remember the last time you had an earache? Whether you were 5 or 50, that insidious little ache is something you never forget. It feels as though an alien something-or-other has landed in your ear and is trying to colonize the planet. And that, more or less, may be what is happening.

EARACHE

Many adult earaches start when mucus secretions, resulting from cigarette smoke or an allergy, block the eustachian tube that leads from your ear to your throat, explains Dudley Weider, M.D., a clinical professor of otolaryngology at Dartmouth Medical School in Hanover, New Hampshire. The problem is that air within the ear is drawn into the ear's tiny blood vessels when the tube is blocked. This creates a vacuum within the ear itself, says Dr. Weider, and as soon as this happens, the result is a stab of pain.

Unfortunately, in some cases that's only the opening thrust in what is about to become an infection. The body always feels a need to fill any vacuum, says Dr. Weider, so fluid begins to collect within the ear. This creates a homey environment for any stray bacteria from your nose or throat that want to establish a new colony. The resulting pressure changes from the growth of this colony will literally push your eardrum outward.

Not only is this a painful experience, adds Dr. Weider, but if you do not start antibiotic treatment fairly soon, the pressure on your eardrum may cause it to bulge and then burst.

Of course that's exactly what used to happen frequently in the days before antibiotics, says Dr. Weider. The eardrum would burst, the fluid would drain, and the person who was attached to the ear would not hear quite as well as before. And the infection might or might not trigger the whole painful episode once again.

Fortunately, says Dr. Weider, once you're on antibiotics, both the pain and the danger of a perforated eardrum will evaporate within hours.

To avoid this whole sorry mess to begin with, says Dr. Weider:

Avoid smoky rooms. Since smoke causes the eustachian tubes to malfunction, try to avoid it whenever you can. For example, always request a seat in the nonsmoking section of restaurants.

Take care of your allergies. With your doctor's guidance, select an antihistamine or decongestant nasal spray that will prevent allergies from closing down your eustachian tubes.

Live an upright life. Try to avoid lying down while your ear actually hurts. Your eustachian tube is far more likely to open up if you're vertical.

SWIMMER'S EAR

Although some adult ear pain is caused by blocked eustachian tubes and an infection in the middle ear, some is also caused by bacteria-laden water in the canal leading to your eardrum—what doctors usually call *otitis externa,* or swimmer's ear.

Normally, water gets into your ear, earwax repels it, and it drains back out. The ear dries, and the bacteria remain few and under control, says Jan Kasperbauer, M.D., senior associate consultant in otorhinolaryngology (ear, nose and throat medicine) at the Mayo Clinic in Rochester, Minnesota. "These bacteria are common, and they're everywhere," Dr. Kasperbauer says. "But sometimes conditions change that allow them to grow." It could be an overdose of bacteria in the water—as from a polluted lake or river—high humidity, too many showers, a dunking in a not-as-clean-as-it-seems hot tub, impacted earwax or an abrasion to the canal.

Trapped water makes the canal skin soggy, and the bacteria—or sometimes fungi—take it from there. Your ear may first feel blocked and itchy but soon becomes swollen, sometimes swollen shut. A milky liquid may drain out, and the pain can be intense. At that late stage, swimmer's ear can become serious and should be treated by your doctor, who will prescribe antibiotics or even steroids.

STAND BY YOUR EARS

Swimmer's ear is best dealt with before it starts. Fortunately, that's easily done. It's important to start with clean, healthy ears. If you've had recurring ear infections, a ruptured eardrum or ear surgery, have your doctor examine your ears before swimming season starts. He can clean out debris—dead skin, excess wax, even clippings from haircuts—that can irritate your ears and promote bacterial growth. Once this has been done, the following self-help tips should get you through the season swimmingly.

Stick only your elbow into your ear. Yes, you've heard it before, but it's a major-league preventive strategy. People keep sticking cotton swabs into their ears to clean them out. Granted, it can feel good. But that cotton swab also pushes your earwax deep inside your ear, Dr. Kasperbauer says. "It can also break the skin, and because the ear canal isn't straight, the swab bumps against the sides," he says. The resulting abrasion, combined with moisture and bacteria, becomes a breeding ground for infection.

Add oil as needed. Rather than trying to clean out your ears with cotton swabs or whatever little pokey thing seems handy, use mineral oil. "A few drops of mineral oil can keep your earwax soft, and usually debris will come out by itself," Dr. Kasperbauer says. "The mineral oil will also prevent the formation of wax plugs." Apply the drops to your ears for several days in a row. Once the wax is soft, squirt your ears *gently* using a rubber bulb syringe and lukewarm water.

Give your ears a drink. Plain old rubbing alcohol absorbs water, drying out the ear and killing germs, Dr. Kasperbauer says. A few drops in each ear after swimming or bathing will help prevent an infection. And it's a good treatment for the early stages of swimmer's ear, he says. Just wiggle your ear, so that the alcohol will go all the way down, and then turn your head to let it drain out.

Over-the-counter antiseptic drops such as Swim Ear, Ear Magic or Murine Ear Drops can be used for the same purpose.

AIRPLANE EAR

Dumbo the flying elephant never had trouble with his ears, although *yours* may not fare so well at higher altitudes. The problem is air pressure. Generally the human ear is well equipped to handle changes in air pressure, but we haven't yet evolved to the point of being able to ascend or descend at hundreds of miles an hour without our ears making a big deal out of it.

Rapid changes in altitude create rapid ranges in air pressure. Particularly after your pilot announces that you're about to land, rapid descending can create a vacuum in the middle ear, sucking the eardrum inward. This is what causes both the muffled hearing and the discomfort experienced by many flyers, says James Donaldson, M.D., professor emeritus of otolaryngology/head and neck surgery at the University of Washington School of Medicine.

In some rare cases, this pressure on the eardrum may even cause the ear to fill with fluid, a condition that can lead to weeks or even months of discomfort. It may even require medical care.

EARS ABOVE GROUND

There are simple ways to prevent the discomfort of flying and any possibility of complications. Keep these tips in mind the next time you board an airplane.

Don't fly with a cold or flu. Upper respiratory infections make your eustachian tubes swell up, so they can't open and close as they should. Not only may your pain on descending be intense and unrelievable, you may have some pain on ascending. Worse, Dr. Donaldson says, the vacuum created by descending can suck cold or flu germs into your middle ear.

Use a decongestant. Sometimes you may have no choice but to fly with a cold, or maybe you have an allergy that also swells your eustachian tubes. In this case, try taking an oral decongestant an hour or two before you take off, Dr. Donaldson suggests. Or as long as you don't have high blood pressure, spray each nostril with a nasal decongestant containing oxymetazoline (like Afrin) about an hour before your first descent; wait 10 minutes, then take a second spray in each nostril. (Nasal decongestants should not be used by those with high blood pressure.)

Swallow and yawn. Done repeatedly, these are highly effective. "But if pain begins to build and your hearing starts to muffle," Dr. Donaldson says, "take a deep breath, hold your nose, shut your mouth tightly, puff out your cheeks and blow firmly, but not forcefully, to equalize air pressure."

Use the pilot's ear pop. If the above technique doesn't work, the next trick is one used by pilots: Pinch your nostrils shut, take a mouthful of air, and puff out both cheeks (as above). Next use the fingers of your free hand to compress your cheeks, forcing the air into the back of your nose while swallowing. You should hear a loud pop in your ears, signaling success.

Stay awake while descending. You don't swallow as much when you sleep, so your ears won't keep up with the pressure changes. If you must doze off, do it while ascending.

Chew gum. Although it's not as effective as yawning or swallowing, the muscular action of chewing a wad of gum may help open your eustachian tubes.

RUPTURED EARDRUMS

The eardrum is only a few millimeters in diameter and so thin a light can shine through it, but it's essential to your hearing. Sound waves hit it like drumsticks, and the resulting vibrations set the tiny bones of the middle ear into motion.

Too loud a sound—an explosion, for example—can pound a hole into an eardrum. So can a slap to the side of the head, a severe middle ear infection or a cotton swab. One British journalist answered his portable phone in the dark and plunged the antenna into his ear, perforating his eardrum.

If your eardrum ruptures, you may have a partial loss of hearing and a slight discharge or bleeding. While it's usually painful, Dr. Kasperbauer says, a ruptured eardrum doesn't hurt as much as you might think. But it can be dangerous: An infection can spread through the hole to the middle and even inner ear. So see a doctor if you suspect your eardrum has ruptured.

"The majority of ruptured eardrums heal themselves," Dr. Kasperbauer says. "But if the perforation won't heal by itself, a doctor can attach a temporary plastic patch over it or graft a tiny piece of tissue over the area." Healing is usually complete within a few weeks with no hearing loss.

EATING DISORDERS

Thirty years ago Marilyn Monroe had the ideal shape, rounded and full of curves. "Yet if she were alive now and in her prime, she would be considered fat," says psychologist Robert Mann, Ph.D., vice president and clinical director of The Rader Institute, a nation-wide eating disorder clinic with headquarters in Los Angeles. "Thirty years ago the 'ideal' figure was achievable. Not now." Every magazine cover and ad, movie and TV show reminds you of the modern "ideal" body: stick-slender, with a minute percentage of body fat that women are not physiologically destined to attain. Yet try to attain it they do—with fad diets, endless exercise and constant self-critiques in the mirror.

And some people take this body dissatisfaction to such an extreme that it becomes a mental illness—the eating disorders anorexia and bulimia, or a combination of both. "The anorexic sees in the mirror something that isn't there," Dr. Mann says. "She shows you her emaciated arms with bones and joints sticking out and says, 'Look how fat I am.'" To shed that imaginary fat, she starves herself. Most doctors label someone an anorexic who falls to 15 percent or more below her ideal body weight.

The bulimic, on the other hand, says, "I want to look like (insert the name of any currently popular, impossibly thin media star)." She typically cannot be found after dinner—where she's just binged on a king-size filet of beef, a baked potato smothered with butter and sour cream and three slices of ice cream–covered apple pie—unless you check the bathroom. There you'll find her, forcing herself to vomit. Bingeing and purging—either by vomiting or with laxatives—are the classic symptoms of bulimia.

THE ROOTS OF EATING DISORDERS

Why do some people take the normal desire to look good and run amok with it? Some of the cause may lie in their family background, says psychiatrist Joel Yager, M.D., professor of psychiatry at the University of

California, Los Angeles, and senior consultant in the UCLA Neuropsychiatric Institute's Adult Eating Disorders Progam. "Their families often have higher levels of dysfunction," he says. "There's a higher alcoholism rate among the fathers, a higher rate of depression among the mothers. Often there's been a divorce or a chronically unhappy marriage. And physical appearance may be of paramount importance to a parent or sibling." Sexual abuse is common in these families—it has been reported by 86 percent of the patients that Dr. Mann sees in the hospital, admittedly a worst-case setting. Where some people choose drugs, promiscuity or other extremes to dull or forget their psychological pain, others choose food.

Ninety-five percent of people with eating disorders are women between the ages of 12 and 25. Some studies estimate that 4.5 percent of 18-year-old college women are bulimic, while the rate of anorexia is up to 1 percent in females 12 to 18 years old. One study of female professional tennis players revealed 30 percent of them were bulimic, Dr. Mann says. Ironically, he adds, "another huge bulimic population is student dietitians—one study indicated as high as 40 percent."

But anorexia and bulimia are becoming more of an equal-opportunity disorder. "We're seeing an increase in the number of men with eating disorders," Dr. Mann says. " 'Coming out' is more acceptable now, but there is also a rise in incidence. Men are coming under more and more pressure to look good—there's the gym, men's magazines, the same things women have been exposed to for decades."

The starvation an anorexic imposes on herself can kill her. And a bulimic "does murderous things to her gastrointestinal system," Dr. Mann says.

Anorexia is the more dangerous of the two disorders. "Ten percent of anorexics die," Dr. Mann says. Malnourishment can be deadly. Their muscles atrophy and waste away. Their blood pressure drops to dangerous levels. Their periods stop. Abuse of laxatives causes dehydration. They have low resistance to infection. They develop potassium deficiencies, which can cause heart damage and heart attacks. Others become depressed—depression that may be exacerbated by nutritional deficiencies.

But bulimics don't get off easy. "They can test anywhere from healthy to critically ill," Dr. Mann says. Repetitive vomiting lets stomach acid scar the esophagus and throat and erode tooth enamel. Some bulimics habitually take Ipecac, an over-the-counter drug that induces vomiting. "It's sometimes a testament to the resilience of the human body that a bulimic can maintain good health," he says. But he's not talking about good mental health—bulimics also often suffer depression.

Regardless of what led to your anorexia or bulimia, you can learn how to overcome it.

Treatment for bulimia can range from self-treatment to nonprofessional counseling to professional help to hospitalization—a reflection of the wide range of severity typical of the disease. Because they're in more serious mental and physical shape, anorexics need professional help right off the bat, Dr. Yager says.

FLUSHING OUT BULIMIA

If you have bulimic tendencies, Dr. Yager says, understanding what's creating your problem will help in dealing with it. Learn all you can about the disease and consider joining an eating disorders group, where you can get counseling from professionals and those who've "been there."

At the very least, find a good confidant. "It's always good to tell somebody else 'I have this problem, and I'm going to try to get better,'

PROFILE IN HEALING

EDITH MOORE: EATING TO LIVE

Control plays a big part in the lives of people with eating disorders, and Edith Moore was no exception. To see and hear her now—a sweet-voiced, quite attractive, 26-year-old woman just over 5 feet tall and 100 pounds—you'd never know she had been out of control for years.

"I learned to be negative about myself way back in fourth grade," says Edith, now an eating disorders counselor herself. A rough childhood may have contributed to her bulimia, but she doesn't blame any one person or thing. She first purged at age 14, but by then she was already a real problem child. "I made a decision that no one was going to control me. If my parents grounded me or tried to discipline me, I blatantly rebelled. I got into drugs, but they caused even more problems," she says. Thievery, screaming battles with her parents, jail and probation were becoming the pattern. She became a prostitute for a time. "But I retreated back into bulimia. It was a clean, safer way to do the same thing," she says, which was to abuse herself—all the time.

Her parents knew she was bulimic but did little to help. "My mom just told me to clean up the bathroom," Edith says. "I guess my eating problem was less scary for her than drugs."

But bulimia was plenty scary for Edith. Although she would wait at least 20 minutes before vomiting to allow some—"but not too much"—food to get into her system, "it almost ended up killing me,"

---

because then you've made a statement and you feel you have to stick to it," Dr. Yager says.

Check out nutritional counseling, so that you can get back on a sound eating program. Colleges—those hotbeds of bulimia where newly arrived freshmen begin copying the bingeing and purging traits of their dormitory peers—often offer education, peer counseling and student health programs.

Serious cases of bulimia, says Dr. Yager, require more than self-help. "Bulimia is more serious when it's accompanied by depression," Dr. Yager notes, "and if that's the case, the person is better off with professional help. Some depression is a response to bulimia that's out of control, but some bulimia is a symptom of depression." Antidepressants are sometimes prescribed.

---

she says. She was hospitalized twice for dehydration and headaches, two typical symptoms of bulimia. She was sent home with a prescription for pain medication, which resulted in another addiction. She eventually suffered through a bad marriage made worse by bulimia, drugs and alcohol. "It kept me pretty sick. I continued to get tests for every disease, but I didn't know there was any treatment for an eating disorder," says Edith.

In the end, enough was enough. "I finally just accepted that I was kind of a lost soul and I'd better start working on my soul," she says. Edith first got herself into an outpatient treatment program and then checked into The Rader Institute in mid-1985. It was a six-week program. "I gave up," she says. "I told myself 'I don't care if I gain a hundred pounds, I just can't live like this anymore.' I gave up the alcohol and the drugs and bingeing and purging. I just quit beating up on myself."

At Rader she worked on her spirituality, her body image and her relationships with others, particularly her parents. "I learned how to eat," she says. "And of course after I started eating normally, I didn't gain weight. That was a wild discovery. I learned that there were some options to life other than the way that I was going, and they looked rather inviting."

Now she's a counselor for the Rader clinic in Houston. "Sometimes I still go through swings," says Edith, "but working with people helps me through that."

CURING ANOREXIA

The surest cure for anorexia, says Dr. Yager, is through professional help. A professional program usually includes a nutritionist and a psychiatrist, sometimes a psychologist and your family doctor or pediatrician. If you're anorexic, says Dr. Yager, you may have some physical problems, and it's likely your laboratory tests may show all kinds of abnormalities. These have to be monitored closely. It's likely you'll have to be hospitalized, at least for a while. "The reason is that anorexics are really locked into the compulsions of their disease and are much less likely to be either willing or able to turn it around themselves," Dr. Yager says.

There are two main approaches to hospital programs, Dr. Mann says: traditional psychiatric treatment, and the newer 12-step treatment program fashioned after Alcoholics Anonymous.

In the traditional program, Dr. Yager says, an anorexic will be put on a firm meal plan—even forced intravenous feeding in the most extreme, life-threatening cases. "The nurses will literally sit with you during meals and for several hours after the meals to make sure you don't go throw up or exercise it off," he says. "You'll be weighed daily or several times per week; you'll have your activities restricted if you're an overexerciser. And you'll get psychological counseling to try to help you deal with the fright of eating and changing your self-concept—you may have a phobia about having food inside you and get a panic attack, so you need someone to help you through that."

The 12-step program, offered at The Rader Institute and similar private clinics, approaches the disease as a dependency problem similar to alcohol or drugs. "The primary caregivers often are recovering anorexics and bulimics themselves," Dr. Mann says. Counseling is a strong component of the program. Patients are taught to face their problem and control it, step by step. "It requires you to sign on to the 12-step philosophy, which is based on acknowledging and relying on a higher power outside yourself," says Dr. Mann.

A VOTE FOR MARILYN

Like any mental illness, anorexia or bulimia can leave you feeling hollow and alone. It's hard to see your way out. But there *is* a way out—and help can be tailored to fit you, says Dr. Mann. What you have to do is face the facts of your eating disorder, choose your treatment plan and learn how to eat right.

Serious cases of anorexia and bulimia have their roots far deeper than the superficial appeal of trying to look like the ideal woman, yet that false hope serves as the spur for all the physical and emotional torture anorexics and bulimics force themselves to endure.

Dr. Mann suggests a different, more attainable, more rounded ideal: "The best thing to happen to women now," he says, "is the Marilyn Monroe revival."

EMPHYSEMA

Emphysema is the disease that teaches you to never take your breathing for granted. It also teaches—the hard way—that smoking is about the worst thing you can do to your body.

"Emphysema is caused by the body's own white blood cells chewing up the lungs," says Robert Sandhaus, M.D., Ph.D., assistant professor of medicine at the University of Colorado Medical Center in Denver and director of the intensive care unit at Littleton Hospital in Littleton. White blood cells are the shock troops of the body's immune system. When they sense "invading" smoke particles entering the lungs, they descend to gobble them up. "The problem is that white blood cells are sloppy eaters," says Dr. Sandhaus.

As these "sloppy eaters" do their work, they accidentally do serious and permanent damage to the lung's air sacs—the alveoli, which look like bunches of grapes. As the alveoli are destroyed, breathing gets tougher and tougher. Eventually, those with emphysema may run out of breath even walking across a room.

LOVE YOUR LUNGS

Emphysema is almost totally preventable. Given what you know so far, can you guess the number one prevention measure?

Stop smoking NOW. "Of people with emphysema, 99.99 percent are current or former smokers," says Dr. Sandhaus. Smoking tobacco is the cause of emphysema. Stop. Before it's too late.

Avoid secondhand smoke. Breathing in others' smoke may not be as bad as smoking yourself, but it sure isn't going to do your lungs any good. You're perfectly justified in asking smokers to light up far away from you.

Avoid air pollution. The typical pollutants from cars and factories are also irritants to your lungs, says Dr. Sandhaus. Generally, air pollution isn't as dangerous as inhaling cigarette smoke, but you'd certainly be doing your lungs a favor to dodge areas of thick pollution.

Take antioxidants. If you're at risk for emphysema, consider supplements of vitamins C and E, nutrients known as antioxidants. "We don't have good, solid scientific evidence that antioxidants help, but the rationale is solid, and these vitamins won't hurt you. We usually recommend 500 milligrams twice a day of C and 800 units twice a day of E," says Dr. Sandhaus. The rationale to which he refers is that antioxidants may help protect a protein in the blood that can shield your lungs from the damage of sloppy-eating white blood cells. Consult with your doctor if you take supplements of vitamin E, because it has potential side effects, especially if you're taking blood-thinning drugs.

LIVING WITH BAD NEWS

Breathing and exerting yourself become a real challenge when you have emphysema, but then challenges are made to be met. Your doctor can help, and you can help yourself. If you've been told that you have emphysema, slow down further deterioration by quitting your smoking habit *immediately* and by following the other preventive measures listed above. Also follow the tips below. They'll help you to feel better and to retain as much independence as possible.

Avoid cold air. "Cold is a trigger that can make the airways spasm shut," says Dr. Sandhaus.

Exercise moderately. And work up to it gradually. Exercise can be a trigger to make airways spasm, but moderate exercise is essential to strengthen your heart and breathing muscles. The stronger they get, the more work they can do with less oxygen. Walking is probably the best exercise. Mild calisthenics are also good. Work with your doctor on developing a safe exercise program.

Eat properly. Emphysema can make eating difficult, but you've got to keep up your interest in food to keep up your strength.

Drink plenty of fluids. Liquids keep your lung fluids thin and easy to cough up. Check with your doctor before increasing your fluid intake, though. And do not consider alcohol a proper fluid! Alcohol is a central nervous system depressant that can slow breathing.

Avoid sick people. Stay away from people with colds or the flu. A lung infection will hurt you a lot more than it hurts them.

Get organized. Organize your chores to make the best use of your energy. Do things consciously that you used to do unconsciously. Think of your energy as money that you have to invest wisely. Spread big jobs throughout the day. For example, if bathing and dressing give you the vapors, bathe before breakfast and dress afterward.

BLASTING BLEBS AND BULLAE

Emphysema is not a pretty disease—in its final stages, the lungs fill with cysts called blebs and bullae (bullae are big blebs). These masses cut short what little breathing capacity is left. Once a critical mass is reached, death usually comes within a year, unless a lung transplant is performed—and that is an option only for people able to withstand such major surgery.

But a recent technological breakthrough is showing promise at removing blebs and bullae. At the University of California, Irvine (UCI), Medical Center, a 75-year-old man came to the hospital so short of breath he could walk only ten steps before collapsing. He had to use an oxygen tank to breathe, and a lung function test showed his breathing capacity was only 20 percent of normal because both lungs were compressed with bullae. A transplant was out of the question because of his age and general poor health.

The only choice left was to use an experimental laser developed by lung specialist Akio Wakabayashi, M.D., associate professor of surgery at UCI. Threading the tiny laser into the man's lungs through a device called a thoracoscope, Dr. Wakabayashi focused the intense beam of light on the blebs and bullae. The cysts shrank and dissolved under the pinpoint heat. After the treatment, x-rays showed the man's lungs were clear—the cysts had been destroyed.

"This man now walks 3 miles a day and no longer needs to be on oxygen," Dr. Wakabayashi says. The doctor went on to give more than 65 other end-stage emphysema sufferers the laser treatment. "It's amazing," he says. "All of these patients showed significant improvement on both lung function and treadmill tests." Dr. Wakabayashi estimates that thoracoscopic laser surgery will be in wide use by the mid-1990s.

Meanwhile, at least nine drug companies are working on ways to stop emphysema from forming in the first place. "These drugs are certainly on the near horizon, maybe within the next couple of years," says Robert Sandhaus, M.D., Ph.D., of the University of Colorado Medical Center in Denver. "They won't reverse the destruction that has already taken place, but they will prevent additional destruction in people who continue to smoke." One drug appears to survive combustion, so there's even talk of putting it in cigarettes. Of course, smoking would still cause cancer and heart disease.

Breathe deeply. That is, breathe so that your belly, not your chest, expands with each inhalation. (Check yourself with your hand.) And wait a full second after each exhalation before inhaling again. This will help force stale air out of your lungs, so that you can breathe in fresh air.

How Your Doctor Can Help

Your doctor has various treatments that can help you breathe easier and prevent complications. For instance, he or she may prescribe a bronchodilator. "Many people with emphysema have an element of asthma that accompanies it—asthma defined as airflow obstruction that is helped by using a bronchodilator," Dr. Sandhaus says. "The asthma part of emphysema is reversible with a bronchodilator."

You may also be given antibiotics. "Upper respiratory tract infections also make the airways spasm, and they also call white blood cells into the lungs, where they do more damage," Dr. Sandhaus says. "We make sure our patients have a stock of antibiotics at home, so that they can start them at the first sign of a lung infection."

Other medical options might include a flu shot (you don't need the flu of the year attacking your lungs) or various medications. Common drugs include nasal and oral steroid sprays to reduce swelling in the airways and diuretics to get rid of extra fluid. Supplements of the mineral potassium may also be prescribed to replace the potassium lost because of the diuretics. In the very worst cases of emphysema, a portable oxygen tank may be an option.

ENDOMETRIOSIS

Many women expect some aching, heaviness and cramping during the first day or two of their menstrual period. It's a good excuse to duck the nonessentials and curl up with a book. But a normal menstrual period does not wreak havoc on your life.

The symptoms of endometriosis are different from the tweaks and twinges of normal menstruation. "The most common complaint is pain bad enough that it can't be ignored," says Mary Lou Ballweg, cofounder and president of the Endometriosis Association in Milwaukee.

Symptoms include increasingly painful periods, tenderness and swelling in the lower abdomen that may even start two or three weeks before menstruation, pain that radiates into the groin or lower back, pain during bowel movements or urination and sudden, sharp pain during sexual intercourse. "Not every woman has devastating pain, though," says Camran Nezhat, M.D., professor of clinical obstetrics and gynecology at Mercer University in Macon, Georgia, and director of the Fertility and Endoscopy Center in Atlanta. "Symptoms can range from mild to extremely severe."

TISSUE ON THE LOOSE

Why pain in so many places? Because given enough travel time, endometriosis can "invade" the entire pelvic area, an area abounding with nerve endings.

Endometriosis begins when the tissue lining the inside of the uterus, the endometrium, ends up outside the uterus, in the abdominal cavity, explains Robert Barbieri, M.D., chairman of the Department of Obstetrics and Gynecology at the State University of New York at Stony Brook Health Sciences Center. Normally, this tissue is shed each month during menstruation. It flows out through the cervix, into the vagina and out of the body.

In almost all women, small amounts of endometrial tissue are also pushed out through the fallopian tubes and into the abdomen, Dr. Barbieri says. This tissue generally doesn't cause problems—it's destroyed by the body's immune system.

In women who develop endometriosis, though, the stray endometrial tissue is not destroyed by the immune system. (In fact, some studies show immune system abnormalities in women with endometriosis.) Instead, the tissue proliferates and thickens, responding to the female hormone estrogen the same way it does within the uterus. Doctors don't fully understand the interplay between the tissue, the immune system and estrogen, but they do know the consequences. The tissue attaches to organs such as the ovaries, colon and bladder and can actually infiltrate the tissue of these organs, causing painful, constricting scar tissue and hindering these organs' ability to function properly. "This tissue seems to be able to drift anywhere," Dr. Nezhat says.

Serious cases of endometriosis may require removal of sections of the bowel or bladder. In severe cases, hysterectomy (removal of the uterus) may be a possible, if controversial, solution. (See "Is a Hysterectomy for You?" on page 170.) And if stray endometrial tissue blocks the fallopian tubes, preventing the egg and sperm from uniting, pregnancy may be impossible.

Unfortunately, endometriosis, no matter how painful, usually catches a woman by surprise. "Women are conditioned to expect problems with their menstrual cycles," Nezhat says. "They may ignore the early symptoms of endometriosis or, if they've never had normal periods, think the amount of pain they have is normal.

"They simply adjust to more and more pain and problems by taking painkillers or limiting activities, including sex, to the days when they feel better," he says. "Then they suddenly realize they are losing ten days a month to incapacitating pain or that they are having only one good week a month." That's usually when they see a doctor.

REDUCING THE RISK

Your risk of developing endometriosis is above average if your mother or a sister has the condition, if your menstrual flow is heavy or longer than normal (five days is average) or if your cycle is shorter than normal (28 days is average). Some doctors feel that your risk also grows the longer you put off motherhood, giving endometriosis its reputation as a career woman's disease.

If you're at risk, you can help reduce your odds of getting endometriosis by following this self-help advice.

Get regular exercise. Harvard researchers have found that regular aerobic exercise, started early in life, may lower women's risk of developing endometriosis. In one study, women who exercised more than 7 hours a week reduced their chances of developing endometriosis by 80 percent compared with women who did not exercise. If you started exercising later in life, or if you exercise only in moderation, you may not get the same high level of protection. But certainly the added activity will do you no harm, says Dr. Barbieri.

Stay hard and lean. "Leanness—a higher muscle to body fat ratio—means reduced blood levels of estrogen, which may reduce your risk of developing endometriosis," Dr. Barbieri says. (Estrogen is stored in fat, and estrogen makes endometrial tissue grow.) Exercise, along with a low-fat diet, builds muscle and burns fat.

Avoid using an IUD. The use of intrauterine devices (IUDs) is definitely related to heavier-than-normal menstrual flow, which is a risk factor

---

IS A HYSTERECTOMY FOR YOU?

All things being equal, you'd just as soon keep your uterus and ovaries. But you're anxious to get rid of your endometriosis, and you've heard that hysterectomy is one possible way to accomplish that. Is it? And if so, is this a trade-off worth considering?

Most women with endometriosis should consider a hysterectomy only as a last resort, most doctors agree. "If you are diagnosed early and get appropriate treatment, your condition should never deteriorate to the point where you would consider a hysterectomy," says Camran Nezhat, M.D., professor of clinical obstetrics and gynecology at Mercer University in Macon, Georgia, director of the Fertility and Endoscopy Center in Atlanta and advisor to the Endometriosis Association.

The medical community reports a 95 percent cure rate of endometriosis with a total hysterectomy, which involves removal of the uterus, ovaries and fallopian tubes, says Dr. Nezhat. But in one recent study, women who'd had a total hysterectomy as a treatment for endometriosis reported much lower cure rates.

The study, done by Karen Lamb, R.N., Ph.D., director of the Endometriosis Association Research Registry, looked at 189 women who'd had a total hysterectomy for the treatment of endometriosis. Of that group, 56.3 percent reported that surgery had offered relief or a cure, while 13.1 percent said they "didn't know yet" or thought it was "too early to tell." And about one-third (30.6 percent) reported

---

for endometriosis. Some researchers think IUD use may be associated with an increased risk for endometriosis.

EASE THE PAIN

Like diabetes or arthritis, endometriosis is considered a chronic condition. That means it cannot be cured or completely eliminated, even though its symptoms can usually be controlled.

"If it's diagnosed and treated properly early on—at the first realization that something's not right—almost every woman has a better chance of controlling it than when it's diagnosed later in the course of the disease," Dr. Nezhat says. While menopause or a hysterectomy may improve symptoms for most women, neither will completely eliminate the disease in women with endometriosis that has infiltrated the bladder or bowel, he says.

hysterectomy had offered neither relief nor cure. They still had pain.

One possible reason for the lower cure rate: Many of the women in the study had endometrial tissue that had infiltrated their bladder or bowel, which was not removed during the surgery, and that continued to affect the functioning of these organs even without estrogen-producing ovaries. "That's one reason why leading doctors in this field are now doing bowel and, less frequently, bladder resections where appropriate for endometriosis," Dr. Nezhat says. "Even if you have a total hysterectomy, you will continue to have trouble if not all of the disease is removed."

He suggests you find a doctor who can do bladder and bowel surgery, if necessary, along with (or instead of) a hysterectomy. (This could include a general surgeon, urologist, gastroenterologist, gynecological surgeon or colon-rectal surgeon.) Get at least two expert opinions before you make this big decision.

And be aware that hormone replacement therapy (often given after a hysterectomy) may trigger a recurrence of endometriosis, although just how likely this is to happen is uncertain. "Our own study looked at that, and the findings regarding the use of estrogen replacement and continuing symptoms were very unclear," Dr. Nezhat says. "It's possible that the rate of recurrence could depend on how much of the disease is left behind, whether parts of an ovary remain, even the kind of estrogen that is used in replacement therapy. We just don't know."

Home remedies can be appropriate to treat the pain of mild or moderate endometriosis, Dr. Nezhat says. "They won't stop the course of the disease, but they may relieve symptoms well enough to suit some women and may be used along with other treatments," he says. So you may want to try these simple pain tamers.

Take aspirin or ibuprofen. Both are antiprostaglandins, says Dr. Nezhat. These drugs block the chemicals that contribute to cramping and pain. Take as needed, not exceeding the recommended dosages on the label.

Use a heating pad. Placed on your belly or back, a heating pad or hot water bottle may help relax cramped muscles and improve blood flow, reducing pain, says Dr. Nezhat.

Opt for ice. For some women, ice relieves pain better than heat. (It reduces tissue swelling.) Place an ice pack or a plastic bag of crushed ice wrapped in a washcloth on your lower abdomen.

TREATMENT TO THE RESCUE

Home remedies can help comfort you to a point. Beyond that, you'll need your doctor's help. "The progress and symptoms of endometriosis can usually be controlled with a careful balance of surgery and drugs," Dr. Nezhat says.

These days, most surgery for endometriosis is done with a viewing tube inserted into a small slit near the belly button and a laser beam or electrothermal instrument inserted through a second slit near the pubic hairline. Using this procedure, called laparoscopic surgery, or laparoscopy, a surgeon can remove most of the stray tissue growing in the abdomen. The procedure is done on an outpatient basis, requires general anesthesia and can take up to 4 hours if extensive tissue needs to be removed, Dr. Nezhat says.

Because endometrial tissue can continue to migrate outside the uterus, and because surgery seldoms gets every single bit of tissue, the procedure may need to be repeated. "Laparoscopic surgery can be performed as often as a women needs it to control her symptoms," Dr. Nezhat says. Although some women may need to have this procedure done only once, it may be done three, four or more times during the course of a woman's illness. The illness may last from the time she is diagnosed with endometriosis (average age of diagnosis: mid-twenties) until menopause. After menopause, symptoms abate for most women as estrogen levels drop off.

After surgery, there is no standard procedure for treatment. "It depends on a woman's needs," Dr. Nezhat says.

Some doctors recommend the long-term use of low-estrogen, high-progestin birth control pills, unless a woman is trying to get pregnant. These pills are deliberately used to lighten or sometimes even stop periods and appear to help keep stray endometrial tissue from growing, Dr. Nezhat says. Of the drugs used for endometriosis, birth control pills have the mildest side effects, Dr. Nezhat says.

DRUGS THAT BLOCK ESTROGEN

Drugs that suppress the body's production of estrogen may also be used to control endometriosis. "Usually they are used to shrink large tissue deposits before surgery, but some doctors use them instead of surgery, or after surgery to help keep the disease at bay," Dr. Barbieri says.

Danazol (Danocrine) is a powerful drug similar to the hormone testosterone. It shrinks endometrial tissue very effectively, but because of its many serious side effects, including masculinizing effects such as voice deepening, it is seldom used these days, Dr. Nezhat says.

The two most commonly used drugs are derived from gonadotropin-releasing hormone, a naturally occurring brain hormone. They are called gonadotropin-releasing hormone agonists (GnRH-a for short). Nafarelin (Synarel) comes as a nasal spray. Leuprolide (Lupron) is given by injection once a month. Both decrease production of estrogen by the ovaries, and both have menopause-like side effects: hot flashes, vaginal dryness and decreased bone strength.

Based on their studies, the manufacturers of both of these drugs recommend the drugs be used only once during a lifetime—for no more than six months. But many doctors, including Dr. Nezhat and Dr. Barbieri, may put their patients on either of these drugs several times during the years-long course of treatment, with "rest periods" in between to allow for the regeneration of bone.

"For many questions about endometriosis, there are no answers with a capital *A*," Dr. Nezhat says. "There are lots of questions that still need to be addressed. That's why the best thing a woman can do is to become informed, find a knowledgeable doctor, weigh the risks and benefits and make her own decisions about what treatments are best for her."

EPILEPSY

I f you think you can recognize someone with epilepsy just by looking at him, think again.

"There are 2.5 million people in the United States with epilepsy, most of them leading normal lives like you and me, and you don't know it," says Robert J. Gumnit, M.D., professor of neurology and neurosurgery at the University of Minnesota Medical School and director of the Minnesota Comprehensive Epilepsy Program in Minneapolis. "You don't know that your next-door neighbor or your boss or your lawyer has epilepsy, because they don't talk about it. There are sports stars, movie stars and politicians who have epilepsy, and you'll never guess. But what impresses me the most is the woman who can raise a family and work a full-time job despite the fact that she has epilepsy."

Anyone can have epilepsy, and most can still lead a normal life—without the fear that their brain might "misfire" and send them into seizures.

SHORT CIRCUITS IN THE BRAIN

There are many forms of epilepsy, but all have the same cause: Something interferes with the ability of brain cells to communicate with each other through electrical signals. In epilepsy, the electrical charge in one group of cells builds up and suddenly discharges, overwhelming neighboring cells. This is a seizure. Depending upon how much of the brain they invade, seizures can range in intensity from a briefly jerking arm or leg to a blank state that unaware observers may think of as daydreaming to full convulsions. They can occur as seldom as once a year or as often as 100 times a day, and they can last as briefly as a second or as long as 5 minutes. It's likely that you'll have a seizure at some time in your life—one in ten people does—but there are only one or two chances in a hundred that you'll have more than one and be diagnosed as having epilepsy.

Epilepsy has no sexual preference—males and females are equally at risk. Children are more at risk for the milder seizures, which usually disappear by the late teens. Adults are more susceptible to the severe type, which lasts a lifetime.

There's much more to epilepsy than seizures. "There's been a stigma on epilepsy throughout Western history," Dr. Gumnit says. "Society doesn't tolerate a loss of control of behavior. Epilepsy causes social isolation, because people who have it often withdraw. They get frustrated, angry and alienated. That's the so-called epileptic personality, but it doesn't exist." That "personality" is something imposed by an uninformed and intolerant society.

The cause of epilepsy is a mystery in about half the cases. The other half have more than 100 possible causes: The 2 leading known causes in America are head injuries from automobile accidents (a good reason to wear your seat belt) and complications in a developing fetus. Other causes include lack of adequate blood supply to an infant's brain during birth, diseases like meningitis and encephalitis, brain tumors, thyroid problems, hypoglycemia, cerebral hemorrhage and inherited disorders. How epilepsy is treated depends on the kind of seizure, and that's where diagnosis comes in.

TROUBLESHOOTING
THE SHORT CIRCUIT

The milder forms of epilepsy can be very difficult to diagnose, says Ilo Leppik, M.D., clinical professor of neurology and pharmacy at the University of Minnesota Medical School and chairman of the Epilepsy Foundation of America's Professional Advisory Board. "People can have seizures for months without knowing it," Dr. Leppik says. "They don't have any recollection of them, so they don't know what happened unless someone else was around to tell them about it. Doctors often don't find out until mild seizures become major ones."

Once your doctor's involved, he'll most likely interview your family for insights into your seizures. He may induce a seizure in you through sleep deprivation while measuring your brain's electrical pattern through an electroencephalogram. That's how he finds out if you have epilepsy or if some other condition is causing the seizures, says Dr. Leppik.

If the diagnosis is true epilepsy, "the first problem is the patient understanding the diagnosis," Dr. Gumnit says. "They often hear only the word *epilepsy* and leave the office in shock. Then they'll come back in a week with thousands of questions."

LEE STARKEY: ATTITUDE IS EVERYTHING

Lee Starkey had his first epileptic seizure at age 18—but didn't know it. He thought his fainting spell was an allergic reaction to the flowers at a funeral.

That fall, after he went off to college at the University of Tennessee, Lee suffered three more seizures. His father took him to see a neurologist, who tested him and prescribed medication—without anyone telling Lee what it was for. It was seven years before Lee found out that he had epilepsy. Soon after he had quit taking the mystery medication, he had major convulsions in front of his students at a junior college. It was two more years before Lee's father tearfully confessed that he had hidden the truth to protect Lee from the "stigma" of epilepsy, Lee says. "I turned to him and asked, 'What stigma?'"

Lee has an entirely different attitude about epilepsy. "I don't try to hide it. I never have," he says. "I wanted to know everything about something that was going to so profoundly affect my life. I didn't want my life to go down the tubes because of something that I could handle. I was determined to find a way around it."

Find a way he has. He makes sure he sees doctors who are experienced in treating epilepsy. He's had a few problems with too little or too much medication in his system but has always gotten back on an even keel. He had to fight in court for his privilege to drive. Now a marketing representative, he has never had a problem finding work "because my positive attitude is more important than anything. I don't tell prospective employers about my epilepsy. It's controlled, so I don't have to." However, he admits, he sometimes enjoys telling his boss and co-workers after he's been on the job for a while—and learns they never had a clue.

In August 1990 at age 51, Lee had his first seizure in five years. Appropriately enough, it was the exhausting rigor of buying a new car that triggered it. His doctor discovered that Lee needed higher blood levels of medication. And he needed to eat right and get enough rest.

Lee also works with the Epilepsy Foundation of America's Training and Placement Service (TAPS), speaking at job fairs, seminars and workshops for job hunters and employers. His job, he says, is to prove that people with epilepsy can do their work as well as anyone else.

That's good. Go ahead and ask thousands of questions. You need to know everything you can find out about your epilepsy. If your doctor can't answer them, get another doctor. You and your doctor should accept nothing less than total control of your seizures without side effects, allowing you to return to the mainstream of society, Dr. Gumnit says. "This is possible for the great majority of epilepsy patients," he says. And total control is the only option, because even one seizure a year raises fear of another, leading to anxiety and interference with work and driving and socializing. "Everything gets put on hold or distorted by the fear you'll have another seizure," he says.

FINDING THE RIGHT DOCTOR

One of the main problems in treating epilepsy is the attitude and knowledge of doctors, Dr. Gumnit says. "Patients often say that their doctors don't listen, don't spend time with them, don't try to solve their problems. They just renew the prescriptions and say, 'Come back in three months,' " he says.

Much of the problem stems from inadequate medical training, says Dr. Gumnit. Some doctors learn to approach epilepsy negatively and, as a result, get frustrated. And if your doctor is frustrated, think how *you'll* feel. Your doctor's attitude and ability have a dramatic impact on the treatment you get.

"I try to put a human face on epilepsy," Dr. Gumnit says. "You need to find a doctor who understands the special needs of epilepsy and who is comfortable dealing with it."

How do you know if your doctor is treating you right? "You should expect control over your epilepsy within three months," he says. "If that doesn't happen, your doctor should refer you to a neurologist. If your epilepsy still isn't controlled after nine more months, then you need to see a specialist in epilepsy."

There are only a few such specialists in America, and one can be found through epilepsy organizations or university hospitals. But take heart, Dr. Gumnit says: The chances your epilepsy can be well controlled are eight in ten. Maybe 10 percent of the cases will be partially controlled, and surgery can help the other 10 percent.

PLANNING YOUR TREATMENT

Your doctor's job is to create a good treatment plan and stick to it, Dr. Gumnit says: "It's more than drug prescriptions." Beyond diagnosis and drugs, it involves psychological and social support. A conference is a good place to start, calling in the family to discuss the plan with you, your doctor, your psychologist, your social worker and maybe a neurologist. "Everyone needs to understand what is going on," says Dr. Gumnit.

Medication will be the first line of defense, and it has to be tailored to *you,* not to everyone with epilepsy. Which drug you take depends not only on your type of seizure but on your age, lifestyle, whether and how much you drink, other medications you may be taking and how much physical activity you like. There are about 18 medications now available.

Carbamazepine and phenytoin are the first choice, Dr. Leppik says. Other popular drugs are valproate and clonazepam.

All of these drugs can have side effects, so you need to have your blood levels tested regularly. The higher the blood level, the more likely side effects will crop up. "Side effects can be the most difficult part of treatment to manage," Dr. Leppik says. "If the doctor decides you have a low likelihood of seizure, you can probably get by with low blood levels of medication."

The most common side effects are slow thinking, difficulty concentrating, memory loss, sedation and vertigo. "All of these are dose related and can be corrected by lowering the dose," he says. "These drugs are very safe for long-term use."

YOUR PART IN THE PLAN

Yet half of epilepsy patients don't take their medications properly, Dr. Leppik says. It's called noncompliance, and that's the number one reason for a drug not working. A large part of the success of your treatment depends on your doctor, but an equally large part depends on you. After all, you can have the best doctor in the world, but *you're* the one with epilepsy.

Side effects are a main reason you may not take the drug that could be helping you. But you also have to be careful about your thinking. "Some people use illogical thinking," Dr. Leppik says. "They tell themselves 'If I don't take the medication, I don't have the disease.' Others take the medication for a year or so, the seizures stop, and they start thinking 'I don't really need this medicine.'" So they stop taking the drug—often with disastrous results, like a seizure while driving.

Or you may forget to take the drug. Maybe you can't afford to buy it. Maybe you're abusing alcohol or other drugs. "The doctor and patient have to work together to find out the reasons for noncompliance," Dr. Leppik says.

With the proper treatment, you can lead a normal life, and no one needs to know you have epilepsy, says Dr. Leppik. But drugs are key. If you're having a hard time sticking with your treatment plan, talk about it with your doctor. And consider contacting the nearest chapter of the Epilepsy Foundation of America. It can lead you to support groups that can bolster your resolve to control your epilepsy instead of letting it control you.

EYE INFECTIONS

W hose eyes are those, staring back at you in the bathroom mirror this morning? That runny stuff is seeping out and crusting in the corners and along your red-rimmed lids. Once you've un-glued your lids, you see red veins snaking across the whites like highways in a road atlas. Those eyes itch and burn, they're not seeing straight, and for a second, you wonder if you have multiple personalities and one of them is an all-night party animal.

These symptoms are typical of garden-variety eye infections whose names end with -itis, signifying "inflammation": conjunctivitis, blepharitis and keratitis. These can be pesky infections, but simple medical treatment and sometimes self-help can get you through the worst.

CONJUNCTIVITIS

The conjunctiva of your eye is the thin membrane that lines your eyelids and covers the surface of the eyeball. When it gets inflamed, you have conjunctivitis, among the most common eye disorders in America. And the most common form, pinkeye, is usually caused by very common bac-teria, says Gilbert Smolin, M.D., clinical professor of ophthalmology at the University of California, San Francisco, and research ophthalmologist at the Proctor Foundation, which specializes in external and infectious eye diseases. These bacteria—streptococcus, staphylococcus and hemo-philus—are spread like the common cold: coughing, hand-to-eye contact, using the same towels and doorknobs. "It's so contagious that in poorer countries without access to antibiotics, entire villages can be hit by con-junctivitis," Dr. Smolin says.

Irritants are the second most common origin of conjunctivitis, Dr. Smolin says. Pollutants are the most common irritants, expecially in smog-bound cities like Los Angeles and Denver. "If you're exposed to smog all the time, it can be a common cause of conjunctivitis," he says.

Whatever the cause, the symptoms of conjuctivitis are pretty much the same—a discharge that ranges from watery tears to mucus to pus, which is yellow to green in color, Dr. Smolin says. Your eyes may be red, scratchy and irritated. Conjunctivitis is not often dangerous, Dr. Smolin says, "but sometimes it's caused by an aggressive microorganism that, if untreated, can lead to serious changes in the eye or spread and cause bronchitis and even pneumonia." This is because the eyes drain into the nasal passages in the back of the throat. For this reason, it's always best to see your doctor.

GETTING THE RED OUT

Your doctor will probably prescribe antibiotic eyedrops if your conjunctivitis is due to microorganisms. You'll be putting in the drops four to eight times a day. And he'll probably also tell you to apply warm compresses several times a day. "Your eyes should slowly improve over several days to a week," Dr. Smolin says.

Soothe the soreness. Before you see your doctor, you can apply warm compresses to the sore eye. "The warm compress dilates the blood vessels," says Dr. Smolin. "This brings the white blood cells to the area to help kill off the infection. They won't cure it, but they're very soothing." The compresses also clear away the discharge and its crusty buildup.

For relief from allergic conjunctivitis or conjunctivitis due to irritants, Dr. Smolin suggests, try cold compresses and an over-the-counter antihistamine. Or you can use artificial tear drops, also available over the counter at your drugstore. You can suspect you have a case of allergic conjunctivitis if your eyes are very itchy; irritant-related conjuctivitis, if you're surrounded by smog.

STOPPING THE SPREAD

The kind of conjunctivitis caused by bacteria or by viruses may be highly contagious, so make sure you take steps to prevent its spread.

- If your child has infectious conjunctivitis, keep him home from school.
- Don't share towels, washcloths or pillowcases.
- Wash your hands frequently, especially after you touch your eyes.
- Don't irrigate the eye if you suspect an infection—it may only spread the disease.

BLEPHARITIS

This inflammation of the eyelids has two main causes: a skin condition like eczema or dandruff, or a staph infection. "Most people with blepharitis also have dandruff," Dr. Smolin says. In fact, many people have both types, and they have it chronically. "It can go on for years and usually gets worse with age," he says. And blepharitis is very common, he adds: "Up to 50 percent of all people have it."

The symptoms include crusting of the lids, "especially worse in the morning, like sleep in your eyes," Dr. Smolin says. "There's also a scratchy and burning sensation, and your eyes get red easily." Your lashes will be littered with dandrufflike flakes and bits of dried pus. And your eyelids will have a constant pinkish color, a condition undiplomatically called rabbit eyes.

Blepharitis can make a mess of your eyelashes. The infectious type can start in the oil glands of the lids and spread to the follicle of the lash, Dr. Smolin explains. "In fact, if it's chronic, you can lose some or all of your lashes, or the lashes will grow out smaller and maybe even turn white." One of the complications of blepharitis can be a sty—the infected oil gland gets plugged up and develops into a boil.

Very often, the symptoms of blepharitis are so minimal and so chronic that people just live with it, Dr. Smolin says. It's not usually dangerous. The staph bacteria that cause the infectious type are few in number, "far down in the eyelid, just smoldering along for years," he says, and so blepharitis "is not contagious unless it's very severe." If your blepharitis is the infectious type, it may occasionally worsen, and then your eye doctor can prescribe an antibiotic ointment.

REACHING A TRUCE

"Blepharitis is usually very hard to cure, and so what you end up doing is establishing some kind of equilibrium with it. You have to understand that you'll have to treat yourself for years," says Dr. Smolin.

Shampoo your eyelids. With a persistent enemy like blepharitis, a strong offense is the best defense. One of your best strategies is to shampoo your eyelids, which keeps the oil and flakes under control. "Put a little of Johnson's No More Tears Baby Shampoo on a washcloth, mix it with water to make it foamy, close your eyes, and scrub your eyelids," Dr. Smolin advises. "After you scrub real well, keep your eyelids closed for a couple of minutes, and then wash them off." If you're shampooing daily for dandruff, go ahead and shampoo your eyelids daily, too. Or you may be able to get by with a weekly eyelid scrubbing.

Compress and soften. Another extremely helpful weapon is the warm compress, Dr. Smolin says. Apply the compress for 5 to 10 minutes to loosen the crust on your lashes. Then use a cotton swab to clean off the softened crust.

The compress is also the cure for a sty. Apply the compress for an hour a day. The warmth should bring the sty to a head, which then will spontaneously drain.

KERATITIS

A clear, dome-shaped film over your iris and pupil, the cornea is sometimes called the window of the eye. It's your eye's leading edge—where your contact lens rests—and because it sits right out front, it's also subject to injury and infection. Injury and infection cause inflammation, and when the cornea is involved, it's called keratitis.

There are a great many causes of keratitis, Dr. Smolin says. "You can get keratitis if you scratch your eye or from a toxic reaction to irritants in the air—like from someone painting nearby, or from spraying yourself in the eye with hair spray." But infectious keratitis is the most dangerous, because it can scar the cornea and lead to loss of vision.

Each different cause has a different treatment, but no matter what form of keratitis you have, the symptoms will be more or less the same: eye pain, scratchiness, redness, decreased vision, a watery discharge and sensitivity to light.

SIMPLE CAUSE, SIMPLE SOLUTION

No one knows how many people get keratitis each year, because so many cases are so mild that people don't see their doctors, Dr. Smolin says. "They just wait it out," he says. "If your vision is affected, you should see a doctor. But if it isn't, and you know the cause—like dust or sand or hair spray or a little Windex—you can care for it yourself."

Water and rest is best. One good way to care for your eye is to wash it out well with an eyecup, or just slosh saline solution or plain tap water into your eye. Then rest the eye, wearing dark glasses if it helps. "Wait 24 hours," Dr. Smolin advises, "and if it still hurts and looks bad, see a doctor." And you should also see a doctor immediately if you have a chemical burn or a particle embedded in your cornea.

HERPES IN YOUR EYE

At 500,000 cases per year, keratitis caused by the herpes simplex virus is probably the most common form of infectious keratitis, Dr. Smolin says. It's also one of the most potentially dangerous. "If you have one attack, you have a 30 percent risk of having a second," Dr. Smolin says. "If you have a second attack, your risk of a third goes up to 55 percent, and if you have a third, there's a 90 percent chance you'll have a fourth."

If the attacks remain on the surface of the cornea, they're not too serious, he says. But each succeeding attack increases the chance of the virus digging itself deeper into the cornea. The result can be a scarring of the cornea, a partial loss of vision and, eventually, maybe the need for a corneal transplant. "And even after the transplant, you can still get another infection," Dr. Smolin says.

Herpes simplex is the same virus that causes cold sores. "The virus has to be transmitted to your eye, and the eye has to be susceptible," he says. "I often see babies with keratitis brought in by mothers who have cold sores on their lips," Dr. Smolin says. Touching your cold sore with your hand and then rubbing your eye is another easy way to give yourself keratitis. "Once you have it, it's easy to reinfect yourself," he says. "The virus hides out and waits for the right time." If you're under stress or have a fever or a sunburn—all of which lower your immunity—the virus is likely to strike.

Keratitis caused by the herpes simplex virus should clear up without treatment in about two weeks, much like a cold sore, says Dr. Smolin. But your eye is much more delicate and more valuable than your lip, so the condition warrants a doctor's attention. But how do you know if your keratitis is herpes infected? "If you've had a previous attack, you probably will recognize the next one," he says.

The standard medical treatment is debridement—when the doctor first numbs the eye and then literally rubs off the virus with a cotton swab. You also will probably be given antiviral eyedrops, like Viroptic. This treatment usually clears up the infection within a week, he says.

THE CONTACTS THAT ATE YOUR CORNEA

Number two in the infectious keratitis race, and gaining fast, is pseudomonas bacteria. "It's now far and away the most common bacterial cause in America because of contact lens wear," Dr. Smolin says. "It's not very fastidious—it can grow in anything moist and does very well in contact lens cases. And people who wear the extended-wear lenses have a ten times higher risk than daily lens wearers."

The infections usually start off slowly without severe symptoms, Dr. Smolin says. "But the organism grows at a tremendously rapid rate," he says. "In severe infections, we've seen patients come in holding their hands under their eyes to catch the pus. Pseudomonas is particularly virulent—it can even cause loss of the eye—but it's not very contagious."

The treatment is "a very high dose of antibiotic drops as soon as possible," Dr. Smolin says. The keratitis generally clears up in a few days, but severe cases can take weeks.

Keratitis caused by pseudomonas is highly preventable. All it requires is good hygiene when it comes to caring for your contact lenses.

Handle with care. "You have to change your contact lens storage solutions frequently, sterilize your lenses appropriately, handle your lenses carefully and wear them intelligently," Dr. Smolin says. Always wash your hands before you handle your lenses. If your eye is already irritated for some reason, don't put in your lens.

"Some of the lens cases I've seen have been extraordinarily filthy," Dr. Smolin says. "You can see the dirt in them, and I've been able to culture pseudomonas growing right in the case." When you're cleaning your lenses, it's a good idea to clean the case, too, and then let it dry out—that will kill any organisms lurking inside, he says.

And since the extended-wear lenses lend themselves to even more abuse, "I never recommend them for cosmetic purposes," Dr. Smolin says. "Even the throwaways have the same problems."

If you follow these simple steps, it's not likely your pseudomonas keratitis will come back. If it does, it's very likely you didn't learn from your first experience.

WHEN IT'S SIMPLY STAPH

Everybody has staphylococcus bacteria just about everywhere on their body. Usually we just coexist with it, but sometimes when it gets into a wound or an irritation, it can cause an infection. Even the infections are generally mild, because your body's immune system has staph's number and does a pretty good job of stomping it out.

When the infection is in your lids, the inflammation causes keratitis. Staph causes the most common form of noninfectious keratitis, and it is also the least dangerous by far, Dr. Smolin says. Your doctor may give you cortisone eyedrops for the inflammation and antibiotic ointment for the staph. It should clear up within two weeks.

FATIGUE

Your spouse says it's all in your head. You say it's in your head, your neck, your arms, your legs. You're tired down to your toes, and you're tired all the time. Your doctor says it's not chronic fatigue syndrome, anemia, anxiety disorder or any other of the usual instigators of fatigue. So what *is* causing you to feel like you're walking underwater, 5 miles down?

There are many things—a lack of exercise, poor sleep, too much boredom—that can cause long-term fatigue. There are also many diseases and medical conditions that can cause chronic tiredness. For this reason alone, fatigue is a symptom that should not be ignored. But for ordinary, run-of-the-mill fatigue—burning the candle at both ends, so to speak—there are also many things you can try to get your engine started again.

MOVING AND SHAKING

You sit behind a desk all day. You go to bed at 9:00 P.M. You never overexert yourself. Yet you're always tired. How can that be?

Experts agree that not being active can make you feel lethargic and fatigued. "It's common sense," says D. W. Edington, Ph.D., director of the Fitness Research Center at the University of Michigan. "The body at rest tends to remain at rest."

Regular exercise, on the other hand, can make you *more* energetic—not only in the long run but on the spot. What's more, the benefits can last for hours, says Robert Thayer, Ph.D., a California State University psychology professor.

If you've been inactive up until now, consult your doctor before jumping into any exercise program.

Ease into it. The "no pain, no gain" theory has no place with beginners, particularly those already pained by fatigue. If you are experiencing pain—either while exercising or the day after—you're probably pushing yourself too hard. Take your exercise program slowly and advance gradually, says Dr. Thayer.

Choose the right workout. Keep in mind that vigorous exercise can initially wear you out. After a 30-minute aerobics session, for example, you may feel fatigued—the energy-enhancing effects will come an hour later. But a less intensive workout—a brisk walk, for example—can boost your energy sooner.

Make a date. To help you stick to your exercise program, set aside 30 minutes several times a week. How hard should you push yourself? As a guide, try the "talk test." If you can't talk comfortably while you're working out, you're probably working too hard. Of course, if you experience chest pains or dizziness, it's time to get off the track and into your doctor's office.

Beware the midnight oil. Some people can exercise at any hour and still get plenty of sleep. For others, late-night workouts turn into all-night insomnia. So avoid vigorous exercise before bedtime, doctors say.

RUDE AWAKENINGS

You're early to bed, early to rise—and still you're exhausted all the time. Could it be . . . your breathing?

An often undetected cause of fatigue is called obstructive sleep apnea. Most common among middle-aged men, obstructive apnea occurs when breathing is blocked by "collapse" of throat tissues during sleep. This causes breathing to stop for 20 to 40 seconds at a time. Each episode is accompanied by a brief awakening. Multiply this by hundreds of times a night, and you can see why some people with apnea feel so tired all the time.

Besides causing fatigue, obstructive sleep apnea often causes loud snoring as well. So even though *you* may not realize something is wrong, your spouse most certainly will!

If you suspect you have sleep apnea, see your doctor. He may refer you to a specialist in sleep disorders, who may recommend drugs or surgery to correct the problem. However, there are things you can do yourself that may help.

Cut the fat. Doctors agree that losing weight can often reverse obstructive sleep apnea. If you're overweight, extra tissue in the neck and throat, combined with poor muscle tone, can restrict the movement of air through the upper airway.

Ban the booze. Since alcohol works as a depressant on the central nervous system, it increases muscle relaxation and enhances airway blockage. Skipping alcohol can reduce the severity of obstructive apnea. It can also improve the overall quality of your sleep, thus boosting the next day's energy levels.

TOSSING AND TURNING

About 8 percent of Americans—and at least 15 percent of those over 50—experience what doctors call periodic leg movements, or nocturnal myoclonus. These nighttime leg movements can mean anything from a toe flex to a full-fledged kick sure to catch a bed partner's attention!

Sleep disorder experts aren't sure what causes these involuntary movements. Some suspect lower back injuries, while others suspect central nervous system problems. What they do know is that these movements, which can occur hundreds of times a night, may cause fatigue.

If you suspect your legs are doing laps while the rest of you is sound asleep, see your doctor. Periodic leg movements can't always be eliminated, but taking medication can help reduce the number of awakenings during the night, thus reducing fatigue.

(For more on what may be troubling you through the night, see "Sleep Disorders" on page 462.)

NOT ENOUGH STRESS!

Sure, you know stress can make you feel fatigued. But did you know that a *lack* of stress—*excitement* might be a better word—can also make you feel fatigued?

Some researchers suggest there's a delicate balance between boredom and burnout. As excitement level increases, so does performance—but only to a point, they add. If you're stressed too much, performance dips.

"It's sort of like the tension on a violin string," explains Paul J. Rosch, M.D., president of the American Institute of Stress. "If you have too much tension, the string is going to break. If you don't have enough tension, it's not going to make any music."

So how do you get yourself into tune?

Restress. "You have to find out what works for you," says Dr. Rosch. "Some people leave everything to the last minute, so they can get that little surge of adrenaline."

If dashing to the airport minutes before takeoff isn't your style, however, there are other ways to create a helpful edge. For example:

Get involved. A lack of creative engagement can be more taxing than doing too much, says Dennis T. Jaffe, Ph.D., author of *Take This Job and Love It*. Try getting involved in more things, he suggests. Brush up on your Shakespeare. Give a speech at Toastmasters. Take up swimming or tennis.

Help someone else. "I used to write prescriptions for becoming a volunteer," says John Renner, M.D., president of the Consumer Health Information Research Institute in Kansas City, Missouri. "I recommend that you get into something where you are needed. Work with children, work with senior citizens, work with an agency that needs your help." Getting interested in others' lives, he says, can add oomph to your own.

BREATHE AWAY FATIGUE

Some people feel fatigued simply because they breathe wrong. In fact, doctors have suggested that many of their fatigued patients may have a condition called hyperventilation syndrome—a disorder caused by improper breathing.

People with this syndrome hyperventilate—that is, they breathe shallowly and rapidly. This causes an excessive loss of carbon dioxide, making the blood less able to carry oxygen throughout the body. So even though they're breathing quickly, they're really getting less air. Hyperventilation syndrome can cause anxiety and tingling, coldness or numbness in the fingers as well as fatigue.

While hyperventilation syndrome can be caused by many medical problems—these include anemia, diabetes and heart and kidney disease—it can also be caused by stress. It can even be caused by good posture. That's right—good posture. According to Robert Fried, Ph.D., director of the Institute for Rational Emotive Therapy in New York City and author of *The Breath Connection,* people who keep their stomach firmly tucked in when they stand up straight may be tensing the diaphragm muscles, making it difficult to take in a full breath.

Do you have hyperventilation syndrome? Put one hand on your chest and the other on your abdomen. If your hands don't rise with each breath, you may be hyperventilating.

Most people can "relearn" proper breathing techniques, says Dr. Fried. One way is simply to keep your mouth closed. When you breathe through the nose, it's virtually impossible to hyperventilate—the nasal passages are too narrow. Also, relax that tummy! These two simple steps may help you breathe a little easier—and, perhaps, recoup some of your lost energy as well.

CUT THE CALORIES

When you aren't eating well—you're dieting, perhaps, or simply too rushed to eat correctly—fatigue can hit you hard. And why not? You're not taking in enough calories to sustain your body's normal functions.

"The body starts to live off itself," says Manfred Kroger, Ph.D., professor of food science at Pennsylvania State University. "This whole process is abnormal and very stressful to the body, and one of the many symptoms of this type of stress is fatigue."

To lose weight without losing energy:

Forgo the fat. Calories from fat are more easily turned into body fat than those from proteins or carbohydrates. Plus, fats contain more calories per gram of food. So replacing fatty foods with high-carbohydrate foods like fruits, vegetables, grains and pasta can give you an edge in losing weight—without reducing energy.

Lose in moderation. It's reasonable to lose 1 or 2 pounds a week. Any more than that is getting risky. Drastic weight loss, doctors say, only increases your chances for feeling fatigued.

FIBROCYSTIC BREASTS

andra Tudor remembers with perfect clarity the shower she took more than ten years ago. That's when she found the lump in her left breast. "Naturally, I panicked," remembers Sandra, a jewelry designer who lives in Albuquerque, New Mexico. "I was absolutely positive that at the age of 34, I had breast cancer."

Actually, she didn't. What she does have are fibrocystic breasts. Lumps, in other words.

Finding a lump can be a terrifying experience. But fibrocystic breasts, as Sandra soon learned, are not *diseased* breasts. As James E. DeVitt, M.D., wrote in the *Canadian Medical Association Journal,* it "is inhumane . . . to label breasts as diseased when they are only showing expected physiologic variations." In other words, "lumpy" breasts are normal.

THE DISEASE THAT ISN'T

During a woman's childbearing years, it's very likely that she will develop numerous harmless lumps in one or both breasts, a condition often called fibrocystic breasts, one form of benign breast disease. The lumps typically occur in clumps, so your breasts may feel as though there are bunches of peas (or grapes) just under the surface. Sometimes, as in Sandra's case, it can feel like one lump.

Doctors aren't sure what causes fibrocystic breasts, but the condition probably is related to fluctuations of the hormones estrogen and proges-terone during a woman's menstrual cycle. In fact, when women stop men-struating after menopause, the lumps may disappear. Fibrocystic lumps are not dangerous, but they can become quite sore as your period ap-proaches. They may hurt at other times as well.

"The large majority of women have some pain in their breasts before their period starts," says David P. Rose, M.D., Ph.D., chief of the Division of Nutrition and Endocrinology at the Naylor Dana Institute in Valhalla, New York. "It is such a common finding that it really can't be considered a disease."

To understand just how common fibrocystic breasts are, consider this: If ten of your friends had a careful breast exam, at least five might have *detectable* fibrocystic lumps. The others might have fibrocystic lumps too small to be felt. If a doctor proceeded to inspect their breast tissue under a microscope, he might very well find fibrocystic changes in at least nine cases.

This doesn't mean you can ignore any new lump that appears in your breast, Dr. Rose stresses. Statistically, it probably isn't cancer, but you need a medical examination and occasionally a biopsy to be sure.

GETTING THE LUMPS OUT

A diagnosis of fibrocystic breasts doesn't necessarily mean you have to live with pain each month. For starters:

Cut the caffeine. Some researchers suggest that caffeine not only gives you a morning jump-start but also can stimulate changes in your breasts. In one study, for example, 113 women with fibrocystic breasts were asked to forgo their morning brew. After one year, nearly two out of three said they had less breast pain than before.

However, quite a few doctors aren't convinced that coffee makes a difference, Dr. Rose says. "The large studies would suggest that there isn't a relationship between caffeine and fibrocystic breasts. Yet we all know of patients who swear they had trouble with breast pain until they cut out caffeine—which to me is a good reason for trying it," he says.

Forgo the fat, fill up on fiber. Women with high levels of the hormone estrogen may be at risk for developing fibrocystic breasts, Dr. Rose says. "You can reduce the circulating levels of estrogen by going on a low-fat, high-fiber diet," he says.

Vitamin E for aches. Several studies have suggested that daily doses of vitamin E may reduce both the pain of fibrocystic breasts and the size of the lumps. As with caffeine, however, some doctors aren't convinced that it really works. If you decide to give vitamin E a try, ask your doctor to recommend a safe dose—400 international units (IU) a day or less. In large doses, vitamin E can be toxic.

Break in a new bra. Exercise bras, sometimes called jogging bras, can relieve tenderness by giving your breasts extra support during the last days of your menstrual cycle.

OTC relief. On particularly bad days, over-the-counter painkillers such as aspirin and ibuprofen can help.

Only rarely do women with fibrocystic breasts need ongoing medical attention, Dr. Rose says. But if your pain is more than you care to bear, medical intervention can help.

YOUR MEDICAL OPTIONS

The slightest disturbance in your body's delicate plexus of hormones can exacerbate the pain of fibrocystic breasts. There are several drugs your doctor may recommend to help correct your chemistry. For example, some oral contraceptives, and prescription drugs such as danazol and

---

LUMPS THAT AREN'T CANCER

Cancer of the breast kills more women than any other kind of cancer except lung cancer. That's why it's so important that you call your doctor *immediately* if you discover a lump. Fortunately, most lumps aren't cancer, even though you fear that yours is. In most cases, what you're feeling beneath the surface is benign breast disease—harmless lumps, says David P. Rose, M.D., Ph.D., of the Naylor Dana Institute. Sometimes your doctor will only perform an examination in making a diagnosis. Occasionally, a biopsy or mammogram will also be recommended. There are many types of noncancerous breast lumps.

CYSTS. These fluid-filled sacs usually get larger before your period, shrink when it's over and disappear after menopause. Some cysts are too small to feel; others can be a few inches across. If your doctor decides to withdraw fluid from a cyst, it will often collapse like a water balloon with the water let out.

FIBROADENOMAS. These round, rubbery lumps freely slide around inside the breast. Common in younger women, they often get larger during pregnancy and when you breast-feed. Even your doctor can mistake a fibroadenoma for a more dangerous tumor. Your doctor may remove it just to be on the safe side.

LIPOMAS. These small, soft, painless, slow-growing lumps are often found in older women. Consisting of fatty tissue, they slide freely in the breast. Lipomas often are removed or biopsied to check for cancer.

INTRADUCTAL PAPILLOMAS. Relatively rare, these small growths can appear in the lining of the ducts near the nipple and will occasionally cause bleeding. Such bleeding should never be ignored. As with lipomas and fibroadenomas, your doctor may remove them just to be sure they're harmless.

---

bromocriptine, can help relieve the pain of fibrocystic breasts by acting on your body's hormones. Unfortunately, these drugs can also cause side effects such as nausea, headaches and weight gain. "Without question, these drugs should be used only in the worst cases," Dr. Rose says.

Another option, which is used both to diagnose and to treat fibrocystic breasts, is fine-needle aspiration. This is a simple procedure in which a thin, hollow needle is guided through the skin and into the lump. The doctor then removes (aspirates) cells for inspection. In many cases, the lump will simply collapse and disappear during the procedure. If cancer cells are detected, then treatment can be started right away.

Of course, aspirating a harmless lump won't cure the underlying problem; additional lumps will invariably appear, doctors say. In fact, the lumps come and go even without medical treatment. Sandra says it has been happening to her. But now that she knows her lumps aren't cancer, she doesn't worry so much when new ones appear. Of course, she has an annual breast exam as recommended by the National Cancer Institute, just to make sure. "It's just one of those things you deal with," she says. "There are months when I have just a little breast tenderness, and months when I have a lot. But it's less painful than the cramps I usually get."

FIBROIDS

When Ellen was 35 and had recently moved to Sarasota, Florida, she noticed that her periods were gradually getting longer. She was bleeding more, too, sometimes soaking through a dozen tampons a day. "That was the summer I took up roots and started my new job, so I figured I was just stressed out," remembers Ellen, now 40. By the fall, however, she was feeling much calmer—yet the bleeding was still heavy. Finally she made an appointment to see her gynecologist.

"Is something . . . wrong?" Ellen nervously asked.

"What you have are fibroids," her doctor replied. "But don't worry. It's probably not a serious problem."

Also called leiomyomas, uterine fibroids are common tumors that affect as many as one in four women during their reproductive years, says Julia V. Johnson, M.D., an assistant professor of obstetrics and gynecology at the University of Vermont in Burlington. Composed of normal uterine musculature and fueled by the hormone estrogen, fibroids can be as small as a seed or as large as a melon. They grow inside or outside the uterus, sometimes attached by stalks, like mushrooms.

HARMLESS GROWTHS

For many women, fibroids never cause symptoms. In fact, smaller fibroids are often discovered "accidentally" during routine pelvic examinations. But those that grow to look more like melons than seeds can cause a host of problems. For example, some women notice they're getting bigger around the middle, even though they're not gaining weight. Some others have low backaches. "Probably the most common symptoms are pelvic pain and heavy bleeding during the period," Dr. Johnson says.

Fibroids may also worsen during pregnancy. In some circumstances, they can actually obstruct labor. Large fibroids sometimes degenerate or cause acute pain during pregnancy. Conversely, fibroids inside the uterus that distort the uterine cavity (called subserousal fibroids) may occasionally prohibit pregnancy from occurring.

If the word *tumor* makes you think of cancer—*relax.* Fewer than 1 in 200 uterine fibroids ever becomes cancerous. "In fact, it's unknown if fibroids actually turn into cancer or if there just happen to be cancers that coexist with the fibroids," says Dr. Johnson.

THE FAT FACTOR

Since fibroids depend on estrogen for their development and growth, in theory it may be possible to control them merely by watching your weight, says Richard J. Worley, M.D., an associate clinical professor of obstetrics and gynecology at the University of Colorado Health Science Center in Denver. This is because estrogen is produced not only by the ovaries but by fat tissue as well. "Obese women produce more estrogen in fat tissue than do slender women," explains Dr. Worley.

When researchers from Harvard Medical School studied the hospital records of 144 women who had surgery for fibroids, they found that 51 percent were obese. The researchers defined obese as 20 percent or more above ideal body weight. By contrast, only 25 percent of all American women are overweight.

Although doctors aren't yet certain that obesity stimulates fibroid growth, it does appear to be one risk factor that women can control, Dr. Worley says. "Given a genetic predisposition to fibroids, the ability of obesity to add to the estrogen in the system certainly could be a factor."

STRAIGHTFORWARD OPERATIONS

Many women with fibroids will never need treatment. "If the fibroids are relatively small and they're not producing any symptoms, then you may want to just follow them and see if they get worse," says Dr. Johnson. But if they are causing problems, "then removing them is going to be the way to go," he says.

Doctors in the past typically treated symptomatic fibroids by removing the entire uterus, an operation called hysterectomy. While hysterectomy still is the most definitive treatment for fibroids—once the uterus is removed, fibroids can't come back—it obviously won't do for women who still want to have children, Dr. Worley says.

Instead of hysterectomy, doctors often recommend myomectomy, an operation that removes the fibroids while leaving the uterus intact. This is often done by making an abdominal incision to expose the uterus, then opening the uterus to remove the fibroids. This procedure takes about 90 minutes, and women can usually return home within a few days, Dr. Worley says. A relatively new technique for removing fibroids from inside the uterus is even simpler. A surgeon can remove the fibroid by inserting a telescope-like instrument (hysteroscope) through the cervix and into the uterus. Women often return home the same day. "It's quite a straightforward and predictable operation," Dr. Worley says.

For all of the benefits, there is one problem with either kind of technique: The fibroids often come back. "The risk of recurrence can be as high as 30 percent," Dr. Johnson says. For a young woman, this could

PROFILE IN HEALING

JUDITH CALICA: FINALLY, A HEALTHY BABY BOY

When Judith Calica and her husband, Richard, decided to have a baby after nearly ten years of marriage, they didn't anticipate any problems. "I was among that first generation of women who believed you could have ultimate reproductive choice in terms of when, how many and at what intervals," says Judith, a clinical social worker and a board member of Resolve, a national information and support group for people with infertility.

At first her confidence seemed well founded. She conceived right away and started her pregnancy in the autumn of 1976. But then she started bleeding. "I bled for weeks, and one day before my tenth wedding anniversary, I miscarried," she remembers.

Without being sure what was wrong, her doctor suggested she try again. She did, and again she miscarried. This time her doctor was getting worried, more so since x-rays indicated that she had a large, *growing* mass inside her uterus. He admitted Judith to the hospital for exploratory surgery, during which he discovered and removed scar tissue, an encapsulated interstitial pregnancy (a failed pregnancy trapped inside the wall of the uterus) and a uterine fibroid. "He thought the fibroid may have accounted for the interstitial pregnancy by interfering with the egg's implantation," Judith says.

After the surgery, with her uterus cleared both of scarring and of fibroids, she was ready to try again. Again she readily got pregnant. But this time, instead of miscarrying, "I gave birth to a healthy, 6-pound 9-ounce son, and he's everyone's dream," Judith says. Today, her son is 13 years old.

mean having several operations before reaching menopause. But for older women already approaching menopause, the one operation will probably be all they need. (After menopause, estrogen-starved fibroids usually shrink on their own.)

THE DRUG ROUTE

A relatively new option for treating fibroids—at least in the short run—are drugs called gonadatropin-releasing hormone agonists, or GnRH-a. One such drug, leuprolide (Lupron), is currently approved by the Food and Drug Administration for shrinking cancers of the prostate gland in men. In women, it may shrink uterine fibroids.

Leuprolide works by shutting off estrogen production at the ovaries, thus "starving" fibroids of their needed fuel. In a study led by researchers at Harvard Medical School, 124 women with uterine fibroids were given either leuprolide or a placebo. After three months, the fibroids in women treated with leuprolide shrank by more than 25 percent, whereas they *increased* by 16 percent in women taking placebos. In addition, of the 38 women whose main symptom was heavy bleeding, 37 (97 percent) had normal periods after taking leuprolide.

While leuprolide is unquestionably effective, it has serious drawbacks, Dr. Johnson says. "What it basically does is produce a state similar to menopause, so any risks associated with menopause—hot flashes, night sweats, vaginal dryness and bone loss—could occur with leuprolide. Also, when you take people off it, the fibroids grow back within months to the size they were before."

However, researchers are investigating ways to make the most of leuprolide's fibroid-shrinking potential while limiting its side effects. One promising treatment involves combining leuprolide with hormone replacement therapy. In a small study performed at Boston's Brigham and Women's Hospital, five women with fibroids were given leuprolide for three months, then leuprolide plus estrogen and progesterone. After two years, their fibroids had decreased in size by 49 percent, and they showed no significant changes in bone density.

Still, it's unlikely that leuprolide (or other drugs currently in use) will replace myomectomy as a treatment for fibroids, Dr. Johnson says. Not only because of possible side effects but also because of cost: Leuprolide therapy may cost $500 a month or more. But for women approaching menopause, leuprolide can help reduce symptoms until their estrogen supplies shut down. Leuprolide can also shrink large fibroids prior to surgery, reducing blood loss and making them easier to remove, Dr. Johnson says.

FIBROMYALGIA

The best thing you can say about miscellaneous aches and pains— those caused by flu, hard work or sitting in an awkward position— is that they're usually here today and gone tomorrow. Not so with fibromyalgia. This mysterious condition, affecting millions of Americans every year, causes aches and pains to reappear with regularity. For some, they may come and go during an entire lifetime.

The term *fibromyalgia* refers specifically to recurrent aches and pains (which can affect ligaments, tendons or muscles). But doctors often talk about "fibromyalgia syndrome," which is a condition also characterized by disturbed sleep and daytime fatigue. The pain and fatigue often go together. "When you don't get restful and restorative sleep, that causes muscle pain and stiffness," says James J. Curran, M.D., an associate professor of medicine at the University of Chicago Medical Center. In turn, muscle pain and stiffness erode good sleep, causing an "endless cycle of increasing pain and discomfort and decreased mobility," says Dr. Curran.

Another sign of fibromyalgia is the appearance of numerous "tender points"—spots behind the knees, at the sides of the elbows and elsewhere—that are excruciatingly painful when pressed.

BAFFLING PAIN

Though fibromyalgia can be caused by underlying diseases such as hypothyroidism, in the majority of cases, doctors can't pinpoint any one cause. It is possible that the frequent brief awakenings during sleep experienced by those with fibromyalgia may cause increases in the body's levels of substance P, a "pain amplifier" that can cause muscle pain, Dr. Curran says.

Theories abound, but most doctors believe that fibromyalgia may also be linked to stress, exercise (too much or not enough) and poor posture, says Jeffrey M. Thompson, M.D., an assistant professor of physical medicine and rehabilitation at the Mayo Clinic in Rochester, Minnesota.

Women are affected five to ten times more often than men, Dr. Curran says, "probably because they face tremendous amounts of pressure" at work and home. "In general, people with fibromyalgia are hardworking individuals," he adds.

PROFILE IN HEALING

RUTH BUZARD: RELIEF AFTER 20 YEARS

Thirty-one years ago, when Ruth Buzard was in her mid-twenties, she had a car accident that changed her life. With bruised muscles and fractured bones, she began the slow process of healing, looking forward to the day the pain would end.

It never did.

Ruth didn't know it then, but the accident triggered fibromyalgia syndrome, a mysterious disorder that causes sleep disturbances, daytime fatigue and nearly constant aches and pains. "I hurt all over," says Ruth, a registered nurse and president of the Fibromyalgia Association of Central Ohio. "When I walked, my knees and hips would hurt. When I moved my arms, my shoulder, neck and arms would hurt. When I got up in the morning, I was so stiff I couldn't even move."

For the next 20 years, Ruth went from doctor to doctor, but no one knew what was wrong. By chance, a colleague noticed how tired she looked and suggested she see a specialist. Ruth did, and the diagnosis was clinched. That's when her life, after so many years, took a turn for the better.

Her doctor put her on a regimen of massage, heating pads and electrical treatments to relax her painful muscles. More important, he put her on an exercise program. It was exercise, Ruth soon discovered, that was to make the biggest difference.

"Every day I take a lot of walks and do stretching exercises," she says. "I get the blood circulating, and that gives me a really good overall feeling." It took years of perseverance and practice, but finally Ruth got a pretty good hold on the disease.

There isn't a cure for fibromyalgia, and Ruth still has days when the fatigue, aches and pains catch up with her. But by breaking the pain *cycle,* she can do the things she only dreamed of before. "Before, the kids were always saying 'We can't disturb Mom, she's sick.' Now they say, 'Mom, you're doing too much.'"

RESTORING REST AND RELAXATION

Treating fibromyalgia—or preventing it—can be daunting. "No one knows exactly what causes it, so no one can say for sure that it can be prevented," Dr. Thompson says. Once symptoms appear, however, restoring lost sleep is one place to start. Your doctor can help.

Sure, you *could* take over-the-counter sleeping pills. These, however, often make things worse, because in the long run, they tend to make you groggier than you were before. But a class of prescription drugs called tricyclic antidepressants—for example, amitriptyline (Elavil) and cyclobenzaprine (Flexeril)—helps restore normal sleep with few side effects, Dr. Curran says. "People sleep better, they feel better, and their fibromyalgia symptoms decrease."

You don't want to stay on the medications forever, though. The goal, says Dr. Curran, is to escape the pain/fatigue/pain cycle.

Also important in breaking the cycle is learning to relax more during the day. One effective technique is biofeedback, which teaches the body to relax in response to mental cues. In one study, people with fibromyalgia were given 15 sessions of biofeedback. Of the 15 people in the study, 9 had "significant improvement" in their symptoms. Indeed, 4 of them felt improved a year after they left the study.

Talk to your doctor about finding a biofeedback instructor near you.

IMPROVED MOVES

There isn't a once-and-for-all cure for fibromyalgia, but there are many things you can do that will help, says Dr. Thompson. For example:

Watch your posture. If you walk hunched over or spend entire days scrunched over a computer keyboard, you're setting the stage for muscle pain. Walk erect, and sit at a desk and chair right for your height. "With your elbows relaxed at your sides and your forearms level, the surface of your desk should be slightly higher than your hands," says Dr. Thompson.

Alternate tasks. Repetition—pulling weed after weed from your flower patch, for example—can make fibromyalgia flare. Don't spend too long doing any one activity.

Hit the track. Or the aerobics class, swimming pool, even the dance floor. People who participate in aerobic exercise—exercise that boosts your pulse rate for sustained periods of time—often have less muscle pain and fatigue.

In one Canadian study, 42 people were assigned to two groups. Those in one group were given stretching exercises, while those in the other got their hearts pumping with aerobic exercise. Twenty weeks later, both groups reported improvement, but those in the aerobics group reported having less pain compared to those in the flexibility group.

Aerobic exercise is thought to be helpful for several reasons. One, it stimulates the release of chemicals—for example, cortisol and endorphins—that are the body's natural painkillers. In addition, exercise is an excellent stress buster, adds Dr. Curran. "If there's a stress component to the disease, exercise may relieve your stress."

Lay on the heat. Many people say that heating pads, hot packs, whirlpools and massage can give welcome, if temporary, relief.

FOOD POISONING

Candles cast a soft glow on the anniversary roses, and soft music ushered in the oysters, shrimp bisque and succulent bay scallops. Then Harry and Sally went dancing, and he whispered the sweet nothings she loved to hear. A perfectly romantic evening—until Harry, all at once, turned an unromantic shade of green. His stomach churned. "It's the blasted scallops," Harry moaned, as he headed for the men's room.

Harry's rush to the men's room was precipitated by eating bad scallops—food poisoning, or as Harry's doctor called it, gastroenteritis.

By some estimates, at least 24 million cases of food poisoning occur in the United States every year. And that doesn't count the stalwarts who simply stay at home and suffer in silence.

But gastroenteritis rarely is serious. Sufferers may feel *so* bad they think they're going to die, but in most cases, they're better after one to five days. Even Harry, poisoned by his expensive supper, was up and courting by the end of the weekend.

Just about everyone, at one time or another, suffers from some form of gastroenteritis, says David L. Swerdlow, M.D., a physician with Community Disease Control in San Diego. And except for the really nasty kinds—botulism, for example, or mushroom poisoning—it will usually go away on its own. This is because our bodies quickly expel the offending poisons and bacteria that make us sick. Furthermore, the treatment—time plus plenty of liquids—is quite effective.

The bacterial varieties of gastroenteritis are extremely common, Dr. Swerdlow says. "We estimate there are millions of infections every year. But a lot of people with gastroenteritis don't see their doctors," he adds. "We only hear about a fraction of the cases."

INVASIONS AND INTESTINAL POISON

Basically there are two types of gastroenteritis. One type occurs when invading organisms burrow right into the intestinal wall. The now-inflamed intestine, to protect itself from this onslaught, exudes large quantities of a protective, watery discharge. Bacterial invaders such as shigella often cause frequent (and copious) diarrhea. It can get pretty uncomfortable.

On the other hand, when gastroenteritis is caused by bacterial *toxins* (and not necessarily by the bacteria themselves), people may have vomiting and diarrhea—sometimes at the same time. Here's how food poisoning begins.

Unlike people, most bacteria prefer their meals at room temperature. So when Harry's scallops were left on the restaurant counter all afternoon, waiting bacteria lined up for the buffet. First they feasted; then they multiplied. By the time their population had reached hundreds of millions of organisms—by bacterial standards, a not-unusual occurrence—they were producing poisonous by-products in sufficient quantities to spoil Harry's evening—and, quite literally, his scallops.

Just about any food, if left out long enough, will attract marauding bacteria. But red meat, eggs and poultry are particularly susceptible, Dr. Swerdlow says. "Contaminated eggs have been a big problem in recent years, but outbreaks have been associated with cantaloupe and tomatoes that have been sliced and left out without adequate refrigeration."

GUT-LEVEL RELIEF

For people with garden-variety gastroenteritis, there's usually no reason to go to the doctor, says Andrew K. Diehl, M.D., professor of medicine at University of Texas Health Science Center at San Antonio. Of course, there are times when it's best to play it safe, he adds. "I would be concerned if someone was passing blood in the stool or had a fever, or if they were having so much diarrhea and vomiting that dehydration could occur." Generally, people who continue to feel sick for longer than five days, Dr. Diehl says, should probably see a doctor.

But most people will benefit from some simple home treatments, he adds. You still won't feel good, but you will feel better.

Fill up on fluids. This is the first—and most important—treatment for all types of gastroenteritis, Dr. Diehl says. This is because prolonged vomiting and diarrhea will drain life-sustaining fluids from the body. If these fluids aren't replaced, dehydration can occur within days or, in extreme cases, in even just a few hours.

Water—and plenty of it—is what you need most, Dr. Diehl says. However, don't drink gallons all at once—that will only make your diarrhea worse. Drink it slowly and often. One level teaspoon of table salt plus 4 level teaspoons of table sugar in 1 quart of water will help your body absorb the necessary minerals as well. If you don't feel like drinking water, juices or tea with sugar will also do the trick. Commercial fluid replacement solutions containing sugar, salt and electrolytes are also available without a prescription in many stores, Dr. Diehl says.

Slow it down. Doctors agree that it's often best to let diarrhea run its course. But when you simply need a break from the bathroom, "several tablespoons of Pepto-Bismol every half hour to 1 hour may be effective for reducing diarrhea," Dr. Diehl says.

Sodium bicarbonate (baking soda) not only helps to settle the stomach but also replenishes the body's sodium that is lost in diarrhea. When you're thirsty, mix 1/4 teaspoon in an 8-ounce glass of water and drink it down.

POISON MUSHROOMS AND BOTULISM

While doctors do their best to reassure people that food poisoning rarely is something to worry about, they hasten to mention some extremely dangerous exceptions. For example, poisonous mushrooms found growing wild: If you eat them, you can die—sometimes in just a few hours. In fact, more than half of the people who eat certain species die within eight days. The surest way to prevent it is to leave mushroom picking to the experts. Buy yours in the supermarket.

Then there's botulism, probably the most dangerous of all the food poisonings. Caused by a microbe that flourishes in airtight environments, botulism has been found in canned goods, baked potatoes and even on oil-covered cloves of garlic. The poison is so strong, scientists say, that 1 gram could possibly kill between 100,000 and 10 *million* people.

Fortunately for its victims, botulism isn't likely to be confused with other, milder forms of food poisoning, says David L. Swerdlow, M.D., of Community Disease Control in San Diego. People with botulism *know* they need a doctor. "The symptoms begin with an inability to speak and an inability to swallow," Dr. Swerdlow says. "Things go wrong with your cranial nerves and then your respiratory muscles." If botulism isn't treated, Dr. Swerdlow says, its victims will simply stop breathing and die.

In the past, more than 60 percent of the people contracting botulism did die. Today, with the aid of antitoxins and techniques for helping people breathe, the death rate is less than 10 percent—*if* you receive treatment. Botulism is rare and can be prevented by avoiding suspicious-looking foods such as bulging cans, inadequately canned homemade goods and foods with foul odors. If you even suspect botulism, says Dr. Swerdlow, rush to the emergency room.

Stay out of the kitchen. Even if you're one of those people who feeds a cold and stuffs a fever, your insides won't take kindly to food. A gut with gastroenteritis needs its rest, Dr. Diehl says. "It's usually recommended that people take clear liquids," he says. "You want something that will be easily absorbed from the gastrointestinal tract."

Once you start feeling better and can handle food again, wean your way back to your normal diet. Stick with easy-to-digest foods such as broth, soft eggs and cooked vegetables at first. Usually you can return to a regular diet within a day or so.

A WORD ABOUT DRUGS

There are occasions when doctors will knock the starch out of gastroenteritis with antibiotics, Dr. Diehl says, but it's not a common practice. Most people, by the time they drag themselves to the doctor, already are getting better. In addition, not all antibiotics are effective for all infections; it can be tough to choose the right one. Finally, some people have dangerous reactions to antibiotics. Why go to all that trouble, Dr. Diehl asks, when the problem will probably go away on its own?

Dr. Diehl says antibiotics are probably most helpful to those with fever or bloody diarrhea. He says he sometimes prescribes drugs to stop vomiting and diarrhea, but they aren't always the best bet. For one thing, people with gastroenteritis need to eliminate intestinal infections, not retain them. Besides, not all vomiting and diarrhea are caused by gastroenteritis. Masking the symptoms can delay the diagnosis of some real problems—cancer, for example, or inflammatory bowel disease.

"Gastroenteritis is a condition that usually cures itself, so I try to give medicines that are pretty low power," Dr. Diehl says. "Besides, I don't have many patients who get terribly upset about it. They just see it more as a nuisance than as anything else."

FOOD OR FOE

Doctors agree that the germs that poison our suppers are everywhere; they can't be eradicated. On the other hand, there's a lot you can do to avoid food poisoning. Here's how.

Keep it cold. Do you remember that infamous Fourth of July when every guest spent the evening—and the next two days—throwing up? The culprit was Aunt Mae's egg salad. As it warmed in the summer sun, it became the promised land for untold millions of bacteria; the smallest serving delivered a three-day punch. But most bacteria don't reproduce when they're cold. Refrigerate leftovers right after you eat. On picnics, keep your lunch in an efficient cooler. And because many types of bacteria are especially fond of eggs, you might want to leave the egg salad (or any egg-based food) at home. Aunt Mae will understand.

Cool it fast. Even in the refrigerator, large pots of hot stew, soup or gravy take a long time to cool—long enough for bacteria to multiply. To rapidly bring hot foods to safe temperatures, first put them in the freezer. Or transfer the contents of big pots into several smaller containers. This will allow them to cool more quickly.

Thaw meat slowly. It's certainly faster to thaw meat on the countertop than in the refrigerator. It's also more dangerous. To keep that steak (or fish, chicken or Thanksgiving bird) from becoming a breeding ground for hungry bacteria, keep it cold until you turn on the oven.

Egg beaters. Had Julius Caesar dined on his favorite salad the day of his demise, his final words might have been "Egg, too, Brute?" Foods such as Caesar salad, uncooked hollandaise sauce, and homemade mayonnaise—all of which require raw eggs—are notorious for transmitting bacterial gastroenteritis. Cook custards and French toast all the way through. Scramble eggs for at least 1 minute; fry them, covered, for 4 minutes; boil them for 7 minutes.

Scour the counters. Even if your cutting boards look safe, they can hide whole conventions of bacteria in microscopic pores, cracks and knife cuts. What's more, all those visiting microbes will feast on the bread crumbs, steak slices and lettuce leaves you leave behind. Scrub your cutting boards with plenty of soap and hot water. Adding a little bleach to the water will help prevent cross-contamination.

Pass on the sushi. Raw or undercooked fish can be an intestinal time bomb. Not only can fish harbor the bacteria that cause cholera, some types—tuna, mackerel and bonito, for example—can produce scrombroid poisoning, a particularly virulent variety of food poisoning. Worse, these poisons aren't inactivated by cooking or freezing. Keeping your catch cool will help keep you safe.

Cook it well. Few bacteria can survive high heats. Cook beef to at least 140°F, pork to 170°F and chicken to 180° to 185°F.

If you touch it, scrub it. Bacteria flourish in our gastrointestinal tracts. Good hygiene is perhaps the best way to prevent them from spreading—and from making you sick. Wash your hands before you start cooking. If you're working with chicken or other meats, wash before you move on to the salad and vegetables.

DISEASE
FREE

FOOT PROBLEMS

The average person takes between 5,000 and 10,000 steps a day. Over a lifetime, that can add up to some 115,000 miles—more than four times around the earth. To make things worse, many of those miles are walked in high heels, tight boots and sweltering athletic shoes. No wonder foot problems often get a toehold!

In the following pages, we'll discuss some common foot and toe woes and look at some of the things you can do to keep your feet from walking all over you.

ATHLETE'S FOOT

You probably remember your mom warning you never to walk barefoot on locker room floors. But athlete's foot—a flaking, scaling, itching, downright ugly fungal disease—can be picked up just about anywhere, says Ronald C. Savin, M.D., clinical professor of dermatology at Yale University School of Medicine. "The fungus that causes athlete's foot is on everybody's floors, on everybody's walls, in everybody's bathroom," he says. "You're going to be exposed to it no matter where you go."

Athlete's foot, however, does thrive in locker rooms and other places—the insides of your shoes, for instance—where the air is warm and humid. And once it takes hold, it can be frustratingly difficult to get rid of, Dr. Savin says. A little prevention can save your feet from a whole lot of itching.

HOT SPOTS

Keeping your feet dry and cool is the first step to fungus-free feet. So if athlete's foot is a problem for you:

Change your socks—often. By replacing damp socks with a dry pair, you reduce the humidity that athlete's foot needs to thrive, Dr. Savin says. While you're at it, be sure you wear socks made from cotton, polypropylene or other absorbent fabrics that "breathe" easily.

Let in the air. Shoes made from vinyl or rubber also trap heat and moisture. Doctors often recommend leather or canvas shoes, which help keep your feet dry by allowing perspiration to escape.

Let them rest. Since all shoes will retain moisture from your feet, it's a good idea to let them dry for 24 hours before wearing them again.

Dry your feet. Particularly between the toes, where athlete's foot often goes. To dry hard-to-reach places, taking aim with a hair dryer (set on low) can also help.

Footloose (and fungus-free). The best way to prevent athlete's foot is to give your feet plenty of air, Dr. Savin says. In summer, don sandals instead of tight shoes. Even better, go barefoot now and then. "It's been hypothesized that athlete's foot is a disease of civilization," says Dr. Savin. "It's likely that Tarzan never had athlete's foot."

Pad your toes. Putting small bits of cotton between the toes helps absorb fungus-friendly moisture. By slightly separating the toes, this trick also allows air to circulate, keeping them even drier.

Stop the sweat. This can be as simple as rolling an antiperspirant on the bottom of your feet. If you've tried antiperspirants and your feet still drip at the end of the day, talk to your doctor. There are prescription solutions available.

Fight back with fungicides. There are many over-the-counter sprays, powders and creams that can kill the athlete's foot fungus, Dr. Savin says. Those containing miconazole (Micatin) and tolnaftate (Tinactin), applied twice a day, will sometimes eliminate athlete's foot in a few weeks or months.

High-powered help. The problem with over-the-counter medications is that the fungus often returns as soon as you stop using them. For serious bouts of athlete's foot, your doctor may recommend a prescription oral drug called griseofulvin, which knocks out the infection from the inside out.

Even with griseofulvin, however, you may need several months of treatment before your feet are clear again. "It's just not easy to knock out athlete's foot," Dr. Savin says. "It often comes back, and we're not sure if that's because people catch it again or they really hadn't killed it in the first place."

BUNIONS

Normally toes grow in straight out (more or less). But if you have an inherited condition called *hallux valgus,* your big toe doesn't know *which* way to go. The tip grows inward, the joint bulges outward, and the result is a knobby joint called a bunion, says Bruce Lebowitz, D.P.M., director of the podiatric clinic at the Johns Hopkins Francis Scott Key Medical Center in Baltimore. By themselves, bunions aren't necessarily painful. "But when you stick your foot into a shoe, particularly if it's a snug fit, you put a lot of pressure on the bunion, and that causes the pain," Dr. Lebowitz explains.

Because women's fashions often call for tight-fitting, high-heeled shoes, women are ten times more likely than men to have painful bunions. "A man's shoe looks like a foot, a lady's shoe looks like a triangle," says Dr. Lebowitz.

MAKING SPACE

Occasionally people with bunions have surgery to realign the bones. But most people can benefit just by giving their toes some breathing room. For example:

Avoid toe jams. Tight shoes exert painful pressure on this tender prominence. Give bunions a break by investing in shoes with generous toe room, Dr. Lebowitz says. "In many cases, you can reduce virtually all the symptoms by changing shoes."

Stretch your wardrobe. Rather than buying new shoes, take shoes you already own to a shoe repair store. For a small fee, the toe space can be stretched from the inside out to make it larger.

Slip into sandals. Weather permitting, open-toed footwear is ideal for giving bunions room to move, Dr. Lebowitz says.

Try some soft sneaks. Athletic-type shoes made from soft fabrics that "give" are less likely to rub your bunions the wrong way than shoes made from tough leather or vinyl.

Put in a patch. "You can put a bunion shield over the bony protuberance, which helps reduce the friction inside your shoe," Dr. Lebowitz says. These are available in your drugstore, or your doctor can make one for you.

CORNS AND CALLUSES

Formed from thick layers of skin on the toes, heels or soles, corns and calluses are your body's armor. They're meant to protect you from painful friction. But sometimes they get sore themselves. Then, like well-meaning friends who have overstayed their welcome, all they do is rub you the wrong way.

You can often prevent corns and calluses (a corn is merely a small, compact callus) by eliminating the source of the friction. So:

Move into roomier shoes. When you wear tight shoes, the constant pressure can give rise to painful corns and calluses, Dr. Lebowitz says. Look for shoes that have an abundance of toe room yet aren't so loose that they slip at the heels. Wearing open-toed shoes and sandals (in warm weather, of course) can be ideal.

Go flat. High heels pitch your weight forward, putting callus-causing stress on your feet and toes. Flat heels are better because they distribute your weight more evenly, Dr. Lebowitz says. This doesn't mean you have to abandon high style altogether. Use flats for your everyday shoes, and bring out the heels for those special occasions—banquets, for instance—when you'll spend most of the evening sitting down.

Insert a shock absorber. Over-the-counter pads and cushions made from foam rubber and other materials are an inexpensive way to reduce pressure on the bottom of your feet. These quickly lose their "spring," however, and should be replaced fairly often, doctors say.

Order orthotics. These prescription, custom-made inserts can cost hundreds of dollars but can make a big difference when corns and calluses are caused by skeletal misalignment.

Rub them out. To eliminate a painful corn or callus, just soaking it can help, Dr. Lebowitz says. "Soak it in warm water, then rub it gently with a pumice stone after bathing. That can help reduce the size somewhat."

Get plastered—carefully. There are many over-the-counter plasters, creams and lotions that contain salicylic acid, which can help "dissolve" corns and calluses. These remedies must be used with extreme care, Dr. Lebowitz warns. "The acid doesn't know the difference between the callus and the skin. If it's not put on exactly right, it can start eating away normal tissue." This can be particularly perilous for people with diabetes, who may have diminished sensations in their feet. So if you have diabetes or other circulatory problems, stay away from acids and see your doctor instead.

PLANTAR WARTS

Unlike corns, plantar warts—*plantar* means "the bottom of the foot"—aren't caused by friction. They aren't caused by toads either. What causes plantar warts is the papilloma virus. When it gets under your skin, it builds itself a protective house—the wart. "Warts are an infection, and they're often difficult to get rid of," says Mark B. Taylor, M.D., a clinical instructor of dermatology at the University of Utah School of Medicine in Salt Lake City.

They're also contagious. You can catch warts in public showers and locker rooms. And by touching your own warts, you can spread them to different parts of your body. Some plantar warts will disappear on their own within months, while others persist for years, Dr. Taylor says. But if you don't feel like waiting, you can give nature a helping hand.

WHIPPING YOUR WOES

There are many over-the-counter wart remedies to choose from. Most contain salicylic acid, which can help whittle small warts down to size, Dr. Taylor says. "But the wart often grows as fast as the salicylic acid can remove it," he adds. To speed things along, see your doctor, who may prescribe acid compounds that are more potent than the over-the-counter varieties.

A quicker way to remove warts is with a technique called cryosurgery. *Cryo-* means "cold," and the liquid nitrogen used in cryosurgery is very cold indeed. When a wart is swabbed or sprayed with liquid nitrogen, it

---

PICKING THE RIGHT SHOES

If people would think more about comfort and less about fashion, there would be fewer sore feet in the world, says Bruce Lebowitz, D.P.M., director of the podiatric clinic at Johns Hopkins Francis Scott Key Medical Center in Baltimore. To buy shoes that are good for you *and* your feet, experts recommend the following.

Shop in the afternoon. Your feet expand during the day, so shoes that fit at 9:00 A.M. may be uncomfortably snug at noon. Do buy later in the day, when your feet have expanded to their maximum size, says orthopedic surgeon Ian J. Alexander, M.D., of the Crystal Clinic in Akron, Ohio.

Put your bigger foot forward. It's normal to have one foot that's bigger than the other. Make sure you measure both feet, so that you can buy the larger size.

Bigger is better. Scrunching your feet into pointy toes virtually guarantees foot problems, Dr. Lebowitz says. Allow 1/2 inch between the tip of your big toe and the end of the shoe. And make sure your toes can wiggle freely without being crushed against the sides of the shoe.

Forget the high high heels. Sure, they look great, but they push your feet into all sorts of uncomfortable angles, Dr. Lebowitz says. Wear shoes with lower heels. Your feet will thank you for it.

---

freezes solid, blisters and falls off, taking the troublemaking virus with it. The procedure takes just a few minutes, although you may have throbbing pain for an hour or more.

Just as cryosurgery uses intense cold to remove warts, electrosurgery uses intense heat. With an electrical instrument shaped something like a soldering iron, the doctor burns the wart, which then blisters and falls away. As with cryosurgery, electrosurgery can be somewhat painful, says Dr. Taylor.

Yet another technique for wart removal is called immunotherapy, which stimulates the body's natural defenses. First a chemical patch is applied to your skin. This sensitizes your body, triggering an alert response in the body's immune system. The same chemical is then applied repeatedly to the wart. The immune system responds by "attacking" the wart, just as it would any foreign invader, Dr. Taylor says. "Immunotherapy works extremely well."

As a last resort, warts can be excised—surgically removed—with a scalpel or laser. Warts can return after any therapy, and of course, there's no guarantee that *other* warts won't crop up.

HEEL PAIN

Often caused by an inflammation in the bottom of the foot called plantar fasciitis or by growths of bone called heel spurs, heel pain can take you off your feet in a hurry.

While most heel pain is mild, it can sometimes be unbearable. For severe cases, your doctor may recommend an injection of steroids, powerful drugs that will quickly quell inflammation. But the injections themselves can be terribly painful, says Ian J. Alexander, M.D., an orthopedic surgeon at Crystal Clinic in Akron, Ohio. This remedy usually is recommended only as a last resort.

Your best bet is to try these self-help measures first.

Stretch it out. Some of the same exercises that stretch the Achilles tendon also stretch the muscle at the bottom of the foot (the plantar fascia). Done regularly, stretches can help prevent heel pain, says Dr. Alexander.

The stretches are simple. Place the ball of your foot on the edge of a step and gently let your heel drop down as far as it will go. Hold this position for about 20 seconds, then repeat. Or while seated on a chair or the edge of your bed, place the ball of your foot on a footstool. Again, let your heel drop as low as it comfortably can. At the same time, press down on the top of your knee to maximize the stretch.

If you're already in pain, don't wait to do the stretches, Dr. Alexander adds. "Doing it right off the bat can help a lot."

Pad your heel. Wearing foam rubber inserts in your shoes can help ease painful pressure. Similarly, devices called heel cups can help prevent the protective layer of fat on the bottom of your foot from flattening out and losing its cushioning ability.

Put up your feet. Just giving your heels a chance to rest will help the healing process, doctors say. So rent some old movies, put your feet up, and take it easy.

Ease the pain. Over-the-counter painkillers—aspirin, acetaminophen or ibuprofen—may be all that you need for quick relief, says Dr. Alexander.

INGROWN NAILS

Imagine a long, sharp spike pressing deeply into your big toe—not for a second, not for a day, but for week after agonizing week. That's what an ingrown toenail feels like.

Often caused by careless trimming, ingrown toenails are bits of nail that grow downward into the skin instead of outward over the toe. "It's like a spike that grows under the skin, and when that spike in there begins to fester, it can be terribly painful," Dr. Alexander says.

Once a nail is ingrown to the point that you're in constant pain, your doctor will have to remove it to get you some relief. But before you get to that stage, the following two prevention techniques can help.

Cut them long. By cutting your nails straight across and no shorter than the end of your toe, they will always grow out of harm's way, Dr. Alexander says. Incidentally, cutting a V-shaped wedge in the middle of the nail *won't* encourage the two sides to grow toward the middle. Nails grow from back to front, however you cut them.

Loosen up. Since tight shoes can force the nails downward, make sure you buy shoes with ample toe room, Dr. Lebowitz advises.

FOOT ODOR

There's something in the air—something with an air of mystery, of power, of . . . Limburger cheese.

Foot odor is caused by bacteria. And the more your feet sweat, the more bacteria you have, says Dr. Savin. To eliminate foot odor, therefore, you need to keep your feet dry and clean. For starters:

Rub-a-dub daily. Washing your feet once a day probably is enough, although people who perspire heavily may want to wash them more often. The cleaner you keep your feet, Dr. Savin says, the fewer problems you'll have with foot odor.

Change your socks. Bacteria that love your hot, sweaty feet are going to *adore* your hot, sweaty socks. Change your socks at least once a day. And if your shoes are machine washable, give them an occasional wash as well.

Roll on protection. The same antiperspirant you put under your arms will help keep your feet dry, too. The less you sweat, remember, the less opportunity there is for bacteria to threaten your social life.

Odor beaters. Your local drugstore stocks many pads and powders that help absorb perspiration and the foot odor that goes with it, says Dr. Savin. Experiment until you find one that works for you.

GALLSTONES

Freida liked to tell her friends that her favorite fast food was fritters. (A poet at heart, Freida loved *F* words *almost* as much as those fabulous fried delights.) But her fancy changed one fateful night when the Frackville firefighters fired up their annual fritter fundraiser. Freida ate and ate and ate—she filled her face with fritters—and when she went home that night, she had a ferocious fit of indigestion (or so she thought). "It's from that fiendish fat!" Freida moaned. "I'm all frittered out—for sure!"

A GALLING PROBLEM

Fortunately, Freida's feeding frenzy wasn't fatal. The problem, her doctor told her the next day when she asked for advice, was gallstones—troublesome little deposits in the gallbladder that sometimes cause symptoms that *feel* like indigestion but aren't. Here's what happens.

The gallbladder is a small, pear-shaped organ that stores the bile (gall) produced by the liver. During meals, the gallbladder squirts some of this greenish brown fluid into the small intestine, where it helps with digestion. Trouble begins when gallstones—they're not really stones, of course, but hard deposits of cholesterol and calcium that often form in the bile—drift into one of the ducts leading to the small intestine. "If there's a stone that gets lodged, the pressure builds up behind it, and that causes the problems," says Henry Pitt, M.D., director of the Gallstone and Biliary Disease Center at Johns Hopkins University in Baltimore.

Gallbladder attacks often occur at night or after meals, when the gallbladder is most active, Dr. Pitt says. That's one reason people often confuse gallstones with indigestion. The symptoms—abdominal pain, nausea and sometimes vomiting—also resemble indigestion. In more serious cases, however, the resemblance ends. If enough pressure builds up behind the stone, the gallbladder can burst, a very rare but potentially deadly complication.

But of the approximately one million Americans who develop gallstones every year—women are three times more vulnerable than men—

most have "silent stones," without symptoms. If you've already had one attack, however, there's a very good chance you'll eventually have another—and another and another. To prevent future problems, your doctor may suggest you eliminate the stones—with drugs, surgery or one of many stone-busting techniques. Even better than removing stones, Dr. Pitt adds, is preventing them. Here's how.

SKIPPING STONES

Research has shown that people who are overweight are considerably more at risk for gallstones than their thinner counterparts, Dr. Pitt says. To keep stones at bay:

Shed some weight. For four years during the 1980s, researchers from the Harvard School of Public Health kept tabs on 88,837 women who had filled out detailed dietary questionnaires. The women who were slightly overweight, the researchers discovered, were 1.7 times more likely to develop gallstones (and related symptoms) than were the women of normal weight. Those women defined as "very obese" were *six times* more likely to develop symptomatic stones.

Clearly, keeping your weight down is one of the best ways to reduce your risk for gallstones, Dr. Pitt says. On the other hand, crash dieting can have the opposite effect; losing weight too fast can stimulate the liver to release extra amounts of cholesterol into the bile, possibly causing gallstones. If you're overweight, ask your doctor to recommend a diet that's right for you.

Cut the cholesterol. Not only can diets high in cholesterol lead to weight gain, the cholesterol itself also may be a problem. At Johns Hopkins, prairie dogs fed large amounts of cholesterol began to develop gallstones in just a few weeks. "The fact that we're so easily able to cause gallstones in the animals makes me think that cholesterol probably is one of many factors responsible," Dr. Pitt says.

However, these findings relate only to the prairie dogs, he stresses. Further studies are needed to determine if people are similarly affected. But since diets high in cholesterol are known to contribute to *other* health problems—high blood pressure, for example, and strokes and heart attacks—cutting the cholesterol is just good sense.

Put some fish on the grill. When the prairie dogs at Johns Hopkins were fed fish oil along with their high-cholesterol feed, gallstones failed to develop, Dr. Pitt says. Again, it's too early to tell if fish oil will have a similar protective effect in people, but adding a little fish to your diet certainly can't hurt. Mackerel, salmon and tuna are among the types highest in fish oil.

Fill up on fiber. Doctors aren't sure whether (or to what extent) a high-fiber diet can ward off gallstones. After evaluating the diets of 4,730 women, researchers at the National Institutes of Health concluded that dietary fiber could have a "small protective effect" against the development of gallstones. At the very least, eating more fruits and vegetables will leave less room for those high-fat foods that *can* cause problems.

SURGERY GOES HIGH TECH

Every year, more than a half-million Americans have their gallbladders removed. Until recently, this common operation not only was painful but also put you out of commission for quite a while. After a month to six weeks, *maybe* you'd feel normal again. And the scar—the 3- to 6-inch medical equivalent of "Kilroy was here"—was a permanent reminder of what you went through.

Things have changed. Today, surgeons can remove the gallbladder through a hole the size of a dime. With a procedure called laparoscopic cholecystectomy, people can have the operation on Monday, go home the next day and return to work the following week, says Henry Pitt, M.D., of Johns Hopkins University's Gallstone and Biliary Disease Center.

Here's how it's done. First the surgeon makes a 1/2-inch incision inside the belly button. Into this incision he slips the laparoscope—a narrow tube fitted with a miniature camera. When he flips the switch, your insides spring to life on one or more television screens in the operating room. For a better view, the surgery often is performed in a darkened operating room.

Into three or four small holes beneath the breastbone and ribs go the instruments: forceps, scalpels, perhaps even a laser. Some surgeons use only two holes; others may use four. During the surgery, the doctor will rarely look at you. He's watching TV!

After he separates the gallbladder from the liver—the instruments, on TV and magnified many times, look immense, like a giant's toys—he pulls the gallbladder up through the hole in your belly button. Sometimes it comes up intact, bulging like a beanbag. If it's especially large, he may cut it into smaller pieces first.

As this procedure becomes safer and more efficient, the nonsurgical treatments for gallstones rapidly are becoming second choices, Dr. Pitt says. "Now that we have laparoscopic cholecystectomy, many of the alternatives that leave the gallbladder in are falling by the wayside."

Since as many as one in ten Americans has gallstones, you shouldn't be surprised if you get them, too. But don't be alarmed, Dr. Pitt says. Gallstones are easily controlled.

OTHER OPTIONS

If you have gallstones that are causing you trouble, your doctor may say that it's time to eliminate them. And most likely, he may suggest you have your gallbladder removed. Called cholecystectomy, gallbladder surgery is the second most frequently performed operation in the United States. (The first is cesarean section.) It's also the gold standard for beating the pain of gallstones.

Like the appendix, the gallbladder is entirely dispensable. Once removed, the bile simply goes straight from the liver to the small intestine. "The vast majority of people do fine without it," Dr. Pitt says. In fact, once you're free from the pain of a *malfunctioning* gallbladder, you'll do better without it, he adds. And without a gallbladder, it is extremely unlikely you'll ever get another gallstone.

If you're not so sick that you need surgery, your doctor may prescribe drugs that can dissolve stones inside the gallbladder. This process, called oral dissolution therapy, is used primarily for smaller stones and is quite safe, Dr. Pitt says. It's also slow, and it may take up to two years before the stones finally break down. Of course, once you stop taking drugs such as ursodeoxycholate, new stones are likely to develop.

In another procedure, methyl-tert-butyl ether (MTBE) is injected directly into the gallbladder. An octane enhancer for gasoline, MTBE will dissolve most stones in hours or days instead of years. But the procedure is more complicated to use than the oral drugs and is more likely to cause side effects, including nausea, vomiting and knocking you out cold, Dr. Pitt says. Apart from a few specialist centers, MTBE rarely is used.

Another option for removing gallstones is lithotripsy. Taken from the ancient Greek, the word means "stone crushing," and that's exactly what it does. Pioneered in the 1950s for crushing kidney stones, lithotripsy pulverizes stones inside the gallbladder with electrically generated shock waves. While quite safe and often painless, the procedure is effective only for crushing small, single stones—a minority of the cases, Dr. Pitt says.

Despite these new techniques, surgery—particularly a type of surgery called laparoscopic cholecystectomy (see "Surgery Goes High Tech" on the opposite page)—often is the preferred method for eradicating these recalcitrant stones. Just ask Freida. She had her gallbladder out Friday and was home the next day. In the future, Freida says, she'll forgo the fritters and feast on flounder instead. "I'm finally frittered out," she says, "and that's a fact."

GASTRITIS

The pain started when he moved from Tulsa to Albuquerque in the early 1980s, John remembers. Perhaps it was the Southwest's spicy foods, or the cigarettes he smoked, or the late nights spent in clubs. Even stress seemed to fan the smoldering coal in his chest into burning flames.

The first few times it happened, John didn't worry about it at all. "I figured it was just a little indigestion. I'd just take an antacid after lunch, and it would usually start feeling better." Eventually, though, the burning pain in his gut started coming on more often, and he started to worry a little. Then he started to worry some more—enough to get him to ask his doctor: "Is there something wrong with my gut?"

GUT TROUBLE

What John called indigestion his doctor called gastritis—a painful but rarely serious inflammation of the stomach's lining. In fact, just about everyone suffers from occasional bouts of indigestion or heartburn, says Frank L. Lanza, M.D., clinical professor of gastroenterology at Houston's Baylor College of Medicine. For most people, it doesn't amount to more than a few minutes of discomfort every now and then. But for some people like John, any number of things can bring it on—and bring it on often.

Dr. Lanza says gastritis can be brought on by several things: heavy drinking, certain medications, spicy or acidic foods or just too many tacos—or pizza, hot dogs or egg rolls—at lunch. And it's most unpredictable. It sometimes causes painful flare-ups for hours, days or weeks at a time. Occasionally gastritis will indicate a more serious problem, such as an ulcer. But in most cases, Dr. Lanza says, gastritis is nothing more than an irritated stomach getting even.

"People come in with heartburn, with bloating and discomfort, with indigestion and dyspepsia," Dr. Lanza says. "We do all the tests and find nothing wrong except a little redness in the stomach. So you say, 'Ah, they've got gastritis.' It's a diagnosis of exclusion."

It's also a difficult diagnosis to make. After all, an inflamed stomach lining isn't as obvious as a black eye or a broken leg. To diagnose gastritis, doctors go inside. Often they take a peek with an endoscope—a viewing instrument that slips down the esophagus and into the stomach. Sometimes they remove tissue samples for analysis. "If the stomach looks a little red, a little irritated, that's gastritis," Dr. Lanza says.

COMMON CAUSES

Aspirin and other nonsteroidal anti-inflammatory drugs such as indomethacin can be particularly hard on the stomach, Dr. Lanza says. Not only can they erode the stomach's lining, but also they impair the stomach's ability to secrete its protective mucus. This means the stomach, in effect, starts digesting itself.

People who party hearty discover that their stomachs, like little Carry Nation, get mighty upset when the drinks start flowing. As you might expect, high-octane drinks such as whiskey and gin can cause the most irritation, but even beer and wine, for some people, will generate painful bouts of gastritis, Dr. Lanza says.

If you're at the mercy of a sensitive stomach, you can depend on late nights, family fights and occupational plights to occasionally trigger painful, but short-lived, bouts of gastritis.

GASTRIC RELIEF

The good news about gastritis is that the symptoms can disappear as quickly as they come on. In fact, the stomach can recover from almost everything, says Dr. Lanza, including all the hot tamales John wolfed down while he lived in New Mexico. When he left the state (and its spicy cuisine), he said goodbye to his daily indigestion. Here's what you can try to help get rid of yours.

Take the acid test. As John can attest, antacids almost always work at relieving the pain. As their name suggests, antacids work by neutralizing stomach acids, which gives the inflamed stomach lining a chance to heal.

Most doctors agree that liquid antacids are more effective than tablets. Take 1 or 2 teaspoonfuls when symptoms flare.

Go on the milk wagon. At one time, doctors thought milk soothed a sore stomach. But now they know better. Milk actually *increases* the acid in the stomach. "As soon as milk's buffering effect is gone—that takes 20 to 30 minutes—the acid will just be roaring," Dr. Lanza says.

This doesn't mean you have to give up milk forever just because you have gastritis, doctors say. You can drink low-fat or skim milk, which should be easier on your insides than whole milk. But when symptoms are flaring, it's best to avoid it altogether. Reach for water instead.

Try a new painkiller. More than most drugs, aspirin is hard on your stomach, Dr. Lanza says. "Generally, people who take the enteric-coated aspirin have less gastritis than the people who take plain aspirin," he says. He also recommends that people take aspirin with meals; food in the stomach acts as a natural buffer. Or ask your doctor about aspirin substitutes such as acetaminophen.

Cut the fat. No matter what you eat, your stomach churns out acid to digest it. The bigger the meal, the more acid it produces. And when you eat foods high in fats, your stomach produces even *more* acid. That's good for digestion; it isn't good for gastritis. "For people with chronic indigestion, I put them on a low-fat diet," Dr. Lanza says. It's also better to eat smaller meals more often, he says, than to pack in a day's worth at one sitting.

Avoid acidic foods. If you ever tried to eat an orange when you had a mouth ulcer, you know it can sting like crazy. Well, acidic foods can also be tough on your digestive tract. If eating oranges, lemons, limes or tomatoes gives you grief, look for less painful ways to get your vitamin C—in peas, for example, and broccoli and brussels sprouts.

Change your bad habits. If wassail makes your stomach wail, try celebrating with softer drinks. Dr. Lanza always advises people with gastritis to drink less alcohol, stop smoking cigarettes and avoid coffee (especially black) and other caffeinated drinks.

SEEKING SOMETHING STRONGER

For most cases of gastritis, these self-help measures should help you stay symptom-free, says Dr. Lanza. If, however, you find you're taking seven or eight doses of antacids a day and not getting much relief, it could be a sign of something more serious, such as an ulcer. You should make an appointment to see your doctor.

Even if you don't have an ulcer, your doctor may decide that what you need is stronger medication. A prescription ulcer medication such as cimetidine (Tagamet), which reduces the quantity of acid in your stomach, can be used to relieve gastritis, says Dr. Lanza. Some people take anti-ulcer drugs *and* antacids, a combination that seems quite effective, he says.

But gastritis can be controlled. Just ask John. After letting up on the drinking, giving up smoking and forgoing overly spicy foods, John says his stomach pain rarely returns.

But John admits he'll always have to be careful what he eats. "I love orange juice, and grapefruit juice, too, but sometimes they kill me—they absolutely kill me."

GOUT

G us kicked off his shoes and collapsed on the bed. What a day! He started it right with a couple of his favorite jelly-filled doughnuts. Then he donned his checked pants and mushroom cap and met his buddies on the links for a leisurely 18 holes. In the clubhouse, they celebrated the weekend with double martinis, double helpings of kidney pie and thick slices of chocolate cake. They followed *that* with more cake, more stories and toasts all around.

"What a night!" Gus mused as he contentedly fell asleep. But an hour later he snapped awake, cursing and howling with pain. His toe—his poor, throbbing, red-as-a-beet big toe—was pounding like a fire alarm. Gus fell out of bed with a groan. "Owww! It's the blasted gout!"

THE DISEASE OF KINGS

Nearly 2,000 years ago, the Greek physician Galen identified, more or less correctly, heredity, intemperance and debauchery as the causes of gout. A type of arthritis (it's sometimes called gouty arthritis), gout historically was thought to afflict the well-heeled, mainly in the big toe. While the poor aren't immune to gout, it does have a penchant for middle-aged men like Gus—men who drink, are overweight and are fond of rich foods such as liver, anchovies and sweetbreads. Here's why.

Your body normally produces a chemical called uric acid that flows in your bloodstream. If you produce too much uric acid, or if too little is excreted through the urine, then tiny crystals, collectively called tophi, begin to form. Most of the time, these crystals, like sugar dumped in a cup of tea, fall harmlessly to the bottom—the "bottom" being the skin, the kidneys, the outer portions of the ear and other parts of the body.

When they settle in one of your joints, however—the big toe is particularly vulnerable—the immune system slams into action. "The crystals tend to be intensely inflammatory," says John G. Fort, M.D., a rheumatologist and clinical assistant professor of medicine at Thomas Jefferson University Hospital in Philadelphia. "The attacks can be very painful, very disabling."

They're also unpredictable. Some people are plagued every month, every other month or twice a year. Others will have one attack but never a second. In general, the higher your uric acid levels, the more often you'll have attacks, Dr. Fort says. But gout doesn't have to keep you down, he adds. By watching your diet, controlling your weight and, sometimes, taking the right drugs, you can toss gout right out of the joint!

ROYAL RELIEF

Since gout only gets the upper hand when you're supersaturated with uric acid, the trick is to dump the surplus. For example:

Can the sardines. And the anchovies and kidney pie. These and other foods—organ meats top the list—are high in purine, a compound your body converts to uric acid. While a low-purine diet won't necessarily cure your gout, it can reduce your risk for long-term problems, Dr. Fort says. (See "Prune Purines from Your Diet" below for a list of purine-containing foods.)

Trim the fat. On average, people with gout are 15 to 30 percent overweight, and heavy people simply have more uric acid than their lighter counterparts. They also tend to have high blood pressure, and some blood pressure *medications* can boost uric acid, Dr. Fort says. While some people

---

PRUNE PURINES FROM YOUR DIET

While most gout sufferers don't need to stick to strict diets, it's still a good idea to limit, if not eliminate, your purine intake. To avoid a possible flare-up, you should avoid the following foods, all high in purine.

- Anchovies
- Brains
- Gravies
- Kidneys
- Liver
- Meat extracts
- Sweetbreads

This next group of foods contains less purine but still may cause problems. Limit your intake to three to five small servings a week.

- Dry beans
- Dry peas
- Lentils
- Meats
- Oatmeal
- Poultry
- Seafood
- Spinach

---

have cured their gout by dropping a few pounds, losing too much weight too fast can actually trigger attacks. Ask your doctor for a sensible weight-loss program.

Eschew the brew. Alcohol, like those extra pounds, is trouble. Beer is double trouble, because it has a higher purine content than other alcoholic beverages. Not only can alcohol boost your production of uric acid, it also slows the excretion. You don't have to be a teetotaler just because you have gout, but moderation certainly is in order, Dr. Fort says.

Fill up on water. The more water you drink, the more you urinate, and the more you urinate, the more uric acid you expel. Again, this may not cure your gout, but it can help prevent some of the uric acid crystals from settling in your kidneys and urinary tract.

Protect your toes. Injured joints are particularly vulnerable to gout, and the big toe wages war daily with curbs, sprinklers and table legs. It's a good idea to keep your shoes on. Just be sure they're *comfortable* shoes; high heels or too-tight pumps can cause a serious toe jam.

Give cherries a try. There's no scientific evidence to show that eating cherries can relieve gout, but according to folklore and some gout sufferers today, the fruit works. Some have speculated that a natural agent in cherries may reduce levels of uric acid in the blood.

RELIEF FOR THE TERRIBLE TOES

In the days when gout really was the disease of kings (or at least of the upper crust), the treatments were less than royal. In fact, except for forgoing anchovies and liver with onions, there wasn't much they could do. The disease often progressed in unpleasant ways. For example, some people developed visible lumps in their ears, palms and fingertips. Gout could actually destroy an entire joint, sometimes bursting through the skin with a small eruption of white, needlelike crystals.

Even today, people with gout are about 200 times more likely to have kidney stones than are people without the disease. And even if they lose weight, eat the right foods and steer clear of beer, sometimes they are clouted with gout. But gout, Dr. Fort says, is "eminently treatable with drugs."

Today's drugs can relieve both the pain and the complications of gout, he says. One of the most popular drugs is colchicine, which can quickly quell most attacks. However, colchicine works best when used within 12 hours of an attack, Dr. Fort says. If you wait a day or two before getting treatment, it will be considerably less effective.

As with many drugs, however, colchicine carries side effects: Nausea, vomiting and diarrhea are most notable. To avoid these side effects, some doctors now prefer the nonsteroidal anti-inflammatory drugs (NSAIDs). Like colchicine, drugs such as ibuprofen and indomethacin work best when given soon after—or even before—an attack begins, Dr. Fort says. "After a while, people know when the attacks are coming. If they begin taking the NSAIDs before the redness and inflammation occur, they might be able to abort the attack."

A third choice for treatment is steroids, powerful drugs that can safely be given for two to three days to relieve pain and swelling. However, steroids can also cause side effects. For example, *rebound* attacks of gout will sometimes occur after the first attack was suppressed. For the most part, doctors use steroids only when colchicine or the NSAIDs don't do the trick.

While each of these drugs can beat the symptoms of gout, they won't cure the disease. If your attacks are frequent or unusually severe, your doctor may recommend drugs that will actually prevent them. For example, a drug called allopurinol, when taken every day, can lower the uric acid levels in your blood and in your urine, thus preventing further attacks.

Of course, using drugs for prevention can get expensive. It also puts you on medication—permanently. For most people, it's better simply to treat the symptoms, Dr. Fort says. "Gout is not that serious a disease. If you're having two attacks a year, it probably isn't worth taking pills every day just to prevent them."

Gum Disease

For people over age 35, gum disease outranks boxing, car accidents, ice hockey, hard candy and saltwater taffy as the leading cause of tooth loss. Three out of four adult Americans will have either the mild form of gum disease—gingivitis—or the severe form—periodontitis, or periodontal disease—at some point in their lives.

Despite such statistics, nine out of ten cases of gum disease could be prevented with simple, regular care, says William Clark, D.D.S., professor of oral biology and director of the Periodontal Disease Research Center at the University of Florida College of Dentistry.

We'll tell you exactly what proper care of your gums entails, but first, a brief explanation of how gum disease does its dirty work.

THE PLAQUE ATTACK

Gum disease starts with plaque. Plaque is a particularly loathsome, sticky concoction of mucus, food particles and bacteria that forms in the tiny spaces between your teeth and the gum line. Left to sit long enough, plaque can harden into a rock-hard substance called calculus.

In gingivitis, the plaque or calculus irritates and infects the gums. Your body's natural defenses against infection make the gums swollen and shiny, and they bleed easily when you brush or floss. As the gums swell, pockets form between the teeth and gums, providing a cozy home for even more plaque.

Gingivitis may lead to periodontitis, a severe form of gum disease caused by bacteria. In good health, the tiny culprits inhabit your mouth in very low numbers. However, poor oral hygiene gives them the green light to multiply, says Dr. Clark. They move into the pockets caused by gingivitis, and your mouth becomes a battleground. The bacteria try to gain a foothold, releasing toxins and enzymes to battle the fighter cells created by your own immune system.

The ongoing war eats away at your bones, gums and connective tissue, and over the years, your teeth loosen in their sockets. Cementum, the sensitive tissue enveloping the roots, becomes exposed, and you feel pain when you eat hot or cold foods. Occasionally an abscess will form in the pocket, and the infection will destroy yet more bone.

In both forms of gum disease, one telltale sign is bad breath. Periodontitis also brings a bad taste in the mouth.

PREVENTING GUM DISEASE

Ask anyone with dentures: Real, healthy teeth are better than false ones. Prevent gum disease, and you should keep your teeth forever. It's no so hard to do.

Brush daily. Let's see, when did you first hear this one? Brushing gently after every meal is best, Dr. Clark says, "but you probably don't need to take your toothbrush to work." (Still, it's a good idea, so at that important meeting you're not caught with broccoli between your teeth.)

Is brushing best done with a plain old toothbrush, with an electric one or with a more expensive gadget that shoots water into your gums? It really doesn't matter. "Electric toothbrushes are no better for most people, but they may help if you have trouble with dexterity," says Dr. Clark. An electric toothbrush may be more entertaining to use, so you may find yourself brushing more often—which is good. Thinking about the money you shelled out may also encourage you to brush more often!

Floss frequently. "At least three or four times a week is usually enough for most people, although flossing every day is best," says Dr. Clark. Floss cleans between teeth, where bristles often can't go.

Get regular professional cleanings. Even with good brushing and flossing, plaque can still form below the gum line. A visit to your dentist once every six months should be enough to keep the plaque at bay. "If your gums bleed when you brush, or if they're puffy looking, you may need cleaning more than twice a year," says Dr. Clark.

Try a mouthwash. This is purely an extra for your arsenal. Mouthwash can kill bacteria, but it's no substitute for brushing, flossing and cleaning.

Use a toothpick. Especially handy when you can't brush or floss, a toothpick can get rid of the big hunks of food and stimulate your gums. Be very gentle, though, to avoid stabbing your gums.

Stop smoking. One study says smoking doubles your risk of gum disease. While there's no proof smoking actually *causes* gum disease, there's plenty of evidence that it suppresses the immune system, "and that makes it harder for your body to fight the infection and makes the infection more resistant to treatment," says Dr. Clark.

TREATING PERIODONTITIS

Periodontal disease is irreversible, at least for now. "But if you have it, you can keep it from getting worse," says Dr. Clark. With the kind of treatment outlined below, you may be able to stop your pain—and save your teeth.

Pocket probing, which can measure the space between gum and tooth, shows your dentist how deep your pockets are (periodontitis-wise, not money-wise). But the traditional manual probe is slow and imprecise. You may benefit from the newer computerized probe in which a slender wire is inserted into the pocket and withdrawn in one-tenth of a second. The computer-aided probe is quicker and able to make more accurate measurements than the old-fashioned manual kind.

Planing and scaling—a *very* thorough cleaning of plaque and calculus from tooth and root—is the first line of attack in halting existing gum disease. One form of the procedure works best on front teeth, using anesthesia to go deeper than usual. This method can take 10 minutes per tooth but usually causes less gum shrinkage than surgery. For planing and scaling to have a chance to work, you have to follow up with your own commitment to faithful brushing and flossing.

Fiber-optic probes can be used instead of surgery for moderate periodontitis. Entering an incision so tiny that it doesn't need stitches, the probe pushes gum tissue aside and shines a light on the root surface, enabling the dentist to scrape off calculus. You might call this "scraping-edge" technology.

Antibiotics are often used in conjunction with cleaning or surgery, says Dr. Clark. Oral tetracycline is the most commonly used antibiotic, and more severe cases often call for amoxicillin. One new form of tetracycline comes in plastic fibers that are placed under the gum line, slowly releasing the medication over ten days, killing bacteria while reducing pockets.

Surgery may be needed in more advanced cases of gum disease. The doctor makes tiny incisions around the neck of the tooth to expose the root and bone, enabling a more thorough cleaning, removal of diseased tissue and a possible reshaping and even grafting of damaged bone and gums.

HAIR LOSS

Baldness, like blue eyes, is for many a result of hereditary potluck. It's a condition that affects about half of all men by age 50, says David A. Whiting, M.D., medical director of Baylor University Hair Research and Treatment Center and a clinical professor of dermatology at the University of Texas Southwestern Medical Center in Dallas.

The strands we leave behind in our hairbrushes are proof that what's hair today may be gone tomorrow. The average person loses 50 to 100 hairs a day. But virtually all of that grows back. Since we have approximately 100,000 hairs, losing 100 here and there doesn't amount to much anyway. But once a man passes his teens, the male hormone testosterone begins to affect his hair follicles. If he is genetically predisposed to baldness (and some men keep their hair forever), he will lose more hair than he replaces. The result is a condition called *androgenetic alopecia,* or simply male-pattern baldness.

HEADING BACK BALDNESS

For centuries men have sought remedies for lost hair, and always they've been disappointed.

As early as 4000 B.C., balding Egyptians were salving their scalps with exotic fruits, oils and animal parts in vain attempts to grow hair. But man's luck changed in the 1970s when doctors discovered that minoxidil, an oral medication for high blood pressure, also makes hair grow—on the head, arms, legs and face. Scientists lost no time in reformulating minoxidil as a liquid and testing it as a remedy for baldness.

"Minoxidil works by pushing hair back into anagen, which is the growth phase of hair," Dr. Whiting says. (The resting phase is called telogen.) "In due course, some hairs will grow longer and thicker and become more pigmented."

However, while minoxidil works for some men, it won't work for everyone, Dr. Whiting warns. "I tell my patients that it will produce hair growth you can see in one-third of the cases, it will produce some fuzz in about one-third of the cases, and it will do nothing in about one-third." What's more, he adds, the benefits are temporary: When you stop using minoxidil, your hard-earned hair will disappear in just a few months.

Minoxidil seems to work best for young men who have just started to lose hair. And it works much better on balding pates than on receding hairlines. But if you're already bald, it's probably too late. "This stuff is a much better preventive than restorative," concludes Dr. Whiting.

PLUGS INSTEAD OF RUGS

Apart from donning a wig, the fastest way to put hair on the roof is with a hair transplant. Assuming you still have an ample supply of your natural hair around the fringes, a trained surgeon can move it around to

---

BALD IS BEAUTIFUL

Some men worry that thinning hair represents lost youth and vitality. But there are a few guys—some 25,000, at least—who firmly believe that less is quite a bit more.

"The good Lord created only a few perfect heads, and the rest he covered with hair," says John T. Capps III, founder of Bald-Headed Men of America (BHMA), an international group that dedicates itself to helping the hairless.

BHMA got its start in 1972 when John lost a sales job because, the boss said, he looked too old. "I figured if it happened to me, it possibly happened to a lot of others." So John began asking his bald friends if they'd like to band together for mutual support. They said yes, and today BHMA has members in 50 states and 39 foreign countries.

Not surprisingly, the group is headquartered at 102 Bald Drive in Morehead City, North Carolina. Members attend an annual convention where they participate in self-help sessions and regale themselves with bald jokes. On a more serious note, they visit hospitals and pass out "Bald Is Beautiful" buttons, T-shirts and balloons to children who have lost their hair during cancer treatments.

John acknowledges that there are a lot of men in the world who are embarrassed to be bald. "There's a billion-dollar industry out there, and it plays on the vanity of those individuals." But the men in BHMA, he says, "don't believe in drugs, plugs or rugs."

---

help cover your bald spots, says Karen Burke, M.D., Ph.D., a dermatologic surgeon and clinical member of Scripps Clinic and Research Foundation in La Jolla, California.

Hair transplants have come a long way in recent years. In the past,

---

TREATMENT BREAKTHROUGH

THINGS ARE LOOKING UP

Today, even the miracle drug minoxidil often can't restore hair to anything resembling its former glory. But tomorrow, things could be different.

Eager to share the bonanza of profits now being enjoyed by Upjohn, other companies are competing to be next with a baldness breakthrough. Some promising research is under way.

One drug, called Tricomin, was tested at the University of Rheims, France. Doctors aren't sure how it made bald men start to grow hair, but they speculate that Tricomin may cause new blood vessels to form in the scalp and boost the pate's production of collagen, a natural protein that keeps skin healthy and supple.

Some researchers say the future of baldness treatment lies in deactivating or blocking male hormones in the scalp that cause follicles (from which hairs sprout) to shut down. Theoretically, any drug that blocks these hormones could control hair loss, and a number have been tried. The trick is to isolate their effects on the scalp without unsafely throwing off the hormonal balance elsewhere in the body.

Researchers at the University of Miami have made some exciting breakthroughs. According to Marty Sawaya, M.D., assistant professor of dermatology and leader of the research, we may see successful hormone treatments for hair loss by the year 2002.

And last, a number of Canadian tests are looking at electrical stimulation as a way to prevent or treat hair loss. The treatment consists of sitting under a helmetlike hood that painlessly bathes the head with a mild current. "The method sounds quackish, but the research being done is legitimate," says Harry Roth, M.D., clinical professor of dermatology at the University of California, San Francisco.

Whether you're thinking of investing in pharmaceutical stocks or a new hairbrush, you might want to exercise caution, says David A. Whiting, M.D., of Baylor University. Although a new miracle baldness treatment *may* be on the horizon, it could be some years before anything significantly better than minoxidil comes along, he says.

---

large tufts of hair were taken from the back of the head and grafted to the bald area, leaving the patient with an artificial "doll's hair" look. But today, with new microsurgical techniques—using minigrafts as small as a single hair—doctors can give you a much more natural-looking hairline.

Most transplants require two to four office visits of about 3 hours each. It depends on how much transplanting you need. Some doctors will suggest using minoxidil to help the transplants start growing.

Unlike your old, undependable hair, transplanted hair can last forever, Dr. Burke says. "A completed transplant looks fabulous," she adds. "Unless you're looking at it from very close, it really can look perfect."

COVERING UP

While drugs and surgery both are effective, there are easier ways to change your looks and improve your (remaining) locks, says Maurice Stein, owner of Cinema Secrets in Burbank, California, and makeup artist to the stars for more than 30 years. Some suggestions:

Cut it short. Short hair can make bald spots less obvious. "The shorter you wear it, the fuller the hair will look," says Stein.

Paint your pate. Have you ever noticed how movie stars, even those you *know* are older than you are, still have young-looking heads of hair? "It's scalp makeup," Stein says, "and it comes in black, dark brown, medium brown, light brown and gray. You just pat it right on the scalp, and it will dry in 15 to 20 seconds."

Get a wig. Shop around and find yourself a quality wig, preferably made from artificial fibers, because they are more durable, Stein says. "You can take it off at the end of the day, dip it in the sink, rinse it out and hang it up to dry." While you're at it, try some different styles, he adds. "Get several of them, and don't wear the same one every day. Treat it like a sports coat. I mean, all your sports coats aren't tweeds, so why should you wear the same hair every day?"

Hands off. "The less you fiddle around with your hair, the better," says Dr. Whiting. "I tell people to stop brushing and combing it all the time—the idea of 100 brush strokes a day is ridiculous," he says. Such overattention can only result in *quicker* hair loss.

HEADACHE

Y ou overslept. The kids fought over the last serving of breakfast cereal. You lost the car keys. Your husband spilled coffee on your blouse. That's when the pain began—a throbbing ache that escalated from a minor nuisance to a major-league skull buster. Now you are thinking about only one thing: finding relief.

Not all headaches are debilitating, of course. For the 40 to 50 million Americans who get headaches every year, the attacks usually are mild. But even a mild headache can make your head pound like a jackhammer, and more serious attacks such as migraines can make you physically ill. What's causing all this pain? Frankly, doctors aren't sure, says Robert S. Kunkel, M.D., head of the Section of Headache in the Department of Internal Medicine at the Cleveland Clinic in Cleveland. While some headaches are caused by tumors or head injuries, the majority aren't so easily diagnosed. "We have some pieces of the puzzle, but we really don't know what causes them," Dr. Kunkel says.

According to the International Headache Society, there are 12 categories of headache, including tension headaches, migraine headaches, cluster headaches and sinus headaches. Some people even get sex headaches, which strike precisely at the moment of orgasm.

THEMES AND VARIATIONS

The tension-type headache is by far the most common, affecting as many as nine out of ten people. Despite the name, these aren't always caused by emotional tension. They can also be caused by muscle strain, poor posture, even tired eyes. While tension-type headaches can be painful, they rarely cause serious, long-term problems, Dr. Kunkel says.

Migraine and cluster headaches, on the other hand, can cause very serious problems. "Migraine probably is the most disabling headache because of the nausea, vomiting and disability that accompany it," says Dr. Kunkel. "Cluster headaches are the most painful."

Both migraines and cluster headaches are called vascular headaches. Doctors suspect that insufficient levels of a neurochemical called serotonin set off the process by causing blood vessels in the brain to constrict (clamp down). The constriction reduces blood flow, which for some people causes the migraine "aura"—nausea, dizziness and altered vision—that may precede attacks. Following constriction, the affected blood vessels dilate (expand) to restore adequate blood flow. The expanded blood vessels press against adjoining nerves, causing migraine pain—a throbbing headache on one side of the head that can last for hours or even days.

Cluster headaches also are accompanied by changes in cranial blood flow. Unlike migraines, however, they are short-lived, lasting less than an hour. Whereas migraines can occur at any time, cluster headaches occur in predictable "clusters," three- to eight-week periods during which they may strike several times a day. "They're sometimes called 'suicide headaches,' " Dr. Kunkel says. "I've known people who broke their hands because they hit the wall during attacks."

FOOD FOES

Although doctors aren't sure what causes migraines, they have identified migraine triggers—conditions or substances that put the process in motion. "Migraine is an inherited condition, but many foods can trigger it," Dr. Kunkel says. In fact, approximately half of all migraine sufferers say that certain foods—chocolate, for example, or the food additive monosodium glutamate (MSG)—stimulate attacks.

MSG often is a headache trigger, says Jack A. Klapper, M.D., director of the Colorado Neurology and Headache Center in Denver. Laboratory studies have shown that when blood vessels are exposed to MSG, they steadily contract.

Because MSG often is used in oriental cooking, the term "Chinese restaurant syndrome" was coined to describe MSG-related headaches. MSG is found not only in chop suey, however, but in frozen foods, lunch meats, canned and dry soups and many other processed foods as well. You have to be something of a detective to avoid it. It may be listed on labels as "hydrolyzed vegetable protein," "natural flavor" or simply "flavoring."

A class of chemicals called nitrites can also trigger migraines, even in small amounts. Used to preserve bacon, sausage, canned ham, smoked fish and other meats, nitrites can cause blood vessels to dilate, sometimes producing throbbing headaches within a half hour.

"Many people who suffer from migraines will get a headache when they drink red wine," adds Dr. Klapper. Along with foods such as cheddar cheese and pickled herring, red wines contain tyramine, a chemical compound that can ring the headache bell.

Other foods to watch out for include peas, chocolate, navy and lima beans and fresh bread. "But migraine rarely is caused by one food alone,"

Dr. Klapper says. To discover which food (or combination of foods) is giving you trouble, try keeping a headache diary, Dr. Kunkel suggests. When you feel a migraine coming on, make a list of everything you ate in the last 24 hours. In time, you'll learn which foods you can enjoy—and which to avoid.

THE TENSION CONNECTION

Muscle tension is one cause of headaches. So is plain old tension. Stress, worry, anxiety—these can make your head pound right when you lack the emotional strength to fight back.

PROFILE IN HEALING

MARY HENNEBERGER: SHE'S IN CONTROL

After talking with Mary K. Henneberger of Hamilton, Ohio, it's hard to imagine that this cheerful, energetic woman has spent nearly half her life battling the relentless pain of migraine headaches. "They could last as long as two days, and the pain was intense," says Mary. "They became an awful cross to bear."

Although Mary has had headaches ever since she was a child, they got progressively worse after the birth of her first son. As time went by, they occurred more and more frequently. "I was teaching English at Miami University in Oxford, Ohio," she remembers. "I didn't miss many classes, but on weekends I would collapse on the couch for three days. It just seemed like my whole life was made up of pain."

Mary went from doctor to doctor, but nothing they recommended seemed to help. Then in the mid-1970s, she checked into the Diamond Headache Clinic in Chicago. Doctors there put her on propranolol (Inderal), a blood pressure drug that also helps prevent migraines. At the same time, they laid down some strict rules. "I was told to eliminate from my diet things that are suspected of causing headaches, such as chocolate, alcohol and aged cheese. I also learned to practice biofeedback," she adds.

The treatments helped, and today, 15 years later, Mary is back in control. She still gets headaches. "But I'm no longer the person on the couch with the ice bags," she says. Indeed, she now writes a column for the National Headache Foundation newsletter. "I want to help people who don't know they can get help."

Don't give up. Studies have shown that people who practice relaxation techniques—for example, biofeedback—can reduce headaches by as much as 80 to 90 percent.

It takes time (and assistance from your doctor) to learn biofeedback, but the results may last forever. "Once you learn to relax your muscles with biofeedback, you'll find it's not something you actively have to do," says Barry A. Reich, Ph.D., director of the Comprehensive Pain Program at the Nassau Pain and Stress Center in Westbury, New York. "It becomes an almost automatic response."

In one study, 703 headache sufferers were treated with hypnosis, biofeedback, transcutaneous electrical nerve stimulation (TENS) or a combination of these treatments. At the beginning of the treatment, 88 percent were taking prescription headache medication. After 15 weeks of once-a-week treatments, only 11 percent still needed the prescription drugs. What's more, benefits still were evident *three years* after people left the program.

"With some types of biofeedback, what you're training the person to do is regulate blood flow throughout different parts of the body," Dr. Reich explains. "I think biofeedback often should be the primary treatment for both migraine and tension-type headache."

HEAD OFF HEADACHE PAIN

Apart from food and muscle tension, there are many factors—stress, menstruation, even weather changes—that can trigger headaches. "If a woman is coming up on her period and the weather is changing, those are two factors," Dr. Kunkel says. "Then if she takes a little wine or too much salt or eats some cheese or chocolate, she might get a doozy of a headache."

To disarm the headache bomb:

Keep regular hours. It's not unusual for people to get headaches when their normal schedules are disrupted—while traveling, for example, or keeping late hours on weekends. "Many people will do better by keeping a regular schedule of eating, drinking and sleeping," Dr. Kunkel says.

Loosen up. If you go through life with a stiff upper lip and a clenched jaw, there's a good chance some of that tension will migrate into your head. "It's very important that you try to identify what it is in your life that's causing your muscles to contract," says Dr. Reich.

At work, pounding on the computer all day can make the muscles in your neck and shoulders lock up. High heels can throw your whole body out of alignment. Even using a chair that's too high or too low can cause trouble. Once you identify the tension makers in your life, Dr. Reich says, you can begin relieving the problem—and the resulting tension head-aches—as well.

Head for the workout room. "Exercise seems to be a wonderful headache reducer," Dr. Reich adds. By relieving tension and anxiety, exercise can help relieve tension-type headaches as well. It has also been found to boost the body's production of certain chemicals—endorphins, for example—that can help dull headache pain.

Say no to joe. Caffeine is yet another chemical that can make your blood vessels constrict and dilate. If you suspect that headaches are brewing at the percolator, switch to decaf or herbal tea instead.

Reach for the aspirin. This potent painkiller—or its herbal equivalent, white willow bark—has been used for thousands of years to quell

---

DRUGS THAT HELP

If you have migraines that are both frequent and severe, your doctor may recommend that you take daily doses of antimigraine drugs. While not a cure, these drugs can help prevent headaches from controlling your life.

Commonly used for treating high blood pressure, a class of drugs called beta-receptor blockers—beta-blockers for short—can help prevent migraines by inhibiting dilation of the blood vessels. At the same time, they affect the brain's absorption of serotonin, a neurochemical that is integrally involved during attacks and that may trigger the entire migraine process, says Jack A. Klapper, M.D., director of Denver's Colorado Neurology and Headache Center.

While effective, beta-blockers such as propranolol (Inderal) and nadolol (Corgard) can cause side effects—weight gain and increases in cholesterol, for example—so they're typically prescribed only for people who have frequent attacks, says Robert S. Kunkel, M.D., head of the Cleveland Clinic's headache section.

A related class of drugs called calcium-channel blockers also helps prevent migraines by blocking painful changes in blood vessels. As with beta-blockers, however, they can cause side effects and generally are used when necessary.

A third class of drugs, antidepressants, has been found to be very effective in heading off headaches. Taken in low doses, drugs such as amitriptyline (Elavil) and nortriptyline (Pamelor) are thought to help by boosting serotonin levels in the brain and perhaps by dulling the brain's perception of pain as well.

headache pain. Americans consume more than 80 million aspirin tablets a day, along with aspirin "substitutes" such as ibuprofen and acetaminophen. Not only does aspirin work as a painkiller, it also helps prevent clotting agents in the blood from sticking together. This can help reduce the arterial "pounding" that causes headaches, Dr. Reich explains. "It just makes everything in the blood flow easier."

PRESCRIPTION RELIEF

When headaches strike, everything else stops. To put you on the move again, your doctor may recommend prescription drugs to quell the pain.

For example, to stop migraines already in progress, doctors often recommend prescription drugs called ergotamines. By constricting blood vessels to the brain, these drugs help "shut off" the pulsations that cause the pain, usually in less than an hour.

Unfortunately, ergotamines can cause serious side effects, which limits their usefulness, Dr. Klapper says. Not only do they stimulate the brain's vomiting center (with predictable consequences), but they can cause nausea and chest pain and decrease circulation to your limbs as well.

Less problematic is naproxen, a prescription nonsteroidal anti-inflammatory drug (NSAID). "In some head-to-head studies, the ergotamines and the NSAIDs have been found to be equally good," Dr. Klapper says. In one study, researchers at the Menninger Clinic in Topeka, Kansas, gave people with migraine either naproxen or an ergotamine compound. While the treatments were equally effective, people taking naproxen experienced less nausea and vomiting. "In my practice, and I would suspect in some others, the NSAIDs are putting the ergotamines in second place," Dr. Klapper says.

HOME REMEDIES

There are no "magic bullets" that will stop headaches cold. However, there are things you can do to lower their firepower.

Put it on ice. At one headache clinic, people with migraine and cluster headaches were given either medication or medication plus a cold pack. Although the cold packs didn't take the headache away, 71 percent of the people using them said that they helped reduce the pain. This traditional remedy is worth a try, Dr. Kunkel says. By constricting arteries in the scalp, cold compresses can help relieve painful throbbing as well.

Heat it up. A long, hot shower or bath, by relaxing muscle contractions in the neck, back and scalp can help relieve tension-type headaches.

Rub it away. Wrestlers long have known that if you decrease the flow of blood to the brain by pressing on the carotid artery under the ear, you can make your opponent pass out. No, you don't have to go three rounds with Ivan the Mangler to beat migraine pain. "What you can do is press on the temple right in front of the ear," Dr. Kunkel suggests. "If the artery

---

TREATMENT BREAKTHROUGH

STOPPING MIGRAINE HEADACHES COLD

The prescription "Take two aspirin and call me in the morning" probably was written for headaches. It's sound advice, but *slow*. In fact, there has never been a shortcut to headache relief.

That's about to change. Researchers have been investigating a drug that appears to stop headache pain at the source—apparently within minutes.

Called sumatriptan, this drug helps the brain absorb a neurochemical called serotonin. "Serotonin is all over the body—in the gut, in the liver, in the heart," says Jack A. Klapper, M.D., director of Denver's Colorado Neurology and Headache Center. However, should serotonin levels in the brain decline, there may be a corresponding *increase* in pain-causing chemicals—substance P, for example—that set the migraine ball in motion.

Researchers long have known that injections of serotonin quell headache pain. But they also cause vomiting and diarrhea. What's needed, Dr. Klapper explains, is a drug that boosts serotonin uptake in the brain *without* the side effects.

Enter sumatriptan, an experimental drug that research has shown to be extremely effective in aborting migraine and cluster headaches. "The advantage of sumatriptan appears to be that it affects only cranial serotonin receptors—it's very specific," Dr. Klapper says. You don't get the side effects you get with other drugs.

In one study, German researchers treated 23 people (and 25 migraines) with 2 milligrams of sumatriptan. Within 10 to 20 minutes, in 71 percent of the cases, the pain was completely relieved. What's more, the drug caused fewer side effects than other antimigraine drugs.

"In the future," Dr. Klapper says, "there will be many more drugs like sumatriptan."

is dilated and pounding and you reduce the blood flow by pressing it, it's not going to throb as much."

Fight it with feverfew. In a British study, migraine sufferers were given one capsule a day of the herb feverfew, a member of the daisy family. Feverfew reduced their attacks by 24 percent and helped reduce the accompanying nausea and vomiting as well. Many health food stores carry feverfew capsules.

HEARING LOSS

*B*OOM! BOOM! BOOM! "So how's Henry doing?" *WHAM-WHAMWHAMWHAMWHAM!* "Yes, it is good, isn't it?" *SKREEEEEEEEK!* "Oh, I'm sorry to hear that." *BOOMSKITCHABOOMSKITCHABOOMSKITCHABOOM!* "Huh?" *ARF-ARF-ARF-ARF-ARF-ARF-ARF-ARF-ARF-ARF-ARF!* "Oh, I agree completely." *RATTARATTARATTARATTARATTARATTA!* "Yes, well, uh ... nice *(BANGBANGBANGBANG!)* talking to you." *ROAR-ROARROAR!*

Ah, yes, nothing like a good conversation to bring us closer together. If only we could hear above the noise of the neighborhood, the factory, the rifle range, the power drill, the pile driver, the boom box, the road crew's jackhammer, Henry's new chain saw, the neighbor's dogs, the jets taking off, the 18-wheelers barreling down the freeway . . .

A DEAFENING SOCIETY

Hearing loss is mainly about noise. Noise is making us deaf before our time, which, in the best of all worlds, would never come. Add up all the other causes of hearing loss—aging, injury and congenital problems top the list—and they still amount to only a fraction of the damage caused by noise, says John S. Turner, Jr., M.D., head of otolaryngology at Emory University in Atlanta and chief of otolaryngology–head and neck surgery at the Emory Clinic.

Take aging. "It's to be expected that as you age, you'll have physical changes in your ears, nerves and brain that will begin to impair your hearing," Dr. Turner says. "After age 70, you begin to lose hearing steadily. It's unusual to reach your late seventies without some degree of hearing impairment, and most people at that age could use a hearing aid, although they often won't admit it. But most of the impairment should be minor,

cy end of the hearing spectrum. That means
th women and children, who have higher-

1 tribespeople of northern Africa shows that
e well into their eighties—hear as well as ten-
r says. That's because they don't have to hear
g and camels grunting and children playing.
ost of the major losses of hearing are related
ialized society," Dr. Turner says. "Men are
f their jobs and recreational activities." From
gunshots at the rifle range to the chain saws
their ears almost nonstop.
nage to get away from it all for a while doesn't
dditive," Dr. Turner says. "It builds up over
g your sense of hearing."
and above—overstimulates the cells in your
d to the auditory nerve. "It exhausts the
urner says. "If it's just a brief exposure, the
ise lasts a few hours, the damage is perma-
l—they've done so much work they burn
unters who have lost much of their hearing
of shotguns."
...bers and more? A screaming child can hit 115, and a
jackhammer, 120; a jet engine at 100 feet blasts out 130, a firing gun, 140,
and a firecracker, 160.

THE BIG TURNOFF

Since noise is the number one cause of hearing loss, it only makes
sense that turning down the volume can save your hearing. Hearing loss
is preventable, Dr. Turner says. Here are the best things you can do to get
rid of deafening noise.

Wear ear protection. Earplugs and earmuffs have become standard
equipment in many noisy jobs. But if you're exposed to loud noise for long
periods of time off the job—using a power mower, weed whacker or chain
saw is a good example—make ear protectors a habit. Don't worry that you
won't hear what you have to: Ear protectors can sometimes *improve* hearing in a noisy environment by filtering out extraneous noise.

Protect your head. Head injuries—from car, motorcycle and bicycle
accidents—are a common cause of hearing loss. "The impact compresses
the inner ear fluid, which then squeezes against the hair cells so strongly
it damages them," Dr. Turner says. So wear your seat belts and helmets.

Beware of rock in your head. Rock musicians are known to suffer hearing loss, but fans are falling victim, too, Dr. Turner says. Long hours listening to music in a headset at high volume can definitely damage your hearing, he says. Most experts consider 80 decibels the cutoff point for hearing safety, but a survey of music headset users found that their listening volumes ranged up to 102 decibels. If you can't carry on a normal conversation while wearing a headset, it's too loud—on a scale of 1 to 10, the maximum setting should not be above 4.

Smoke gets in your ears. The carbon dioxide in smoke restricts the flow of oxygen to the cells of the inner ear. Johns Hopkins University researchers found that rats simultaneously exposed to carbon dioxide and noise suffered permanent hearing loss averaging 20 decibels.

Don't be a fathead. Saturated fat can block the tiny arteries feeding your ears just as it does the big arteries that feed your heart. The inadequate blood flow that results keeps your ears from recovering from noise damage as quickly as they should. Watch your diet, for your heart *and* your ears.

Eat a balanced and varied diet. Eating well goes beyond cutting back on fat. Zinc, calcium, magnesium and vitamin A all have been shown to benefit the sense of hearing. These nutrients are readily available in a healthy, balanced diet.

Keep the top up. People who drive long distances with convertible tops down or windows open or on motorcycles get blasted with wind noise, which can reach the 80- to 90-decibel range, Dr. Turner estimates. While that's within the range of safety set by the Occupational Safety and Health Administration, those standards are general, and your ears may be more sensitive.

TINNITUS: DON'T ANSWER THAT

It's not really the phone. It's your ears. And for some people with tinnitus, the ringing seldom stops. Dr. Turner estimates that one in ten Americans between the ages of 65 and 74—about 25 million people—has tinnitus.

"Tinnitus is a monumental problem, even more than hearing loss, because there's very little that can be done to help," Dr. Turner says. "There's no medical or surgical treatment. There's no safe drug—some help tinnitus but put you at risk of heart arrhythmia [irregular heartbeat]. The only proven thing you can do is prevent it, because noise is the most common cause. (Head trauma is second.) It's the most frustrating problem ear doctors face."

And think how the victims feel, going through life with bells in their heads that no one else can hear. "It's with you day and night," says Dr. Turner. "It ranges from merely an annoyance to, in about 15 percent of the cases, real interference with work and life."

Tinnitus is often a sign of deterioration of hearing, although you can have one without the other, Dr. Turner says. "We don't really know what's

---

PROFILE IN HEALING

ELEANOR SCHWARZ: HEARING LIFE AGAIN

As a 54-year-old teacher, Eleanor Schwarz realized she was hearing less and less when her students would laugh when she answered questions—or *thought* she answered questions. "I soon realized I was answering something they hadn't asked," she says. "I was having trouble hearing them."

No doctor was ever able to tell her what was causing her increasing deafness. "As a child, she had many ear infections and abscesses," says her husband, Maurice. "And those were the days before antibiotics. She feels it may have contributed to her hearing loss, but that's pure conjecture."

For years, Eleanor got along with hearing aids, but her impairment increased. "I had only 4 percent of my hearing left," she says. She was beginning to take sign language instruction and was increasingly isolated from husband, family and friends.

But American high technology—in the form of a cochlear implant—saved Eleanor from the kind of social isolation only not hearing can create. Unlike hearing aids, which magnify sound to reach the inner ear, cochlear implants have tiny wires with electrodes that are surgically inserted into the cochlea of the inner ear to transmit sound energy.

The recipient of the implant has to learn how to use it—the sounds coming across are not normal, so there are a lot of new interpretive skills to be learned. Cochlear implants are not for everyone with hearing loss and are also very expensive.

Eleanor got the implant in December 1988, when she was 68. "And it has made all the difference in the world," she says. "I stopped having to learn sign language. I can talk on the telephone now, although it's hard to understand strangers. I do still have to use lipreading, but now I can hear people talking when they're behind me. I can hear birds, rain, water running. You don't realize what you've lost until you regain it."

happening in the ear when it's ringing," he says, although one theory says that the inner ear's sensitive hair cells get so overwhelmed with the work of transmitting noise that they start misfiring.

Although there is no cure for tinnitus, there are a few things you can do to mask the noise.

Turn up the white noise. White noise is a kind of sound you hear when the TV station you're watching signs off for the night. There are machines that duplicate this sound, which masks the ringing of tinnitus in about 50 percent of the cases, Dr. Turner says.

Try a hearing aid. It's been known for some time that a hearing aid can reduce tinnitus noise—studies show up to two-thirds of people who've tried them reported reduction or total elimination of tinnitus. Why? No one knows for sure, but it may be that amplified outside noise masks the inner noise. Or at least for people whose hearing is normal or near normal, the noise produced by the hearing aid's electronic circuitry may cancel out the tinnitus.

Mask the noise with more noise. This is essentially what a tinnitus masker does. The device looks like a hearing aid but produces either a wide or narrow band of noise. You can control how wide the spectrum is and the volume. This manufactured noise drowns out the noise of tinnitus, and although it's still noise, it's external, which may be more tolerable than the internal noise of tinnitus. It has been proven effective for up to half of the people who've tried it, but the only way to know if it will work for you is to try it yourself. Your doctor can prescribe a unit, and you should be given a monthlong trial to see if it's the right one for you. Some of the people who use maskers find that they have what's called residual inhibition when they don't wear the masker—a period of time when the tinnitus is totally gone. Then it gradually reappears.

Give your tinnitus some feedback. Biofeedback training can teach you to relax to the point that your tinnitus may become more tolerable. Studies show that the majority of tinnitus sufferers benefit from biofeedback; they sleep better and need fewer tranquilizers and antidepressants.

Pack away the cigarettes. "The relationship of smoking to tinnitus is much less direct than that of noise," Dr. Turner says, but the association is there nonetheless. "We think it may constrict the blood vessels feeding the inner ear, which would harm the nerve cells," he says. "And smoking definitely aggravates existing hearing problems."

Rethink your drinks. Caffeine is a well-known constrictor of blood vessels and should be used in moderation by those with tinnitus. Limit your coffee, tea and cola. Besides caffeinated drinks, red wine, tonic water (quinine) and grain-based spirits may also aggravate tinnitus. To find out which drinks affect you, try keeping a diary of what you drink and how it relates to tinnitus attacks.

Keep tabs on your medications. "Aspirin is the leading cause of hearing loss and tinnitus when it comes to medication," Dr. Turner says, "but it's strictly individual. Some people with arthritis have to take large amounts before they get any tinnitus or hearing loss, while my wife can take just one and get ringing in her ears." When you stop taking aspirin, or so much aspirin, the tinnitus usually disappears, and your hearing returns to normal. If you think aspirin may be causing your problem, Dr. Turner advises switching to ibuprofen or acetaminophen.

Check with your doctor. Tinnitus sometimes has a medical cause—an aneurysm or a narrowing in blood vessels, high triglycerides in your blood or even excessive earwax. It's best to check with your doctor to get a proper diagnosis.

Above all, don't give up hope. Up to three-fourths of people with tinnitus say it improves over time.

HIGH-TECH HELP

Some experts say that hearing aids may soon become as common as glasses, as people grow more comfortable with admitting their hearing isn't what it used to be. These people will come from the ranks of baby boomers, who grew up in the world's noisiest civilization. In fact, our rock and roll culture has dropped the average age for first-time hearing aid wearers from 60 to 50.

So if you can't hear normal conversation clearly, it's time to listen up: Have your doctor first check you out and then recommend an audiologist.

Try the new-wave hearing aid. It's the digital revolution in music technology that has provided the most recent advance in hearing aids. New digitally programmable aids use a computer-generated signal and are adjusted like the finest stereo equipment—for more bass, more treble, a "warmer" tone, filtering out background noise. You can use a small remote control device—like the one controlling your TV—to adjust them, so no one has to see you fiddling with your ear. These are the most expensive hearing aids, but as with all new technology, their prices should eventually go down.

Stick it in your ear. In-the-ear aids are favorites, because they're hard for others to see. They are small and fit into your ear canal. Because of their minute size, in-the-ear aids may be difficult to manipulate and care for. Their batteries are tiny and hard to change, so people with arthritis in their hands may have a particularly difficult time. In-the-ear aids are not as expensive as digital aids but cost more than behind-the-ear and on-the-body aids.

Stick it all over your ear. Well, not exactly. Behind-the-ear aids have an earpiece molded to fit in the bowl of your outer ear and a power pack worn behind the ear. They're large and moderately powerful for moderate to profound hearing loss. So who cares what they look like? Hearing is more important than appearance.

Wear it. The most powerful hearing aids connect the earpiece to an amplifier you carry in your clothing. All that juice is best for the most profound hearing loss.

For more information on hearing aids, contact the National Hearing Aid Society at 20361 Middlebelt Road, Livonia, MI 48152, or call their help line at (800) 521-5247.

TREATMENT BREAKTHROUGH

AND THE DEAF SHALL HEAR . . .

If you lose your hearing in the 21st century, chances are that scientists will be able to do something about it, say researchers at the Johns Hopkins Center for Hearing and Balance in Baltimore.

Most people lose their hearing because noise, age, ototoxic drugs (drugs that poison the ear) and head injuries combine to destroy the ear's hair cells, explains Bill Brownell, Ph.D., a researcher at Johns Hopkins whose work is defining the cutting edge of otology. Scientists had always believed that once these cells were destroyed, hearing was gone forever. The cells could not grow back.

But recently, researchers discovered that these hair cells can regenerate in animals, says Dr. Brownell. "The question now is, can we regenerate them in man?"

It's a big question, admits center director Murray Sachs, Ph.D. But if researchers can find the genetic factors that turn off cell growth after the ear is formed in the womb, they may well be able to restart the growth process and regenerate damaged cells.

The result? In a sense, scientists may one day be able to grow you a "new" pair of ears.

HEART DISEASE

Bubba's a little anxious. He just hit 59, the same age his dad was when he dropped dead from a heart attack back in 1964.

You could say that Bubba has something to be anxious about. Although he admits he's "a little" overweight, in truth, Bubba's clothing size has increased over the years from jumbo to family to oh-my-God-it's-coming-toward-us! His blood pressure is an outrageously high 220/120, and he smokes so much that he goes through two lighters a day. The only exercise Bubba gets is lumbering back and forth between the television set and the kitchen.

Bubba knows that his bacon-crunching lifestyle puts him at an increased risk for heart disease. But Bubba doesn't think it matters much. "It's the genes that are gonna get me anyway, just like they got the old man," he says. "What difference does it make what I do?"

The truth is that what Bubba does or doesn't do makes a *big* difference—bad genes or not.

"There's no way you can avoid the genetic inheritance that predisposes you to heart attack, but you have abundant opportunities to overcome other risk factors that multiply your inherited risk," says Edward D. Frohlich, M.D., vice president of academic affairs with the Alton Ochsner Medical Foundation in New Orleans and an official of the American Heart Association.

Approximately one in four Americans has some form of cardiovascular disease (*cardio-* refers to the heart, *-vascular* to the blood vessels). In one recent year, these diseases claimed one American life every 32 seconds— that's nearly one million Americans, one out of every two deaths in the nation. And even though the death rate from heart disease is dropping— by almost 25 percent in the decade between 1978 and 1988—it is still the number one killer in America. It's a startling statistic when you consider there's so much *you* can do to prevent heart disease. But to best understand how to avoid it, you need to understand how you get it.

Public Enemy No. 1

Atherosclerosis—deposits of cholesterol, calcium and scar tissue and cellular growth in the coronary arteries—leads to heart disease by restricting blood flow to the heart muscle. Hardening of the arteries is responsible for most heart disease in America and for more than 90 percent of all heart attacks, says Virgil Brown, M.D., president of the American Heart Association and professor of medicine at Emory University in Atlanta.

The first noticeable sign of atherosclerosis is often an angina attack—a crushing, burning or squeezing pain in the chest that radiates to the left arm, neck, jaw or shoulder blade. The pain comes when the heart needs more blood—after exertion, a large meal, emotional excitement or exposure to cold—but has difficulty getting it because the arteries are too "hardened" with other debris to allow for the free flow of blood. Angina often makes its victims think they're having a heart attack. But angina is usually only a warning. A real heart attack—in which there's sufficient blockage of blood to actually kill part of the heart muscle—may be on the way.

Such serious blockage does not occur overnight. It's the long-term result of atherosclerosis. Year after year, the coronary artery narrows as those deposits grow along the arterial wall. Finally, one unhappy day—Plunk!—the tiny remaining tunnel gets stuffed up with a blood clot. No blood reaches a part of the heart, and that part begins to suffocate. Next thing you know, you're in the hospital or the morgue.

Although you don't have symptoms of atherosclerosis until it's pretty far along, there's no reason to let it sneak up on you. And don't even *think* that clogging of the arteries is a normal expectation of aging, says Dr. Brown. In cultures where risk factors are low, people live to old age without significant clogging in their arteries—and as a result, these people have healthier hearts. "In fact, most people in our own culture can live into their nineties without heart disease if they live right," says Dr. Brown.

10 Ways to Prevent Heart Disease

There are lots of things you could do for your heart, but according to one poll of hundreds of top cardiologists, among the most vital heart-saving measures are those listed here. Depending on what you're already doing, you can choose what to add to your own strategy.

Cut your cholesterol. There's a one in three chance that the amount of total cholesterol swimming around in your blood is borderline high—between 200 and 239 milligrams per deciliter—and that level hikes your risk of dying from coronary heart disease (the kind of heart disease caused by clogged coronary arteries) by 70 percent. If your cholesterol level is 240 or more, as it is in one in four Americans, your death risk goes up a terrifying 200 percent. At those levels, you'd have plenty of company at the morgue: The federal Centers for Disease Control in Atlanta estimates that high cholesterol levels alone cause more than 300,000 needless deaths each year, making it the number one contributor to fatal heart attacks in America.

According to the National Cholesterol Education Project, you should aim for a total cholesterol level of less than 200, but many doctors say you should aim even lower. "Clearly 150 would be much better, because about four billion people on this earth have a cholesterol level of 150, and they don't get cardiovascular disease," says William Castelli, M.D., director of the landmark Framingham Heart Study in Massachusetts.

How do you lower your cholesterol level? Start with cutting down on the two things in your diet most related to high blood cholesterol—cholesterol-rich foods, and foods high in saturated fat. Fortunately, the two are often one and the same and mostly fall into the category of fatty meats, dairy products and junk foods. (For a full program on lowering your cholesterol level, see "High Cholesterol" on page 288.)

Get up and go. Experts say that inactivity is the number two source of fatal heart attacks in America—205,000 in 1985 alone. By virtue of being an American, there's a better than one in three chance that you're not getting the exercise you need, and that a sedentary lifestyle gives you a 90 percent better chance of dying from a heart attack.

We can hear moans wafting from the TV room already. But cheer up—you don't have to go to extremes. "The message has been confused," says Thomas Kottke, M.D., a cardiologist at the Mayo Clinic in Rochester, Minnesota. People think they won't get anything out of it if they do less than a marathon. In fact, a brisk walk 20 minutes a day would make a major impact. "The average person is so sedentary that any exercise other than flipping through the channels or cracking a beer is great," he says.

Blow off that excess blood pressure. Chances are one in eight that your systolic blood pressure (the top number) is between 140 and 159, and that level gives you a 70 percent higher chance of developing a blocked coronary artery that can lead to a heart attack. The odds that your systolic blood pressure tops 159 are one in six, and that high a level raises the odds against surviving a heart attack by almost 200 percent. That makes high blood pressure the number three cause of fatal heart attacks in America.

The time to start controlling your blood pressure is no later than age 20, and the place is your doctor's office—you should have your blood pressure checked at least every 2 1/2 years, more often if it's on the high side. The first three steps to normal blood pressure are controlling your weight, cutting down on dietary sodium—as many as one in three people are sodium sensitive, says Dr. Frohlich—and reducing your alcohol consumption to no more than two drinks a day. (For lots more on lowering high blood pressure, see "High Blood Pressure" on page 277.)

Lose your excess baggage. China has more people, but America probably weighs more. We Yanks are fatsos. More than two-thirds of us are overweight. Those who are 30 percent or more overweight have double the chances of dropping dead from a heart attack. And just because you're only 10 or 20 percent above your ideal weight is no cause to rejoice: You're giving a heart attack a 50 percent better chance to kill you. Excess weight, say the experts, is the number four cause of fatal heart attacks in the nation.

Stop smoking. In 1989, heart disease from smoking killed 115,000 Americans—9,000 more than smoking-caused lung cancer. If you're a

---

PROFILE IN HEALING

BOB FINNELL: LIFE BEFORE LIFESTYLE

Bob Finnell was living what some people might call the American dream: a high-powered executive controlling millions of dollars, with more frequent flyer miles than a Canada goose, gourmet meals complete from soup to dessert, 40 extra pounds of fat, heart attack . . .

The attack came on a Labor Day 1985 hike in Yosemite National Park, but he didn't think the wooziness and weakness was a heart attack. "I kept walking until we were off the mountain," he says, "then I had a beer and nibbled on chips while a friend drove us to our lodge. The next morning I flew back to New York and went back to work."

A couple of weeks later, he went to see his doctor. He was given several tests and was just about to hop on the treadmill when his EKG results came in. "Don't let Finnell take his treadmill!" the doctor shouted. The EKG showed a large area of dead heart muscle. Bob's life was changed forever.

Only he didn't know it. The doctor recommended immediate bypass surgery. "I scheduled it to happen in late 1985, between board meetings," says Bob. But after he saw a picture of his own heart blockage on the doctor's high-tech equipment, Bob began to study up on heart disease.

His studies convinced him that his heart disease had multiple causes, particularly his high-fat, high-cholesterol diet. Bob's research

---

smoker, you're about twice as likely to have coronary heart disease and heart attacks—and you have a 70 percent greater chance of dying from a heart attack. One study of 120,000 women traced half the heart attacks in middle-aged women to smoking. Doctors think that breathing in smoke makes your blood clot more easily. In addition, smoking adds to the likelihood that you'll have high blood pressure and high cholesterol. If, however, you can quit your habit, the benefits come very quickly. But don't fool yourself into thinking you can "cut down," cautions Dr. Brown. "Saying 'I smoke only five cigarettes a day' is like saying 'I drive 120 miles per hour only one or two times a week.' " That is, cigarettes are too dangerous to play games with.

Stop smoking smokers' smoke. They call it passive smoking, but it really does an active job on your heart. Secondhand smoke kills over 35,000 Americans a year via heart disease, estimates Stanton Glantz, Ph.D., professor of medicine at the University of California, San Francisco. "Non-

---

also convinced him that he was a poor bypass candidate. "I realized that if I went through the bypass, I could very easily go back to the same old habits," he says. "I'd end up having a scholarship named after me before 1990." Instead, he got into an experimental study on reversing heart disease supervised by Dean Ornish, M.D., assistant clinical professor of medicine at the University of California, San Francisco. Dr. Ornish taught Bob a completely different lifestyle.

The new lifestyle included a diet that cost him about $5 a day. "That wouldn't have paid for my appetizers before," he says. It also included lots of exercise and relaxation. More than a half decade after he could well have died, Bob still sticks to the program. "I followed it 100 percent for four years, and now I follow it 99.9 percent," he says. "I miss a day of yoga occasionally, I have part of an avocado now and then, or a little caviar, a sliver of cheese." He walks for 1 hour five or six mornings a week. He does yoga and relaxation every day for 60 to 90 minutes. He is at his army-discharge weight, travels for pleasure, takes his time in all things.

Bob's life, in some ways restricted (he can never return to full-time work), has expanded in others. "I read much more, I've learned languages, I travel for leisure, I spend time with friends," he says. The only vestige of Bob's former lifestyle is a 1,000-bottle wine cellar, which he still dips into—but only on occasion.

smokers married to smokers have a 30 percent increase in risk of dying from heart disease over nonsmokers married to nonsmokers," she says.

Take aspirin. Aspirin is rapidly becoming a mainstay in preventing heart attacks. By making blood platelets slippery instead of sticky, aspirin cuts down on clotting. In one study, just one 325-milligram aspirin taken every other day was shown to reduce the incidence of heart attacks in men by 44 percent. And now researchers say women may benefit as well. A six-year study of 88,000 female nurses found that the risk of a first heart attack was 25 percent lower in the women who took one to six aspirin per week than in those who did not take aspirin, says JoAnn Manson, M.D., assistant professor of medicine at Harvard Medical School and associate physician at Brigham and Women's Hospital in Boston.

Preliminary evidence now shows you may be able to benefit from much less aspirin: Richard Milani, M.D., a cardiologist at the Ochsner Clinic in New Orleans, says that your optimum protection can come from half a baby aspirin taken daily or from a whole one taken every other day.

But don't go blithely popping aspirin and think that will solve your problem. "Aspirin should serve only as an adjunct to controlling other risk factors, like smoking, cholesterol, diabetes, high blood pressure and over-weight," Dr. Manson cautions. "And nobody should start treating themselves regularly with aspirin without first consulting their doctor." Although aspirin is usually safe, for some it's potentially dangerous—particularly for people with stomach problems (especially those with ulcers), hemophiliacs and people already taking blood-thinning medications. Aspirin's ability to make your stomach upset or bleed can be reduced by taking it with meals or with a full 8 ounces of water and by using coated aspirin.

Keep your arteries open with omega-3. Several studies have documented the positive effects of this unique fat on arteries. It's been found to lower total cholesterol and LDL ("bad" cholesterol) levels, reduce the blood's clotting ability and possibly help lower blood pressure. Fish are the most common source of omega-3. Experts recommend three fish meals a week. Cold water fish, like salmon and mackerel, have the most omega-3, but all fish have some.

The only rich nonfish source of omega-3 is flax seed. This grain seed offers double-barreled benefits, says North Dakota State University agronomist Jack Carter, Ph.D., president of the Flax Institute of the United States. "Flax seed is about 35 percent oil, and more than half of that oil is omega-3—more than you can get from fish," he says. Flax seed is also loaded with soluble as well as insoluble fiber. Soluble fiber—the kind found in the current darling of fiber boosters, oat bran—is known to bind to cholesterol and to whisk it, eventually, down the drain. Flax seed, says Dr.

Carter, has every bit as much soluble fiber as oat bran has.

Dr. Carter gets his daily dose of omega-3 by stirring 3 heaping table-spoons of flax-seed meal into his morning orange juice. He also bakes the meal into muffins and breads, which gives them a pleasant, nutty taste. You can buy the whole seed in health food stores, but the meal must be kept in the freezer. Cold-pressed flax oil is also good for salads but is too sensitive to heat to be good for cooking.

Live longer with love. In a *Prevention* magazine survey, 64 percent of the cardiologists polled said learning to enjoy love and friendship was "important," "very important" or "extremely important" in preventing heart disease. "Emotions play a powerful role in affecting your body and especially your heart," says Dean Ornish, M.D., assistant clinical professor of medicine at the University of California, San Francisco. "I believe that it's not enough to ask people to change their behavior without also addressing the emotional factors that underlie behaviors." For example, depression can make you feel like sitting in front of the tube all day, eating potato chips until you become one huge potato yourself.

Robert Rosenson, M.D., co-director of Preventive Cardiology at Rush Presbyterian Hospital–St. Luke's Medical Center in Chicago, has added a therapist to his staff to come to his patients' emotional rescue. "I have patients who are overweight and inactive and resist positive lifestyle changes," he says. "And there may be some depression or low self-esteem there that I can't do much about as a cardiologist."

Consider hormones. If you're a woman who's past menopause, that is. Estrogen seems to have a positive effect on keeping arteries clean by keeping cholesterol levels in check. Postmenopausal women are more at risk for heart disease because they stop producing estrogen.

Estrogen is a potent substance—it can do your heart good (and is a proven method of preventing osteoporosis), but it can also increase your risk of breast cancer. "We're not ready yet to make a blanket recommendation that says all postmenopausal women should take estrogen," says Frank Sacks, M.D., assistant professor of medicine at Harvard Medical School. You should make the decision to take estrogen only after consulting with your doctor about your particular needs, especially weighing the benefits for your heart and bones against your risk of breast cancer.

REVERSING HEART DISEASE

Bubba learned too late what he needed to do to prevent heart disease. Now he's got it. And judging by the frequency of his angina attacks, he's revving up for a heart attack. Mrs. Bubba is afraid he'll collapse one day in a doughnut shop, powdered sugar and crushed peanuts slathered over his chin and overalls. Clearly Bubba has to do something.

You're probably thinking that Bubba's only chance is to undergo a serious operation or to take megadoses of potent drugs. These may indeed be options—but certainly not his only ones. Studies done by Dr. Ornish have given sound reason to believe that heart disease can be reversed without surgery or drugs. But to do that, Bubba's going to have to change his attitude not only about doughnuts but also about a whole lot of things.

Can you really turn back your clock? Dr. Ornish's studies indicate that with diet and behavior changes, you can actually reverse coronary blockages *in just one year.* Some people see Dr. Ornish's program as radical and too difficult for most people. But the medication and surgery used to treat heart disease also have their difficult moments, to say the least. With medications, it's nasty side effects; with surgery, of course, the difficult moments may include death on the operating table. "Isn't it ironic," says Dr. Ornish, "that it's considered 'radical' to exercise, relax and eat a heart-healthy diet and 'conservative' to take potent drugs?"

The catch: Reversing heart disease requires *major* lifestyle changes. But one of the lessons Dr. Ornish has learned is that people can change their habits quickly and completely. "In some ways it's easier to make big changes than little ones," he says. "That's because if you make comprehensive changes, you begin to feel so much better so soon. We don't tell people 'Do this because you'll live longer.' We say instead 'Do this because you'll live better.' "

So you're a skeptic? That's understandable. "I say, maintain your skepticism, just try it for a week," Dr. Ornish suggests. If you have angina and you follow the program carefully, "after one week, the pain will probably diminish," he says. The one-week trial run outlined here should give you a feel for the program and what it can do for you. If you decide to embark, your doctor should be involved. You certainly have nothing to lose and potentially much to gain.

Eat lean. This means no flesh. The heart disease reversal diet is built on a foundation of only 10 percent fat, and going vegetarian is about the only way to get that low. No meat, poultry, fish or cheese. Easy on high-fat vegetable foods, like avocados, nuts and seeds. What *will* you eat? Grain products, like bread, cereal, rice, pasta and tortillas; vegetables and greens; fresh and dried fruits; beans, sprouts and egg whites. You can have high-fat tofu and tempeh in moderation and 1 cup of skim milk or nonfat yogurt a day. Herbs, mustard, salsa and ketchup add flavor and variety. A multiple vitamin and mineral supplement ensures that you meet all your nutritional needs.

Exercise every day. This means *moderate* exercise. ("Oh, thank you, thank you, thank you," Bubba wheezes gratefully.) "According to the latest research," Dr. Ornish says, "the equivalent of walking a half hour to an hour a day causes the greatest reduction in mortality. And beyond that, you really don't get much more benefit."

Go Eastern. This means yoga and meditation. Why yoga? Dr. Ornish's data show that the amount of time spent doing yoga was associated as much as diet and exercise changes with reductions in coronary artery blockages. The slow stretching and breathing techniques relax muscles, Dr. Ornish says, and promote feelings of peace. And no, Bubba, it's not just for Western Hindu wannabes; you can learn yoga at your local YM/YWCA or from any experienced instructor, well-illustrated book or videotape.

Why meditation? Meditation may help relieve your stress. Heart disease, after all, is fraught with worry. But its benefits go deeper than that. "At the end of a meditation," Dr. Ornish says, "you're feeling more peaceful, stronger and happier." Meditation is easier than you might think. There's nothing supernatural about it. In fact, with practice, you'll find it's as natural as eating, sleeping and breathing.

There are many ways to meditate. You can concentrate on your breathing. You can focus on a word or a sound, repeating it silently as you breathe out. Or you may want to focus on an image—say a warm fire, a softly glowing light or a mountain.

Open up. Work on improving communications with your family and friends. Opening up to others helps heart patients get well, says Dr. Ornish.

WHEN THERE'S NO OTHER CHOICE

If you have heart disease, it was a doctor who told you, and you should continue to be under a doctor's care. It's very likely your doctor will tell you to lose weight, exercise and learn to relax, but you may need more. Doctors have a wide range of drugs and surgical procedures to call on to treat heart disease.

The kind of medications for heart disease vary greatly, depending on specific conditions. Many people with high blood pressure, for example, also have high cholesterol levels. The drugs given for these disorders have to be carefully balanced and stringently monitored to prevent or reduce side effects. At all times you must communicate with your doctor. He or she needs your feedback to find the drugs that work best for you and to adjust the dosages.

Sometimes your heart's arteries may be so blocked with plaque that a trip to the hospital may be your only recourse. The three common hospital procedures for heart disease are angioplasty, atherectomy and bypass surgery.

Angioplasty is a procedure in which doctors try to reopen a clogged blood vessel. In balloon angioplasty, they insert a tiny balloon into the

ARTIFICIAL BLOOD VESSELS

They answer the phone with a breezy "Plastic lab!"—but they're not perfecting beach balls. They're letting the air out of synthetic blood vessels, a research advance that could revolutionize the treatment of heart disease.

The "plastic lab" is Duke University's Plastic Surgery Research Laboratories. Duke researchers are working on a way to overcome one of the major stumbling blocks in coronary bypass surgery: In as little as a day or as long as 15 years, the substitute vessels now used to replace the bad vessels can become plugged up themselves. The only solution becomes another operation.

Most people have bypasses using their own vessels, which sets them up for future failure, says physiologist Bruce Klitzman, Ph.D., director of the plastic lab. "The reason for the bypass in the first place is because the person has arterial disease—and it's often throughout their body," Dr. Klitzman says, "so you're replacing a very bad vessel with one that's only a little bit bad." Often another bypass operation is needed.

Synthetic vessels are used when the person's own vessels aren't fit for the job. But synthetics also have a problem: The Teflon material they're made from is 70 percent air. And when blood contacts air, it clots.

So Dr. Klitzman and his team have devised two methods of removing the air from the synthetic vessels: soaking them in acetone, and using pressure to squeeze out the air. Acetone gets rid of 99 percent of the air, while pressure removes 100 percent. This bodes well not only for coronary bypasses but also for bold new forays into artificial organs.

"What called a screeching halt to the artificial heart was clotting," Dr. Klitzman says. "The more we understand about how blood reacts to synthetic materials, the better we can design a variety of artificial organs." This means an artificial heart that won't produce stroke-causing blood clots.

When can you expect to see these advances? Certainly by the end of the century the new synthetic vessels will have made their debut, says Dr. Klitzman. And the new and improved artificial heart won't be far behind.

artery and inflate it. The balloon squashes the deposit against the artery wall, making more room for blood to flow. In cold-laser angioplasty, a laser beam literally vaporizes the plaque. Angioplasty is safer than bypass surgery, but there can still be serious complications. Roughly 1 in 100 angioplasty patients requires emergency bypass surgery because of such a complication.

The "success" rate for both balloon and cold-laser angioplasty is about 96 percent, says James Tcheng, M.D., assistant professor of medicine at Duke University. Success is measured by whether the artery is opened up at all, not by how long the opening lasts. In 30 to 40 percent of the people receiving an angioplasty, the arteries become blocked up again, usually within six months, says Dr. Tcheng.

Atherectomy, like cold-laser angioplasty, is a relatively new procedure. It opens your artery like Roto-Rooter does your plumbing, albeit with more finesse. A motorized device the size of a matchstick with a miniature drill attached to the end is slipped into the artery through a pencil-size plastic sheath. The drill shaves away the plaque on the artery wall. The shavings fall into a little receptacle, which is removed through the sheath.

"Atherectomy holds promise for people with blockages of the largest coronary artery," says Jeff Brinker, M.D., associate professor of medicine at Johns Hopkins Medical Institutions in Baltimore. "It may be able to cut the restenosis [reblockage] rate in half."

Bypass surgery is open-heart surgery. Surgeons take a blood vessel from another part of the body and use it to construct a detour around the blocked artery. Serious business, the bypass should only be done when the heart arteries have multiple blockages or after all other attempts to clear the arteries have failed. In a nonemergency bypass, the risk of a fatal complication is usually less than 1 in 50. Proceed with caution—and always get a second opinion.

HEART INFECTIONS

You'd think that a virus that causes colds and flu would be satisfied with making millions of people miserable every winter. You'd think that two common bacteria would be happy inflicting countless infections and sore throats. You'd think that, but you'd be wrong. Coxsackie virus and strep and staph bacteria will sometimes go the extra mile and infect your heart. The result can be a potentially life-threatening infection that goes by the name *myocarditis* or *endocarditis.*

Fortunately, these infections are not something most people have to worry about. They're as rare as the nasty little microbes are common. Less than 28,000 cases of myocarditis and endocarditis are reported each year, and of these, an estimated 1,000 are fatal—small numbers in a nation of a quarter-billion people. But for those who have them, the infections and their repercussions can be serious.

MYOCARDITIS

Myocarditis is an inflammation of the heart muscle itself. Inflammation—the *-itis*—is a by-product of the immune system reacting to a foreign substance or even to the body itself. The Coxsackie virus is the most common known cause, says Herman Price, M.D., associate director of the Cardiology Section and medical director of the heart transplant service, the coronary care unit and the cardiac intermediate care unit at Ochsner Medical Institute in New Orleans. "But most of the time we don't know for sure what causes myocarditis," he says. "And it's very difficult to diagnose. Probably there are many who get it without being diagnosed."

There are no specific people prone to myocarditis, outside of people with weak immune systems, Dr. Price says. "Young people, old people, middle-aged people—all are susceptible," he says. "There are no preventive measures you can take."

From Flu to Heart Failure

A doctor will suspect you have myocarditis if you have a viral-like illness, followed shortly by congestive heart failure. "If a 25-year-old healthy male had a respiratory illness three weeks ago," Dr. Price says, "and now comes in with symptoms of heart failure—he is short of breath, fatigued, he has a rapid pulse and an enlarged heart, and his cardiovascular tests are abnormal—he may have myocarditis, even if we can't identify a virus or bacteria." Usually there's no heart pain with myocarditis alone, but the infection is often accompanied by pericarditis, a painful inflammation of the membrane surrounding the heart.

"The primary treatment is directed at controlling heart failure, unless the specific cause is known," says Dr. Price. That usually means bed rest and drugs to reduce fluid buildup, inflammation and pain and to maintain blood pressure and proper heart rhythm.

"If the myocarditis is mild or moderate, you may fully recover with no damage to your heart," Dr. Price says. "You can do whatever you want. Your limitations are determined by how you feel. The more physically fit you were before the infection, the better off you'll be after you recover."

ENDOCARDITIS

"Endocarditis is a different kettle of fish," Dr. Price says. "It usually attacks the heart valves instead of the muscle or membrane—and it usually can be prevented."

Strep and staph bacteria are the most common causes of endocarditis, and they may be found anywhere. "But most people are not at risk for endocarditis," Dr. Price says. "The people who are at risk are those who already have a valve abnormality, whether it's congenital or the result of heart damage from another cause. At even higher risk are people who have artificial valves." Fever is usually the first symptom of the disease.

"Endocarditis is always dangerous, because there are so many complications that can occur," Dr. Price says. "Clots that form on a valve can break off and go any place the circulation takes them, such as the brain. There they can block a blood vessel and cause a stroke. In the leg they can block blood flow, which, if not corrected, can eventually cause loss of the leg."

Sometimes endocarditis is caused by slower-growing microbes, and the damage can develop over several months. But a fast-acting form of endocarditis can destroy the valve in a matter of days, Dr. Price says, causing life-threatening heart and organ failure and fluid buildup in the lungs. Surgery to replace the value is often required, he says.

REDUCING YOUR RISK

If you have a valve problem, or if you have an artificial valve, dental work that causes bleeding—cleaning, fillings or extractions—is the most common situation that puts you at risk, says Dr. Price. Bacteria can evade even the most stringent standards of cleanliness and sterilization. Other medical procedures that cause bleeding, like colonoscopy or biopsy, are also risky. Your doctor will most likely order a course of antibiotics before any dental or medical procedure that causes bleeding.

If it's too late for prevention—don't despair. With good treatment, your chances of complete recovery are high, Dr. Price says. Treatment usually is limited to antibiotics, but if they don't work, doctors can surgically replace the infected valve. If the infection didn't spread to the heart muscle itself, Dr. Price says, "a new valve can mean a whole new person."

HEMORRHOIDS

H ere are some things everyone should know about hemorrhoids.
Hemorrhoids are blood vessels. It's normal for them to bleed.
Usually they bleed a little, sometimes they bleed a lot.
Hemorrhoids can protrude from your bottom, making sitting
an uncomfortable experience.

Finally, hemorrhoids are very common, affecting as many as three
out of four people. According to Yale gastroenterologist Howard M. Spiro,
M.D., hemorrhoids "are among the commonest afflictions of man, so ubiq-
uitous as to seem no more an abnormality than gray hair, though sometimes more painful!"

VEINS UNDER PRESSURE

Hemorrhoids are anal veins that, like varicose veins, become distended and engorged with blood. This condition often runs in families, but
the real cause is pressure bearing downward on the veins. This pressure
commonly comes from being overweight or pregnant or from straining to
have a bowel movement. But it can even come from merely walking upright. (Four-legged animals *don't* get hemorrhoids.)

Hemorrhoids, despite their humble location, do have two things going
for them: They're usually harmless, and although some can be painful,
most are not, says John L. Cocchiara, M.D., a general surgeon in Lake
Charles, Louisiana.

The reason most hemorrhoids don't hurt is that they originate inside
the rectum, where there aren't any nerve endings. While these *internal*
hemorrhoids don't hurt, they often bleed, Dr. Cocchiara says. Bleeding is
one of the most common symptoms of internal hemorrhoids, and the most
frightening. Everyone gets nervous when they bleed—they get *very* nervous when they bleed from down under. It's not a pleasant discovery, but
it does get people to their doctor in a hurry.

And seeing a doctor isn't a bad idea. Rectal bleeding can be a sign that something other than hemorrhoids—cancer, for example—is wrong.

External hemorrhoids may not announce themselves with blood. They don't need to, because they are, well, external. Originating near the anus, they can often be felt—or, if you're creative with mirrors, seen. These are the kinds of hemorrhoids that sometimes hurt, because the anus, unlike the rectum, has plenty of nerve endings. Should a blood clot form inside a hemorrhoid—doctors call this condition *thrombosis*—the resulting pain can be excruciating.

As a general rule, hemorrhoids heal with time. Even thrombosed hemorrhoids, given time, will disappear on their own. But when you can't sit down without wincing, waiting for that to happen can be quite unpleasant. Fortunately, you don't have to. With the following tips, not only can you relieve the pain of hemorrhoids, you also can help prevent new ones from forming.

ABSTAINING FROM STRAINING

"More than anything, it's chronic constipation that causes hemorrhoids," Dr. Cocchiara says. "When there's no straining, there's no swelling of the veins and no pushing of the veins out of the anus. If you can correct the constipation, you often can prevent hemorrhoids."

No strain, no pain. The easiest way to prevent both constipation and hemorrhoids is to eat plenty of beans, grains, fruit and vegetables—all foods that are high in dietary fiber, Dr. Cocchiara says. Dietary fiber simply is the indigestible parts of the plants you eat. When fiber enters your digestive tract, it acts like a sponge and soaks up water. This makes your stools larger, softer and easier to pass. The result is less straining—and less pressure on your sensitive anal veins. (For more about dietary fiber, see "Constipation" on page 125.)

Reach for the psyllium. If you want more fiber than you get in your everyday diet, psyllium seeds may be the answer, Dr. Cocchiara says. Nearly pure fiber, psyllium comes in many forms and brands (Fiberall, Metamucil) and is available over the counter in most drugstores and supermarkets. It's a natural way to keep stools soft. Ask your pharmacist to point the way.

Fill your water tank. Your intestines need lots of moisture to keep things lubricated, particularly if you've started your high-fiber diet. To prevent constipation, doctors recommend that you drink *at least* six to eight glasses of water every day.

Sit in a sitz. Sitting in warm water several times a day can help soothe a sore bottom, Dr. Cocchiara says. A handful of Epsom salts mixed into shallow bathwater can help shrink the swollen tissue as well. Gently spread your buttocks and let a gentle stream of warm water do its work. If you don't have a bathtub, use the shower.

Shed a few pounds. When you're overweight, those extra pounds put plenty of pressure on your already burdened bottom. People who lose weight sometimes lose their hemorrhoids, too.

OVER-THE-COUNTER RELIEF

Step into the "Hemorrhoid" aisle of your local drugstore, and you're sure to find two things: a dizzying array of products, and embarrassed shoppers trying to make a selection.

These shoppers spend more than $100 million a year on over-the-counter hemorrhoid remedies, and according to the Food and Drug Administration (FDA), not all of that money is well spent.

Remember that inside the rectum you have no nerve endings. So hemorrhoid remedies that claim to reduce pain or itching are useless for internal hemorrhoids. As for external hemorrhoids, these anesthetics can sometimes give temporary relief, but in some cases, they may cause skin reactions that are more painful than the hemorrhoids, says Dr. Cocchiara.

Preparations that promise to temporarily shrink hemorrhoidal tissue may be helpful, but the FDA doesn't recommend them if you have heart disease, high blood pressure or certain other conditions. Consult with your doctor about any of these products.

BEYOND THE HEMORRHOID AISLE

Ironically, some of your best choices for hemorrhoid relief may not be found in the "Hemorrhoid" section of your drugstore, say the experts. Stool softeners, for example, can be useful remedies, Dr. Cocchiara says. When your hemorrhoids are so tender that having a bowel movement feels like you're passing barbed wire, then drugs such as mineral oil or docusate calcium (Surfak) can make your stools easier to pass and give your hemorrhoids some much-needed relief.

For extra hemorrhoid relief, apply a dab of emollient, suggests Dr. Cocchiara. Emollients protect the inflamed tissue of tender hemorrhoids and help stools slide by with a minimum of friction. There are many commercial preparations, but some doctors say that plain ointments—petroleum jelly, for example—work just as well, and for a fraction of the cost.

A special caveat holds for steroid creams, such as 1 percent hydrocortisone. While steroids quickly reduce inflammation, they can also thin the skin covering the anal veins when used for long-term treatment, making the veins more vulnerable to damage, says Dr. Cocchiara.

Your goal should be prevention, not treatment, Dr. Cocchiara says. "I ask people to try to rely on the bran or the fiber to make the stools softer. Then if they're pushed against the wall, they can use the drugs."

THE BOTTOM LINE

Hemorrhoids sometimes cause more problems than diet or even medications can cure. Internal hemorrhoids, for example, can bleed so profusely that people become anemic. External hemorrhoids can be unbearably painful.

To eliminate bleeding internal hemorrhoids, a procedure called sclerotherapy, or injection therapy, can help. Commonly used to eliminate varicose veins, sclerotherapy is safe and effective for hemorrhoids as well. Your doctor will inject a solution into the vein, which then shrinks and disappears, along with the hemorrhoid. The treatments don't always work the first time, however, and repeated injections may be required.

A technique called ligation, or rubber-banding, will also clear up internal hemorrhoids, Dr. Cocchiara says. A tight band is wrapped around the base of a hemorrhoid, cutting off its blood supply. In approximately a week, the hemorrhoid simply sloughs off, often with little or no pain.

In recent years, doctors have also treated hemorrhoids, internal and external, with infrared photocoagulation (in which a beam of infrared light burns and destroys them), cryosurgery (the hemorrhoids are frozen with liquid nitrogen) and lasers (beams of high-intensity light nearly vaporize them).

Sometimes, for serious hemorrhoids, the best treatment may be a procedure called hemorrhoidectomy. "With surgical removal, you can scoop the whole thing out," Dr. Cocchiara explains. The procedure is performed under a general or spinal anesthetic, and people commonly spend two or three days in the hospital. And once a hemorrhoid has been surgically removed, it never comes back.

HEPATITIS

epatitis is one of the reasons your mother always told you to wash your hands after you went to the bathroom. It is also the reason why restaurants post signs that say "Employees *must* wash hands before returning to work!" in their restrooms.

Unfortunately, employees don't listen to the signs any better than you listened to your mother. And—since hepatitis A is transmitted through what doctors refer to as the "fecal/oral" route—the result is around 31,000 cases of hepatitis A every year.

A BATTLE IN THE LIVER

Hepatitis is actually a liver inflammation that occurs when your body's immune system warriors attack a viral invader that is trying to take over your liver. Because the invader is dug in behind the magnificent cellular fortifications of the liver itself, your immune system ends up torching your liver along with the invader.

The battle ends with the virus dead, your liver inflamed, your immune system on guard against future incursions and your body feeling like you've got a bad case of the flu: Fatigue, aching joints and muscles, headache, loss of appetite, sore throat, nausea, vomiting, fever and swollen lymph nodes are all typical.

You may also feel some pain in the right side of your torso—which is the site of your liver—and you may begin to lose weight. Your urine can also darken. And in some cases, your skin and the whites of your eyes can turn yellow—a condition known as jaundice. All these color changes happen because your embattled liver is temporarily unable to remove all the wastes from your blood.

HEPATITIS A

The invader that launched a frontal attack on your liver can wear any one of at least five different suits of armor. But the one your immune system is most likely to meet—the one that is transmitted by unwashed hands or fecally polluted water—is the virus called hepatitis A.

Fortunately for you, the liver is well able to repair itself after your immune system has defeated the invader. That's why even though you feel like a battlefield casualty, there is no need for medical treatment in hepatitis A (although it does take a doctor to diagnose it), says Gary

---

CIRRHOSIS: THE DRINKER'S DISEASE

Most of us have cleaned enough chicken to know what a healthy liver looks like: a silky smooth, reddish brown organ that shines with health.

Your liver should look just the same. But if you have cirrhosis—a disease caused mostly by alcohol, drugs or hepatitis—your liver is more likely to look like a tough old steak.

Alcohol is by far the most likely agent to cause cirrhosis, doctors agree. Men who imbibe as little as 36 ounces of beer a day over 10 to 15 years are particularly at risk, as are women who drink as little as 18 ounces of beer a day over the same time period. And unfortunately for a society notorious for its fast-food habits, malnutrition seems to potentiate the adverse effects of alcohol on the liver.

Drugs that can cause cirrhosis are those used to treat high blood pressure, tuberculosis, Parkinson's disease and cancer. And any form of hepatitis that burrows into the liver for a permanent stay can cause cirrhosis.

How do you know when your liver's in trouble? As cirrhosis progresses, you may feel tired, weak and nauseated. Your skin may turn yellow, the palms of your hands may become red, and small, spiderlike blood vessels may appear just under the surface of your skin.

Treatment depends upon the cause. Cirrhosis due to alcohol can frequently be stopped if the problem is detected early and no further alcohol is consumed, doctors say. Liver damage due to drugs also can frequently be arrested if the problem drug is discontinued. But cirrhosis due to chronic hepatitis is hard to stop. A liver transplant is frequently the only solution.

Gitnick, M.D., a professor at the University of California, Los Angeles, Medical School and chief of staff at its medical center. The liver itself will regenerate—the only organ in your body known to have that ability—and your body itself will soon be back to normal. In the meantime, however, there are two things you can do to feel better.

Stay home. Don't try to carry on with work or school. Although you may not feel quite so sick after a couple of days, you may still feel pretty tired, since the liver plays a key role in generating your body's energy supply. Besides, if you stay home, you're less likely to infect anyone else. You're still contagious for up to five weeks, says Dr. Gitnick, so wash your hands thoroughly after using the bathroom and avoid sharing food, love or utensils. And once you start going out again, most doctors recommend an easy schedule for several weeks or even months after recovery.

Stay away from drugs. "You should also avoid alcohol, barbiturates and pain medications," adds Dr. Gitnick. "They all have to pass through the liver, and an inflamed liver is in no shape to handle them." In using a drug to feel better, you could end up making yourself worse.

SHOOT IT DOWN

Fortunately, a vaccine against hepatitis A is currently being evaluated, says Brent Burkholder, M.D., an epidemiologist at the federal Centers for Disease Control (CDC) in Atlanta. It will probably be of particular benefit to food service workers, to travelers to parts of the world where sanitation is poor and to both children and adults in day care centers, where there is a high risk of fecal/oral contamination.

Until the vaccine is on the market, however, talk to your doctor about a gamma globulin shot if you're afraid you've been exposed to the virus. A dose of gamma globulin will give a boost to your immune system. "If you get the shot within 7 days, it will almost always prevent you from getting hepatitis," says Dr. Gitnick. "If you get the shot within 14 days, it may not prevent the disease, but it can lessen the severity."

HEPATITIS B

A second form of hepatitis that you may occasionally hear about is hepatitis B. "It's a leading cause of death in China, and it's constantly circulating in Japan, southeast Asia and Africa," says Dr. Gitnick. The infection is contracted primarily through sexual activity with infected partners. In heterosexual prostitutes and male homosexuals, says Dr. Gitnick, hepatitis

B is nearly epidemic. It's also transmitted by infected blood that clings to needles shared by intravenous drug abusers.

The symptoms of hepatitis B are the same flulike complaints of hepatitis A. And unless you develop the chronic form, hepatitis B will also resolve itself without treatment, says Dr. Gitnick.

Unfortunately, a significant number of people do develop chronic hepatitis B. The hepatitis B virus burrows into your liver, your immune system keeps on torching both virus and liver in an attempt to dislodge it, and your liver becomes progressively damaged. Eventually the damage is so severe that your liver becomes vulnerable to both cirrhosis and cancer. (See "Cirrhosis: The Drinker's Disease" on page 268.)

Should you develop the chronic form of hepatitis, you need to be under a doctor's care, says Dr. Gitnick. Some doctors say that injections of interferon, which is actually one of your body's natural immune system warriors, can sometimes control the virus and prevent further damage.

What can you do about hepatitis B?

Stay home and away from drugs. If you develop the disease, give your poor, embattled liver a break, says Dr. Gitnick. Avoid alcohol and drugs, and get lots of rest.

Practice safe sex. Since hepatitis B can be spread like any sexually transmitted disease, you should always use a condom if there's any chance whatsoever that you or your partner may be carrying the disease, advises Dr. Gitnick. If you know you have the disease, you should definitely wear a condom, or better yet, avoid sex altogether until you're healthy again.

Get the vaccine. If you're a health-care worker, get the hepatitis B vaccine and prevent the disease to begin with, says the CDC's Dr. Burkholder. He also recommends that this vaccine be given as a part of routine infant immunizations.

HEPATITIS C

Hepatitis C is slightly rarer than hepatitis B. Years ago, most people got this form of hepatitis through transfusion of bad blood, before blood was routinely screened for the virus. Although some people may still become infected from transfusions received back then, most new cases of hepatitis C will be caused by the sharing of needles by intravenous drug abusers.

About half of the people infected with hepatitis C develop chronic hepatitis, and cirrhosis follows in about 20 percent of these cases. According to Dr. Burkholder, interferon treatment is currently being tried in certain cases of hepatitis C but has met with little success.

HERNIA

The battle of the bulge doesn't necessarily end at the waistline. Sometimes the soft tissue of an inner organ, such as the intestine, will start to bulge through a defect in the muscle wall. This protrusion doesn't exactly announce itself by saying "Peekaboo," but most often, it will create bulging and sometimes tenderness in the groin area.

At the very least, this protrusion, called a hernia, is an uncomfortable nuisance. But it may also become painful and, in rare cases, lead to complications that, if untreated, can even cause death, says Alex G. Shulman, M.D., director of the Litchtenstein Hernia Center in Los Angeles.

A hernia is something like a tear in a piece of fabric. It most often results when the abdominal muscles are strained by doing things such as heavy lifting, having a difficult bowel movement or even coughing or laughing. Those that appear in the lower abdomen are by far the most common, and nearly nine of ten people who get them are men. That's probably because of a potential physical weakness where the spermatic cord passes through muscle in the groin.

STOPPING THE BULGE

The best way to deal with hernias is to never get one in the first place. There are several things you can do to prevent one.

Lift properly. Any type of heavy lifting increases pressure on the abdominal muscles and can cause a hernia, says Timothy Pohlman, M.D., assistant professor of surgery at the University of Washington School of Medicine. Try to use your leg muscles and distribute the weight of the object over your entire torso. Better yet, hire a professional mover or find a friend to help you with heavy objects!

Avoid constipation or straining during bowel movements. "There are people who get fixated on the idea that they have to have a bowel movement at a certain time of the day, even if they have to strain," says Arthur Gilbert, M.D., director of the Hernia Institute of Florida in

South Miami. "Those people predispose themselves to hernias." Eat lots of fiber and drink plenty of fluids—at least six to eight glasses a day—to keep your stool soft and prevent constipation, he says.

Firm your abdomen. Exercises such as sit-ups strengthen the abdomen and are particularly useful in helping to ward off hernias, says Dr. Pohlman. Work up slowly to two to three sets of 10 to 15 sit-ups, keeping your legs bent to avoid back strain.

Quit smoking. Yes, here is yet another reason to give up tobacco. If you're a smoker, you're more likely to have a chronic cough that may strain your abdominal muscles and increase your likelihood of getting a hernia, Dr. Pohlman says.

HERNIA RELIEF

If you think you have a hernia, see your doctor. Several other conditions, including an abscess, muscle strain, an aneurysm, an undescended testicle and arthritis, can cause groin tenderness. Only your doctor can determine the specific cause.

If you do have a hernia, you can wear a truss, an elastic or canvas pad that may keep a small hernia from protruding. A truss can be cumbersome, however, and cause skin irritation. And if the hernia enlarges, a truss may cut off blood to the herniated area.

"Trusses are generally a stopgap measure," Dr. Pohlman says. "Most people will eventually opt for surgery."

That's because hernias almost always get larger and more uncomfortable over time. "Usually, when a hernia first becomes obvious, it's about the size of a golf ball. Then it gets bigger and bigger until it's the size of a tennis ball or softball. They can get as big as a watermelon in some rare cases," Dr. Shulman says.

Although hernias usually don't present emergency situations, call your doctor immediately if you develop severe and constant pain in your abdomen, particularly around the hernia, if you become nauseated and vomit or if the hernia doesn't shrink when you lie down or when you press on it. These are signs that you may need immediate surgery, because a loop of intestine may be trapped in the hernia and may become blocked.

THE SURGICAL OPTIONS

Surgical corrections of hernias are common: About 600,000 such procedures are performed every year in the United States.

If you do have surgery, you and your doctor will have a choice of three basic procedures. The first is the traditional operation, performed since the 1880s. The surgeon makes an incision in the groin and pushes the hernia back into the abdomen. Then the edges of the tear in the abdominal wall are sewn together to prevent the hernia from bulging out again. When the tear is sewn up in this fashion, however, there is tension on the sutures whenever you move your muscles. Should the edges of the tear rip open, the hernia can recur. The procedure may also require several days in the hospital and weeks of limited activity. On the up side, this is a natural reconstruction of the way things were before the hernia developed, Dr. Pohlman says.

A more common option in recent years fixes hernias in something of the way you would fix a tire. The surgeon covers the tear with a patch made from a synthetic material called Marlex. Because the edges of the tear aren't being pulled back together, there is no tension on the repair, and the chances of the hernia recurring are significantly reduced. The operation itself shouldn't have you in the hospital for more than a few hours. Generally you can resume most of your normal activities within three or four days, says Dr. Shulman.

The latest advance in hernia repair is laparoscopic surgery. The surgeon makes an incision near the belly button, then inserts a scope into the abdomen and guides it to the site of the hernia. Mesh is inserted through the scope to repair the tear. By eliminating the need for an incision in the groin, recovery comes fast—you should be back to your normal self in a day or two. The pain is minimal, similar to that of a finger cut. But doctors are still evaluating the effectiveness of this procedure.

HIATAL HERNIA

You don't have to go to medical school to know where your stomach is. It's, well, inside your stomach. At least, that's where it's supposed to be. But if you have a hiatal hernia, part of your stomach pokes upward through your diaphragm and into your chest cavity.

While anatomically "incorrect," hiatal hernias—the word *hernia* simply means "a protrusion"—rarely cause problems, says John K. Shekleton, M.D., a gastroenterologist in private practice in Indianapolis. In fact, as many as 40 percent of all adults have hiatal hernias, and most don't even know it. For some, however, a hiatal hernia causes burning in the chest, a sensation so painful that sufferers may think they're having a heart attack. What they really have is heartburn, the backwash of harsh stomach acids into the esophagus. Here's what happens.

ACID SPLASHES

Between the stomach and the esophagus is a tight, rubbery band of muscle called the lower esophageal sphincter. Normally, this sphincter allows food to drop into the stomach while preventing stomach acid from splashing out. But if you have a hiatal hernia, the sphincter gets little or no support from the diaphragm. It may become too weak to prevent acid from sloshing into the esophagus, a condition doctors call gastroesophageal reflux. The result, of course, is heartburn.

Almost everyone occasionally gets heartburn, and it's rarely a serious problem, says William Ruderman, M.D., chairman of the Department of Gastroenterology at Cleveland Clinic Florida in Fort Lauderdale. But continued onslaughts of stomach acid can damage the lining of your esophagus. In extreme cases, if it backs up far enough, it even can corrode the enamel on your teeth.

If you often get heartburn—say, four or more times a week—you should see your doctor. But don't be surprised, Dr. Ruderman says, if your doctor seems more interested in quelling your heartburn than in locating your hiatal hernia.

Eliminating a hiatal hernia can be difficult, says Dr. Shekleton. But relieving heartburn, on the other hand, is quite simple. For most people, he says, a few simple lifestyle changes can help douse the flames.

Eat less—more often. A meal doesn't have to be of extravagant proportions to cause heartburn. Any time you fill your stomach, it churns out oceans of acid to digest the food. The fuller it gets, the easier it is for acid to splash upward into the esophagus. To prevent heartburn, Dr. Shekleton says, try eating less. "Instead of having one large meal, it might be better to have several small meals throughout the day," he suggests.

Stay vertical. When you flop on the couch after eating, you're making it very easy for stomach acid to enter the esophagus. To keep acid where it belongs, stay upright for a few hours after eating, Dr. Ruderman suggests. By putting your esophagus uphill from your stomach, gravity can work for instead of against you.

Heads up. Another way to keep acid down is to elevate the head of your bed by 4 to 8 inches, says Dr. Shekleton. Do not, however, depend on pillows instead. For one thing, pillows are unstable; it's easy to roll off. What's more, putting a bend in your waist puts extra pressure on the stomach, which in turn can cause stomach acid to squirt upward.

Tighten up. High-fat foods such as chocolate, hamburgers and french fries tend to loosen the esophageal sphincter, which can make it easier for acid to leave the stomach. Smoking can cause the same problem, as can foods or candies containing spearmint and peppermint.

Avoid the acid test. Try to avoid acidic foods such as coffee, tomatoes and citrus juices. "It's like putting salt on a wound—it irritates what's already sore," Dr. Ruderman says.

Take off the pounds. If you have extra weight around your middle, you're putting unwanted pressure on your stomach—and its contents—every time you lie down. Losing weight often is the best way to relieve your heartburn, Dr. Shekleton says.

Find new vices. Smoking cigarettes is known to worsen any kind of heartburn. Now you have one *more* reason to quit! Belting down alcoholic beverages also will likely worsen your heartburn.

STRONGER REMEDIES

"For most people with occasional heartburn, the conservative measures—losing weight, raising your bed, avoiding alcohol and smoking—tend to help," Dr. Shekleton says. But if you still have trouble, your doctor may enlist drugs—and sometimes surgery—to beat the burn.

Antacids often are a good way to relieve heartburn, Dr. Ruderman says. Taken after meals and before bedtime, they quickly neutralize the acid, limiting its corrosive action in your esophagus. Some antacids, however, can cause diarrhea and constipation, which limits their usefulness. Less uncomfortable are the combination antacids—Maalox and Mylanta, for example—that contain both magnesium and aluminum hydroxides, Dr. Shekleton says.

Another brand of antacid, Gaviscon, contains alginic acid and produces a soothing foam that floats on top of the stomach's contents. When acid backs up into the esophagus, the foam precedes it, coating the esophagus *before* it gets burned.

When over-the-counter remedies don't work, your doctor may prescribe a drug called sucralfate (Carafate). Like the alginic acid in Gaviscon, sucralfate can protect the esophagus by laying down a protective coating that blocks the acid.

A class of drugs called H_2-receptor blockers (the H refers to histamine, a neurotransmitter that helps control acid secretion) can be very effective, Dr. Shekleton says. Drugs such as cimetidine (Tagamet) and ranitidine (Zantac), by reducing the amount of acid in your stomach, help prevent surplus acid from surging into the esophagus.

Finally, your doctor might recommend drugs containing metoclopramide, which can add extra tension to the weakened sphincter. It also speeds *forward peristalsis,* the force that drives food through the stomach and small intestine. This is useful because the quicker the journey, the less acid that remains in your stomach to cause problems.

In a minority of cases, when acid reflux is unrelenting and severe, the best way to beat it might be to surgically tighten the sphincter at the base of the esophagus, Dr. Ruderman says. There are many techniques, but the idea, basically, is to tuck the stomach back where it belongs and to tighten the esophageal sphincter. Afterward, the stomach stays in the *stomach.* So does the acid, where it's less likely to cause harm.

HIGH BLOOD PRESSURE

Like poet Carl Sandburg's fog, high blood pressure silently steals in "on little cat feet." It seems to come out of nowhere—and before you know it, you're in its corrosive clutches.

Experts say that nearly 60 million Americans may have high blood pressure, a disease whose cause, for the most part, is a mystery. What's *not* a mystery is the kind of damage high blood pressure can do. Untreated, it can lead to heart problems, stroke and kidney disease, among other afflictions.

The only way to know if you have high blood pressure is to have a blood pressure test. Tests are simple, painless and often free. (You can find blood pressure measuring machines in many department stores and malls as well as in doctors' offices.) Experts say you should have your pressure checked at least once every two to three years (and more often if you've been diagnosed as having high blood pressure).

WHAT THE NUMBERS REVEAL

Your blood pressure measurement has two numbers. The higher number is the systolic pressure, the pressure exerted when your heart muscle beats; that is, when the muscle contracts to squeeze blood out through the arteries. The lower number is the diastolic pressure, when the muscle is relaxed, allowing blood to flow back into the heart. If someone was to tell you that your blood pressure is 110/75, that would mean that your systolic pressure is 110 and your diastolic pressure is 75.

"Normal" blood pressure for one person is not the same as "normal" for another. Your age, for instance, will make a difference (blood pressure tends to rise with age). And so will your state of mind when you take the test (anxiety tends to raise blood pressure).

In general, however, for most adults, a normal blood pressure is a diastolic (the bottom number) reading of less than 85 and a systolic reading of less than 140. A diastolic reading of 85 to 89 is considered high normal.

And a diastolic reading of above 90 clearly qualifies as high blood pressure. On the systolic side, a reading of 140 to 159 is usually considered borderline; above 160 is high. Because of the different factors involved, even a high normal or a borderline reading should be carefully discussed with your doctor.

THE RISKS YOU CAN'T CONTROL

Although doctors can't be certain what causes high blood pressure, there are several risk factors that are closely associated with it. Some, unfortunately, you can't control.

Aging is the number one risk factor. Perhaps more than 60 percent of Americans between the ages of 65 and 74 have high blood pressure. "If you're an adult man, you have a better than one in five chance of developing high blood pressure," says Edward D. Frohlich, M.D., chairman of the American Heart Association's council for high blood pressure research and vice president of academic affairs with the Alton Ochsner Medical Foundation in New Orleans.

Genetics is another uncontrollable risk. High blood pressure tends to run in families, and black families are especially susceptible. "If you're an adult black man, the odds of developing high blood pressure approach 40 percent," Dr. Frohlich says. Whatever your race, if you have a family history of high blood pressure, you should begin to have it checked early in life, he adds.

Then there's gender. Men are more at risk until about the age of 65. But in the golden years, women catch up and then pass men.

THE BIG BLOOD PRESSURE BASHERS

You can't choose your age, gender or family, but there are many things you can do to beat high blood pressure. "High blood pressure is largely a disorder of lifestyle," says clinical psychologist and high blood pressure researcher John Martin, Ph.D., of San Diego State University. The three most important things you can change are your waistline, your physical fitness and your level of stress, he says.

Send those excess pounds packing. Of all the controllable risk factors, body weight is the one most closely associated with high blood pressure, says Dr. Frohlich. If you are overweight and have high blood pressure, losing weight may bring your blood pressure down to normal. Or at least you may be able to reduce your dosage of medication.

The best protection against high blood pressure is to never get overweight in the first place, says Edward Freis, M.D., chief of the Hypertension Clinic at the Veterans Administration Center in Washington, D.C.

Thin people don't develop high blood pressure nearly as often as the overweight. To control your weight, watch your diet, get lots of exercise, and read "Overweight" on page 401.

PROFILE IN HEALING

BOB SCHOENBERG: NEVER TOO OLD TO CHANGE

Bob Schoenberg will always remember Thanksgiving 1989. He spent it in an emergency room recovering from his second heart attack. For 30 years, Bob took diuretics to lower his blood pressure but never managed to get it below 140/90, which was still borderline high. His doctors told him that his high blood pressure was probably linked to his heart attack and that if it remained high, he might have another. But lying on the table in the ER that Thanksgiving, the man from Fair Lawn, New Jersey, made a promise to himself: "I decided right there I was not going to die. I was going to turn it around."

Although Bob has been active throughout most of his 72 years—bowling, hiking and cross-country skiing—he describes his past diet as "typically unhealthy," consisting largely of pizza, cheeseburgers and fried foods. To lower his blood pressure, he learned, he would have to change his diet. He also realized that he would have to de-stress his life.

So over the next six to eight months, Bob changed both his diet and his attitude. He gradually stopped eating meat, most dairy products and salt and gave up caffeine.

Bob also changed his way of viewing the world, with the help of yoga, meditation and deep-breathing exercises. He even went to practice yoga at an ashram, where he learned that something as simple as chewing his food more slowly could have a calming effect. "I look at things entirely differently now," he says.

Bob lost 45 pounds and lowered his blood pressure enough that his doctor took him off diuretics. Without medication, Bob's blood pressure is now 120/70, a healthy 20 points below what it was when he was on medication! (He also lowered his blood cholesterol from over 200 to an impressive 150.) Even better, no one is insisting that he have bypass surgery anymore. In fact, life in general has changed for the better, even in some unexpected ways, jokes Bob. "My concentration is a lot better—and my bowling average has jumped 13 points!"

Get moving. Get up off that BarcaLounger. Get out of that car. Get out of that office chair. Move your body. Walk. Run. Lift weights. Pull weeds and plant tulips. Do *something* physical. For the vast majority of people who have high blood pressure—and for those who want to prevent its onset—being active may be the ticket. Dr. Frohlich says that exercise is good for overall cardiovascular health and may help take off excess weight.

Why does exercise work? Certainly it helps to keep off those extra pounds, but there's more to it than that. "The exact mechanism is not clear, but it may well be that the amount of inactivity many of us have been accustomed to is simply unnatural from a biological point of view," says Dr. Martin. "A certain level of physical movement may be necessary to

WHERE YOU'LL FIND THE SODIUM

The sodium found in salt plays a vital role in body chemistry, especially in the regulation of water balance. But too much sodium may contribute to blood pressure problems in sensitive individuals. American

FOOD	PORTION	SODIUM (mg.)
Salt	1 tsp.	2,300
Dried beef, chipped	2 oz.	1,988
Sauerkraut, canned	1 cup	1,560
Alaska king crabmeat, cooked	1 cup	1,436
Potato salad	1 cup	1,322
Enchilada dinner, beef and cheese	8 oz.	1,260
Spaghetti and meatballs, canned	1 cup	1,220
Ham, canned	3 oz.	1,086
Cream of mushroom soup	1 cup	1,076
Refried beans	1 cup	1,071
Chop suey with beef and pork	1 cup	1,053
Bread stuffing, from mix	1 cup	1,008
Dill pickle	1 med.	928
Tomato juice, canned	1 cup	881
Cashew nuts, dry roasted, salted	1 cup	877

keep the body's blood pressure regulating mechanisms working as they should." Scientists now know, for example, that small arteries can begin to shut down through lack of physical activity and that blood pressure regulating hormones can be adversely affected.

Getting active doesn't mean you have to run marathons. In one study done by Dr. Martin and colleagues at the Veterans Administration Medical Center in Jackson, Mississippi, "the people exercised at levels well within their comfort zone," says Dr. Martin. "That exercise consisted of either walking, jogging or cycling or doing any combination of these activities for approximately 30 minutes, four times a week."

And what happened? These sedentary men—aged 18 to 59, with mild high blood pressure—didn't lose much weight or body fat, but they defi-

adults eat an average 3,000 to 7,000 milligrams of sodium a day— far above the daily allowance of about 1,100 to 3,300 milligrams. The foods listed here all contain substantial amounts of sodium. And table salt is 39 percent sodium.

FOOD	PORTION	SODIUM (mg.)
Cheese pizza	2 slices	811
Creamed corn, canned	1 cup	730
Chinook salmon, smoked	3 oz.	666
Turkey hot dog	1	642
Green olives, canned	5 large	463
Beef bologna	2 slices	460
Parmesan cheese, hard	1 oz.	451
Vanilla pudding, canned	1/2 cup	441
American cheese	1 oz.	406
Carrot cake	1 slice	373
Total cereal	1 oz.	352
All-Bran cereal	1 oz.	320
English muffin with butter	1	310
Pickled herring	1 oz.	262
Pita bread	1	215
Bagel	1	198

nitely lost a few points on their blood pressure readings. In only ten weeks, they took seven points off their average systolic pressure and ten points off their average diastolic—dropping the average from 145/97 to 131/84. "The results suggest that even fairly light physical activity may be more helpful against high blood pressure than previous research has led us to think," says Dr. Martin.

Be aware, however, that other research shows conflicting results. In a study done at Duke University, researchers found no great differences in the blood pressure of exercisers and nonexercisers. Given the controversy, you'd be wise to exercise if you have high blood pressure—but exercise should not be your only action!

Calm down. Whatever your level of blood pressure, stress can only make it higher. One study at Cornell Medical College found that those who experience chronic stress on the job are three times as likely to develop high blood pressure.

Studies have shown that mild high blood pressure can often be successfully treated by using relaxation techniques such as yoga, biofeedback and meditation. Exercise is also a good way to relieve stress. Another option might be to seek professional therapy. A good therapist might teach you a new and calmer way of looking at life. Or you might consider changing your life, like looking for a new, less stressful job.

DIET FOR A LOWER BLOOD PRESSURE

The evidence is mounting that certain nutrients may have an impact on your blood pressure. This evidence is not yet sufficient for a solid verdict, but there is enough to permit specific recommendations.

Watch that sodium. Dr. Frohlich estimates that as many as one-third of people with high blood pressure may be sodium sensitive and may benefit from reducing sodium intake. About 50 percent of dietary sodium comes in the salt we eat. The rest comes in the form of sodium-containing food additives and preservatives such as monosodium glutamate (MSG) and sodium benzoate. "If high blood pressure runs in your family, then you should probably start reducing sodium at an early age," says Dr. Frohlich. Start by tossing the salt and carefully reading food labels.

Load up on calcium. Several studies have shown that adding calcium to your diet can lower your blood pressure. In one study, more than half of the women and a third of the men shaved more than ten points off their systolic blood pressure by taking extra calcium. Because of the interaction between calcium and salt, a diet rich in calcium works especially well if you're salt sensitive.

You can add calcium to your diet by eating tofu, low-fat dairy products such as nonfat yogurt and skim milk and certain fish such as canned sardines and salmon. Do check with your doctor, however, before you start dropping calcium pills—you may be in a small group whose blood pressure actually goes *up* with calcium. A family history of kidney stones may also make you a poor candidate for calcium supplementation.

Reduce the pressure with potassium. Potassium is a natural diuretic, helping your body excrete water and sodium, thus possibly lowering blood pressure. In fact, there's evidence that salt sensitivity may be caused by too little potassium in the diet, says high blood pressure researcher G. Gopal Krishna, M.D., associate professor of medicine at Temple University. Studies have shown that the lower the potassium intake, the higher the blood pressure, and the higher the ratio of potassium to salt, the lower the blood pressure.

Lucky for you, potassium is easy to come by in a normal diet: Fresh fruits and vegetables are rich sources for the 3,000 to 4,000 milligrams of potassium you should be getting each day. Do not take a potassium supplement without first checking with your doctor, though, particularly if you have a kidney disease.

Make sure you're magnesium rich. Magnesium is the fourth member of the mineral quartet that may play an intricate balancing act in regulating blood pressure. Most Americans don't get enough magnesium

UNDERSTAND YOUR DAILY RHYTHMS

Call them your natural peaks and valleys—the variations in blood pressure that occur due to the body's circadian (daily) rhythm, our built-in biological clock. These cyclic changes in blood pressure are mostly harmless, although they may complicate drug treatment in people with high blood pressure.

Overnight, blood pressure drops, usually hitting the lowest point around 4:00 A.M. In the morning, it tends to rise as you wake. "Our hearts beat faster, we breathe faster, and our blood pressure increases as we go about our morning activities," says William Frishman, M.D., professor of medicine and epidemiology at Albert Einstein College of Medicine in New York City. Dr. Frishman suggests that it's this change from low pressure in the early waking hours to elevating pressure as the day progresses that may be a potential problem if you already have high blood pressure. That's why it's key, if you're on blood pressure medication, to make sure you take it regularly—to cover those volatile morning hours, he says.

in their diets (350 milligrams daily for men and 280 for women). Studies say the intake has been dropping steadily over the past 100 years, and maybe it's not a coincidence that blood pressure has been rising during the same time.

Other research shows that people with low magnesium levels often have high blood pressure, especially if they have a family history of high blood pressure. And when people with low magnesium levels and high blood pressure are given magnesium supplements, their blood pressure drops.

Magnesium keeps calcium from making your heart beat too strongly. It may also help regulate sodium levels. This mineral is found in many foods. The richest sources are dried beans, nuts, whole grains, bananas, leafy greens and hard water. Although magnesium is generally safe, too much may actually lower your blood pressure too far or put too much strain on badly working kidneys. Be sure to check with your doctor before taking supplements, especially if you're on high blood pressure medication.

Try C. Vitamin C seems to be recommended for just about everything

---

GUARD AGAINST FALSE READINGS

You pay a visit to the doctor's office. When your blood pressure is measured by your physician, your reading's sky-high. But oddly, when your blood pressure is taken outside that setting, it's just fine. This is "white-coat hypertension"—when you show high office readings, although your blood pressure is fine in everyday activities.

In one study, researchers looked at a group of 292 supposedly hypertensive adults, comparing their ambulatory blood pressure measurements (those taken around the clock by a device they carried along with them) to measurements made by a doctor. Over 20 percent of those who had high in-office measurements turned out to have normal pressure at home and at work.

The culprit in white-coat hypertension is a familiar and insidious one—stress, the plain old anxiety that comes from seeing a doctor. Research suggests that the simple presence of the physician taking the reading can boost blood pressure regardless of the setting. This blood pressure surge in a doctor's office isn't itself the dangerous part. The danger is that the doctor may prescribe medication based on these high readings.

"That's why your doctor should take the average of the high and low readings over time to get a more accurate picture," says Thomas

these days. Some researchers say that C may be important in regulating blood pressure as well. The relationship between the two has not been solidly proven, but "we have a suspicion that it's real," says physiologist David Trout, Ph.D., of the U.S. Department of Agriculture. Vitamin C is part of a healthy diet, and the foods it comes in—citrus fruits, green peppers, potatoes, broccoli, tomatoes, strawberries, cantaloupe, grapefruit and spinach—are also full of other good things, including taste.

VICE ADVICE

What you drink, as well as what you eat, may affect your blood pressure levels. We're talking, of course, about alcohol and coffee. And smoking isn't such a great vice either.

Put the hooch on hold. The more alcohol you drink, the more at risk you are for high blood pressure. Alcohol abuse has been shown to be the most common cause of reversible high blood pressure. Experts say that alcohol use may increase blood pressure by washing calcium out of your system.

G. Pickering, M.D., of the Cardiovascular Center at the New York Hospital–Cornell University Medical Center. An at-home measuring kit would be a big plus for someone concerned about their blood pressure, he says.

If you get a device, though, it's key to check its accuracy against your doctor's measurements. The mechanical aneroid devices are fairly cheap and, when used properly, are usually the most accurate. Ask your doctor or check with your pharmacist for more information.

And research suggests another way to beat white-coat hypertension: Have someone other than a doctor do the measurement. Blood pressure measures have been shown to be markedly lower when taken by a nurse or a medical technician instead of a doctor.

Other factors beyond in-office stress, though, may influence blood pressure measurements, too. One is a full bladder. No one knows why yet, but having a full bladder at the time of a measurement tends to give an abnormally high reading.

Another factor is having a fat arm. If a person with fat arms has their blood pressure taken, the reading may come out inaccurately high. Because of the narrow cuff, the pressure reading may be higher than the real pressure in the arm. To keep from giving a false reading, a wider cuff should be used for plump appendages.

Switch to decaf. The conventional wisdom on caffeine has been that although it does raise blood pressure, the effect is only temporary and even then disappears once you become habituated. But now research is overturning the conventional wisdom.

Twenty healthy young men—regular coffee drinkers all—with normal blood pressure were given three cups of coffee a day in a study at the University of California, Los Angeles. The researchers found that even after 12 hours of overnight abstinence, their morning cup raised the men's systolic and diastolic blood pressure an average of six points. After their morning coffee break, their blood pressure rose more than two points systolic and five points diastolic. The researchers noted that had the young men's pressure been taken 1 hour after drinking the coffee instead of only 10 minutes, the hikes in blood pressure would have been even greater. The conclusion: If you have high blood pressure, consider the caffeine risk.

Take your last puff. Doctors say that smoking doesn't *cause* high blood pressure, only that smoking can *worsen* the condition. In fact, studies have shown that a higher percentage of smokers have high blood pressure than do nonsmokers. Smoking is also a large risk factor for heart disease in and of itself.

WHEN MEDICATION MAY BE THE ANSWER

Not all doctors are in agreement about medication for high blood pressure. Some say that medication is the best and most responsible way to treat all high blood pressure. Others say borderline and mild high blood pressure are being overmedicated. But if your diastolic pressure is 95 or more or your systolic pressure is 160 or more—you need medication, says Dr. Freis.

There are currently four main kinds of drugs doctors can give you. No drug gives you a license to ignore your lifestyle. On the contrary, if you're on blood pressure drugs, it's exceptionally important to watch your weight, follow a diet low in saturated fat and cholesterol, exercise and do everything else you can to help the drugs to do their job.

Diuretics are usually the first drugs given. They work by increasing the excretion of sodium and water by the kidneys (sodium makes the body retain water), thereby reducing the volume of blood and so lowering pressure in the arteries. Their success rate is in the 40 to 50 percent range. Possible side effects include higher cholesterol and triglyceride counts, weakness and sexual dysfunction.

Beta-blockers reduce the amount of work the heart has to do. It's the drug of choice for people who have had a heart attack. A mainstay of drug treatment, they have a 40 to 50 percent success rate—which climbs to 80 to 85 percent when given with a diuretic. Among possible side effects may be insomnia, fatigue, nightmares, sexual dysfunction and depression.

ACE (angiotensin converting enzyme) inhibitors are becoming more popular because they are very effective and their side effects are relatively few. They prevent the production of the enzyme that constricts blood vessels. ACE inhibitors are successful in 60 to 70 percent of people with mild or moderate high blood pressure. Combining them with a diuretic raises the success rate to about 80 percent. They're especially good for people with heart failure or diabetes.

Calcium-channel blockers work by relaxing the blood vessels, thus lowering blood pressure. These medications have a success rate of about 30 to 40 percent. Side effects can include swelling of the legs, dizziness and headaches.

With any of these drugs, your goal will be to take the minimum amount possible to keep your blood pressure in check. To accomplish this, you should work closely with your doctor.

HIGH CHOLESTEROL

You might think that cholesterol, that waxy goo sloshing about in your bloodstream, is all bad. Actually, you couldn't live without it. Cholesterol is a vital ingredient in fat-digesting bile, in all cell membranes and especially in brain and nerve cells. Only when it comes in surplus does the stuff wreak havoc.

You might also think that cholesterol is fat. Actually, it's more related to alcohol. And your doctor has just told you that if cholesterol were vodka, you'd have enough in your blood to see the Russian army through the siege of Stalingrad. In this case, however, it's your heart that's under siege.

"If you could wave a magic wand and change the one thing that would have the most impact in preventing or reversing coronary artery disease, that thing would probably be your cholesterol level," says Virgil Brown, M.D., president of the American Heart Association and professor of medicine at Emory University in Atlanta. "If you look at societies where cholesterol is low, coronary artery disease is low."

And in countries where heart disease is rampant—as in America, where it ranks as the number one killer—cholesterol levels are just where you'd expect them to be: way too high. In fact, it's high cholesterol more than anything else that leads to fatal heart attacks.

WHEN DO YOU HAVE TOO MUCH?

That's not as simple a question as it might seem, because there's good and bad cholesterol, and good and bad testing (see "Checking Your Cholesterol Dipstick"on the opposite page). In a most general sense, your total cholesterol level should ideally be less than 200 milligrams per deciliter (mg/dl), according to the American Heart Association and the National Cholesterol Education Program. Start pushing much above that, especially up around 240, and your risk of heart disease may be getting too high—*especially* if you smoke, are overweight or have high blood pressure.

But your total cholesterol level doesn't give you a complete picture.

There are two specific kinds of cholesterol that you should know about—low-density lipoproteins (LDL) and high-density lipoproteins (HDL). A simple blood test can reveal your levels of both. You want your LDL level to be low and your HDL level to be high. That's because HDL cholesterol works in the opposite direction from LDL, actually carrying potentially dangerous fats and alcohols *out* of the bloodstream.

"LDL and HDL tell a more complete story than total cholesterol," says Dr. Brown. "You should think independently about each, because the things you do to lower LDL may not be the same things you do to raise HDL." Your LDL level should ideally be under 100, says Dr. Brown. "If we all kept it at that level, coronary artery disease would probably be cut by 90 percent."

But that level may be a little impractical, and for many people—especially for those with no other risk factors—it's probably not necessary. "So we tell most people that their LDL level should be below 130," says Dr. Brown. An LDL level of 130 to 159 puts you at borderline high risk,

---

CHECKING YOUR CHOLESTEROL DIPSTICK

You may have had your first inkling of your blood cholesterol level from a finger-stick test at your local mall. Those tests are fine, but the best way to get an accurate cholesterol reading is by following these steps.

Get another test. . . And this time, make it hypodermically drawn and analyzed at a laboratory certified by the federal Centers for Disease Control for testing blood lipids. If the second measurement—which should be made one to eight weeks after the first—is within 30 points of the original reading, then take the average of the two tests as your cholesterol level.

. . . and another . . . But if the discrepancy is more than 30 points, have a third test done in another one to eight weeks. The average of the three tests is your cholesterol level.

. . . and another. If your level is in the high-risk zone—240 or more—you should get a lipoprotein analysis, which will reveal your levels of LDL and HDL as well as your levels of a fat in the blood known as triglycerides (see "What about Triglycerides?" on page 295). For this test, you'll have to fast 10 to 12 hours beforehand. Even if your cholesterol level is *below* 240, you should have this test if a family member has had a heart attack or stroke before age 40. (These tests are expensive, and it's debatable whether you need them if your initial cholesterol count is below 240 and you have no other risk factors.)

while a level of 160 or more is clearly bad news, he says. If, however, you already have heart disease, or if you have other risk factors, an LDL level of only 130 may put you at too high a risk.

Regardless of your LDL level, you should also consider your HDL level. Your HDL, the good cholesterol, should minimally be greater than 35 mg/dl—and should ideally be quite a bit higher. If you are blessed with an HDL as high as 80, despite high total cholesterol levels, you may have little worry of heart disease, says William Castelli, M.D., director of the ongoing Framingham Heart Study in Massachusetts.

Another way to look at this whole messy numbers business is to divide your HDL count into your total cholesterol figure. This gives you your cholesterol *ratio*. If the number on your calculator is 3.5 or less, you may still be in pretty good shape, even if your total cholesterol is slightly high.

CUTTING YOUR CHOLESTEROL DOWN TO SIZE

Let's assume you have just discovered that your cholesterol level is high enough to qualify as a professional bowling score. What do you do? Start with diet and exercise.

"The knee-jerk reaction of most doctors in this country would be to put you on cholesterol-lowering drugs," says Dr. Castelli. "But before you spend money on medication, you should talk to your doctor about investing a good six months in a solid cholesterol-lowering diet and exercise program." Even if your cholesterol level is a sky-high 300 or above (which, in most cases, would be the result of your genetic makeup), Dr. Castelli still recommends an initial drug-free attack plan.

That's because diet and exercise work. Most powerful is the effect of dietary changes on LDL. "LDL is clearly the one that's most out of line in Americans, and it's the one that's linked most clearly to diet," says Dr. Brown. The average American gets 40 percent of his calories from fat, with 13 percent of the total coming from saturated fat—the kind most likely to raise your cholesterol level. Americans also eat too much cholesterol, which comes in nearly all animal products. "The first and safest and only remedy that goes right to the heart of the problem is to lower the amount of saturated fat and cholesterol in the diet," says Dr. Brown.

On Dr. Brown's suggestion, that is where we'll start our three-pronged action plan to lower your cholesterol.

Attack the fat. You may think it's too hard—and not as tasty—to change after a lifetime of hot dogs, corned beef and cheesecake. "As a boy in Georgia, I worked in a grocery store," says Dr. Brown, "and I remember those 4-pound cartons of lard and big slabs of fatback." Most people can cut their fat intake fairly easily—and many who do find they enjoy their food more and have the added benefit of fewer stomach problems. "So this idea that people have to eat a horrible, unpleasant diet to stay healthy is totally wrong. In fact, it's just the opposite," says Dr. Brown.

The American Heart Association suggests a diet limited to 30 percent or less fat, and many doctors say you should shoot for even less. But the *kind* of fat you're eating may be more important than the amount. "Vegans, people who don't eat any animal products at all, tend to get 35 percent of their calories from fat, but it's vegetable fat, and their cholesterol levels are extremely low," says Dr. Brown.

Unless you're going totally vegetarian, for the next two months, try to drop your fat calories to 20 percent. You should also limit the amount of dietary cholesterol you consume. Fortunately, foods high in fat tend to be high in cholesterol, and vice versa. You can avoid both villains by following these guidelines.

- Have no more than one serving of meat, fish or poultry a day, make it lean, and limit that serving to 3 or 4 ounces (about the size of a deck of cards).

ATTITUDE MATTERS

Before jumping into your new cholesterol-lowering lifestyle, consider these few words from the experts on how your attitude can make all the difference.

Set measurable goals for yourself. Like getting a certain amount of exercise and making one dietary change each week. People who do this feel good about their accomplishments, so they want to do more.

Focus on what you can eat. Instead of lamenting the disappearance of bacon and eggs, get your mouth watering over whole-wheat pancakes or French toast made with egg whites and topped with jam or maple syrup or a bagel topped with jelly or low-fat cottage cheese and herbs.

Think about how nice it is to eat more and not hike your cholesterol. Because that's exactly what happens when you follow a low-fat, high-carbohydrate diet. Your food intake isn't limited, so you'll rarely feel hungry.

Do it because it makes you feel good. Not because you're afraid of dropping dead. Fear will motivate you only for a short time, says Dean Ornish, M.D., a leading expert and researcher in reversing heart disease. He emphasizes that people who make positive lifestyle changes stay motivated because they feel so much better.

- Limit red meat to two or three servings a week. Avoid cholesterol-laden organ meats, like liver.
- Have two servings of whole grains, breads or starches (like pasta and potatoes) with every meal—more if you can afford the calories.
- Have at least one totally vegetarian meal each day. Combine pasta, rice, barley and starchy vegetables, such as potatoes, corn and winter squash.
- Each day, substitute two servings of nonfat milk products (such as skim milk and nonfat yogurt) for two servings of fattier ones.
- Each day, use no more than 2 to 4 teaspoons of added fat or oil on foods. When you do, stick with olive, canola, corn, sunflower or safflower oil. Choose margarine with one of these oils listed as the first ingredient. But remember that margarine is made with hydrogenated vegetable oil, which acts the same as saturated fat, so use margarine especially sparingly. Avoid shortening and lard, butter and palm and coconut oils, all loaded with saturated fat.
- Use only low-fat condiments or toppings, like fat-free butter substitutes, nonfat salad dressings, prepared mustard, horseradish, catsup, chili sauce, relish and salsa.
- Eat no more than one egg yolk a week. Cholesterol-free egg substitutes or two egg whites can often be substituted for one whole egg in recipes. Remember that one egg yolk has about 240 milligrams of cholesterol (while experts recommend no more than 300 milligrams for an entire day).

Fill up on fiber. Eating high amounts of fiber, particularly soluble fiber from sources like oat bran and beans, can help lower blood cholesterol, says James Anderson, M.D., famed fiber expert from the University of Kentucky College of Medicine. Soluble fiber works in two ways: It takes its own sweet time going through your digestive tract, so you may feel fuller and won't be inclined to eat as much as you might of other, fat-containing foods. Fiber may also transform in the colon into substances that interfere with the body's production of cholesterol.

Actually, there's some controversy about *how* fiber lowers cholesterol. Some experts argue that people who fill up on fiber are simply going to eat less fat. But whether fiber works because you eat less fat or for more complex reasons is really not important. What matters is that it works. In one study, men asked to eat heaping amounts of foods such as fruits, vegetables, salads, berries and bran were able to lower their total cholesterol by 5 percent in only four weeks.

To avoid digestive upsets, increase your fiber intake gradually, and be sure to drink plenty of water to avoid constipation. Here's how to make sure you get enough fiber.

- Eat a bowl of high-fiber cereal daily, preferably one with oat bran or psyllium. Some research suggests that rice bran may have similar cholesterol-lowering effects. Start looking at cereal labels for total fiber content.
- Slowly work up to having 1/2 to 1 cup of legumes a day—kidney beans, chick-peas, lima beans, lentils, navy beans or pinto beans. A cup of lentils provides about 10 grams of fiber. You'll find that legumes can substitute for the pleasant, full feeling you thought you could get only from meat. Combine legumes with small amounts of meat, chicken, fish, rice or pasta, or add them to hearty salads, soups, casseroles, stir-fries with vegetables or pita-bread sandwiches with sprouts and low-fat cottage cheese.
- Add oat bran to foods whenever you can. One-third cup of oat bran contains about 4 grams of fiber. Try it in low-fat muffin recipes, as a meat-loaf extender, as a thickener in soups and stews, as an ingredient in blender shakes, baked into breads and rolls, in place of bread crumbs, in pancake batter and in casseroles.
- Consider taking a multiple vitamin/mineral supplement containing iron and zinc, since high amounts of fiber can interfere with the absorption of these and other nutrients.

Go aerobic. As is the case with fiber, there is some controversy as to the role of exercise in combating cholesterol. A number of studies have indicated that vigorous aerobic exercise can raise levels of HDL, the good, protective kind of cholesterol. In fact, aerobic exercise is about the only thing you can do to raise your HDL level. It may also help you to lower your LDL and total cholesterol levels.

No one can say exactly what the link is between huffing and puffing and strong blood. But when researchers from the University of Texas looked at a large group of very athletic people (who averaged 9 hours of exercise a week), they found the men had total cholesterol levels 29 mg/dl lower than the average for their age. The women had levels 17 mg/dl lower than average. Just as impressive, both the men and the women had levels of HDL that were at least 15 mg/dl higher than average.

Of course, exercise does a lot more for your heart than help battle cholesterol—it also helps you stay thin, can lower blood pressure and more. Excellent aerobic exercises include running, swimming, biking, cross-country skiing and walking. Walking may be the safest and easiest aerobic activity. Work up gradually to a minimum of 2 brisk miles a day.

GETTING TOUGHER

After two months of following your new diet and exercise program, it'll be time for another blood test. Discuss the findings with your doctor.

By now you should know if the program is working for you. If your cholesterol level has dropped to within healthy range—congratulations! But remember, the lifestyle changes have to be forever, or your cholesterol is going to climb right back up. You have to think in terms of living a new kind of life, not as if this were a temporary change to get your cholesterol down and you can revert to eating in sinful ways.

"One way to stay on the straight and narrow is to have your blood tested regularly for the rest of your life," Dr. Castelli says. "I recommend every three to four months for the first three to four years, then every six months thereafter."

But what if your cholesterol level is *still* too high after two months of diet and exercise? Then you need to take more serious steps. Then you need to go to phase II in your war on cholesterol.

Take a shot of psyllium. Psyllium will give you a hefty soluble fiber boost. A tablespoonful of this crushed seed (available in any pharmacy) boasts about as much fiber as an entire bowlful of bran cereal. Dr. Castelli's advice is to add a daily tablespoon of psyllium to your diet for a month, then have your cholesterol rechecked. If it's still not low enough, double the dose for another month, then check your blood cholesterol again.

Take it easy with psyllium—it's powerful stuff, as your digestion will no doubt tell you. Give yourself time to adapt to its laxative effects, and be sure to drink plenty of water, since psyllium absorbs large amounts of fluid. Don't take more than 2 tablespoons a day. Some people are allergic to psyllium; stop taking it if you experience wheezing, itching or shortness of breath.

If your cholesterol is where it should be after a month or two, says Dr. Castelli, you've found the program that works for you. Keep it up, and keep getting tested.

Go vegetarian. If your cholesterol level is still not low enough, and if you really want to do everything in your power to lower it without medication, it may be time to go on a strict vegetarian diet. Research by Dean Ornish, M.D., assistant clinical professor of medicine at the University of California, San Francisco, and author of *Dr. Dean Ornish's Program for Reversing Heart Disease,* suggests that such a diet, coupled with exercise and stress reduction techniques (plus quitting if you smoke), not only may lower cholesterol but may even reverse existing blockages in the arteries. Other research shows that this kind of very low fat diet is associated with extremely low LDLs, total cholesterol and triglycerides (fat in the blood).

Although it can be tough to follow a strict vegetarian diet, Dr. Ornish thinks it's important that you realize you may have an alternative to drug therapy. Before you choose such an alternative, check with your doctor.

Once you have his approval, here's what you need to do.

- Stop eating all meat, poultry and fish. Let every meal feature vegetables and greens, beans, sprouts, egg whites and grain products such as bread, cereal, rice, pasta and tortillas. Tofu and tempeh, which are high in vegetable fat, are okay in moderation.
- Limit dairy products to 1 cup of skim milk or nonfat yogurt a day. Eat no cheese.
- Use no oil or egg yolks and only a moderate amount of sugar and salt. Eat no butter, margarine, shortening or lard.
- Limit "taste enhancers" to seasonings like herbs, mustard or salsa. Entirely lay off of the mayo and sour cream.

WHAT ABOUT TRIGLYCERIDES?

What with smoking and cholesterol and blood pressure and stress and HDL and LDL and obesity and genes, figuring out your heart disease risk is pretty complicated—so why not toss another risk factor like triglycerides into the picture?

Triglycerides are the principal fat in your blood—in everybody's blood. Most animal and vegetable fat is composed of triglycerides. Now fat is necessary for human life—for energy, insulation, protection of organs, cell membranes, cell metabolism. But like cholesterol, you can have too many triglycerides. There's some evidence that high triglyceride levels may contribute to heart disease. But the evidence is anything but clear.

Among older women participating in the Framingham Heart Study in Massachusetts, those who had heart disease also tended to have high triglycerides. But these same women also tended to be dangerously overweight, making it hard to pin the rap for heart disease on high triglycerides alone, says Virgil Brown, M.D., an official of the American Heart Association.

So do you have to be concerned about your triglycerides or not? A bit—if only because high triglycerides rarely come alone. "High triglycerides are often associated with obesity and several other important risk factors, such as a high-fat diet and sedentary lifestyle," says Dr. Brown. Medical experts generally agree that a triglyceride reading of more than 250 (milligrams per deciliter of blood) is an indication of possible trouble. Triglycerides by themselves may or may not cause problems in your arteries. But when you diet to cut down on cholesterol and saturated fat, you'll also cut down on triglycerides, says Dr. Brown.

- Take a multiple vitamin/mineral supplement to ensure you're not missing any nutrients because of the dietary restrictions.

Yes, switching to such a diet may be a large effort at first, but Dr. Ornish has plenty of now-healthy patients who can attest that adapting to and enjoying this new way of eating is possible for anybody.

PROFILE IN HEALING

PETER WISH: A WISH COME TRUE

Twenty-two years ago, at age 25, psychololgist Peter A. Wish, Ph.D., had a total cholesterol level of 330 and a family that was getting heart disease the way other families get the flu. His aunt had a heart attack at age 37. His father died from a heart attack at age 50. One uncle died at 39, another at 54.

Peter knew that longevity was not something he was going to fish out of this particular family's gene pool. But it wasn't until he developed a fatty bump on his elbow that he finally looked for help.

His family doctor told him that the fatty bump was a symptom of familial hypercholesterolemia—a $12 word that means genetically influenced high cholesterol—and a subsequent blood test confirmed the diagnosis. But his family doctor didn't really know what to do other than prescribe medication that would lower his triglyceride (another type of dangerous fat) levels, which were also high, and suggest that he eat less fat.

Of course, eating less fat 20 years ago meant going from hamburgers, whole milk and cheesecake to a lean steak, 2 percent milk and pound cake. It was a step in the right direction, but it sure didn't lower cholesterol much. And it didn't lower Peter's.

So, determined not to inherit the family shroud, Peter looked around for someone who could help. It wasn't easy back then to find anyone who knew anything about the disease, he says. But down the street from where he worked in Framingham, Massachusetts, he discovered William Castelli, M.D., then associate director—now director—of the landmark Framingham Heart Study.

Dr. Castelli warned Peter that most scientists thought he was a nut. "I'm everything the medical establishment doesn't like," Dr. Castelli reportedly cautioned. "Are you ready to be a guinea pig?"

Since the kind of fatty bump Peter had noticed on his elbow was now appearing on his knuckles as well, his answer was strong and sure: "Absolutely."

WHEN DIET AND EXERCISE AREN'T ENOUGH

It's six months since you started and stuck to your war against cholesterol. But the war isn't going well. Your doctor tells you that there's still too much cholesterol swimming around in your veins. By now you've done

Over the next six weeks, Dr. Castelli put Peter on a cholesterol-lowering drug and a stringent low-fat diet that even today would raise eyebrows: No red meat. No shellfish. Lots of fruits and vegetables. Lots of whole grains.

Peter's friends thought he was as nuts as Dr. Castelli. Every red-blooded American knew you couldn't live without hamburgers and whole milk! What was this doctor trying to do?

Well, what Dr. Castelli *did* was knock Peter's cholesterol down to a heart-healthy level. The bumps around his joints disappeared, and today, Peter has a total cholesterol level of 170.

Not that everything went smoothly. His total cholesterol got stuck around 200 until he "radicalized" his lifestyle even further. He moved toward a more vegetarian style of eating and added exercise to his program—1 1/2 hours a day divided between a treadmill, a stair climber and a stationary bike—before the final 30 points that stood between him and longevity dropped away.

Obviously Peter was highly motivated to make the changes in diet and exercise that he did. But he also had another advantage. As a psychologist, Peter understood that to make any significant lifestyle change, he would have to learn a whole new way of thinking—what psychologists call a cognitive shift. But Peter understood why this shift was difficult: You can't see high cholesterol. You can't feel it, it doesn't cause you pain. So even though you may nod your head, "Yes, I understand"—you really don't.

The way to overcome this handicap and make that cognitive shift, says Peter, is to make the changes so gradually that your body hardly knows what's going on. Implement the changes in bite-size chunks. Set yourself a specific goal—say, a drop in total cholesterol of 50 points—then break it down into small, realistic steps and reward yourself as you accomplish each step.

"This is a lifelong process," says Peter. But it produces a long life.

everything you can to avoid reliance on drugs. You have something to be proud of: You're eating better, and you're healthier, which means you'll likely be able to get by with far less medication should your doctor say you need it.

Once you're on cholesterol-lowering drugs, you must remain on them—forever—or your cholesterol will shoot right back up to where it was, says Dr. Castelli. Since these medications tend to have side effects, "we want you to be on the smallest amount of the drug that will be effective," he says. Possible side effects, such as nausea and constipation, vary from medication to medication and from person to person.

But there's no doubt that medication—cholestyramine, colestipol HCL and lovastatin are most prescribed—works. A large number of studies show that you can lower your total blood cholesterol level by 10 to 35 percent on medication.

Still, says Dr. Brown, drugs are not for everyone. In nearly all cases, he says, "the first therapy is still lifestyle change."

IMPOTENCE

The next time you're at a ball game, take a good look at the men around you—the fans, the umpires, the players on the field. As many as one in eight of those guys has a problem—one he would just as soon keep to himself. "Some men don't even talk about it to their wives. They just stop having sex, and they don't really address the issue," says Stanley Bloom, M.D., a urologist in private practice in West Orange, New Jersey.

The issue is impotence, and it's a lot more common than most men would like to admit. Doctors estimate that there are more than ten million American men, on and off the ball field, who can't get erections. Of course, impotence isn't a new problem. Through the ages, men have sought to restore their flagging sexual potency with substances as varied as oysters, ginseng and rhinoceros horn. Naturally, they rarely were successful. But most men today *can* have erections, Dr. Bloom says—if they get some help.

BASIC MECHANICS

Just as a car needs a smooth flow of gasoline through its fuel lines for the engine to start, a penis depends on a good supply of blood to kick into action. That means during times of sexual excitement, more blood must flow in than out. This is what allows the penis to get longer, fuller and harder. Erect, in other words.

Impotence can occur any time blood flow is interrupted, Dr. Bloom says. "If there is a vascular problem—if arteries are clogged—there may be insufficient blood going *to* the penis. Or there may a venous leak, in which case the blood goes in adequately, but like a tire with a hole, it leaks *out* too fast." Damaged nerves also can prevent erections. So can the brain, the most influential—and irascible—sex organ of all.

The man who gathers his courage, dons dark shades and takes the back stairway to his doctor's office will first be asked some intimate questions. Does he get erections in the morning? Are they hard or soft? Is he happily married? What kind of drugs does he take? How much does he drink? And so on. Answers to these questions can help a doctor decide if the problem might be more psychological than physical.

If the doctor suspects a physical problem, he may measure hormone levels and test the blood flow and nerve impulses that go into and out of the penis. If the problem seems to be upstairs, then counseling might be in order. Often impotence has both physical and psychological causes, and a combination of drugs, therapy and perhaps surgery might be needed, Dr. Bloom says. But for men without serious problems, a little preventive maintenance—check the tires, change the oil—can help avoid a total breakdown and keep occasional malfunctions to a minimum.

A LIFETIME GUARANTEE

You won't have a car you can depend on for very long if you don't take care of it. The same goes for the penis. And like a Mercedes, it's made to last. For a lifetime guarantee, here's what doctors say you should do.

Cut the fat. What's bad for the heart is also bad for the penis. And a fatty diet is high on the list. Some of the penis's blood vessels are smaller in diameter than the head of a pin, and even small obstructions can cause big changes in blood flow. A diet low in cholesterol and saturated fats, by preventing fatty deposits from accumulating, can help keep the arteries open.

Keep the weight down. Men who are overweight are prone to heart disease. They are also prone to diabetes; about half of all men who get diabetes will be impotent as well. What's more, obesity can lead to high blood pressure. That disease, along with the drugs used to control it, may also cause impotence.

Get a workout. A man doesn't have to be a marathon runner to have an active sex life, but regular exercise will help keep the arteries open and ready for business. In one study, researchers found that 78 healthy men who exercised 3 to 5 hours a week had more (and better) sex than the nonexercisers.

Kick butts. It used to be that men smoked after sex, at least in the movies. In real life, they're more likely to smoke *instead of* having sex. This is because tobacco contains substances that cause the blood vessels to constrict, thereby reducing the flow of blood through the penis.

Limit the libations. After the first drink or two, alcohol quickly depresses the central nervous system, with discomfiting—and predictable—results. As Shakespeare wrote in *Macbeth,* strong drink "provokes the desire, but it takes away the performance."

Set the alarm. The sex hormone testosterone rises to its highest levels after a good night's sleep. If the mood doesn't seem right at night, try again in the morning.

Get acquainted with Father Time. You have to realize that you're not as young as you used to be. As a man gets older, it may take longer to get an erection. Also, you might have to wait a little longer to get the *next* erection. This doesn't mean you're on your way to impotence, say doctors. It simply means you need to practice a little patience.

RESTORATION: A NEW YOU

Sometimes a man's problems clearly are psychological—that is, he can get an erection, but not when he wants one. Many men are so afraid of sexual failure—what doctors call "performance anxiety"—that impotence virtually is guaranteed. A technique called sensate focus therapy can help. Basically, couples are instructed to get intimate *without* intercourse or genital contact. If the man should get an erection, the couple is told to ignore it. The point is to focus on each other, not on the penis. Once the pressure to perform is removed, the man's confidence—and erections—can return.

Of course, a man needs more than confidence to get an erection. He needs good blood flow, too. A high-octane drug called papaverine can do the trick. Injected—don't wince—into the penis before sex, papaverine relaxes the blood vessels so extra blood can get in. Erections occur in minutes, usually lasting for 30 minutes to more than 1 hour. Some men use papaverine for years. Of course, men with poor eyesight or shaky hands might do better with treatments a little less pointed.

Yohimbine, for example. Derived from the bark of an African tree, this drug has long been a folk remedy for restoring sexual potency and desire. In one study, nearly one-third of the men who took yohimbine said it improved their ability to have erections. In other studies, however, yohimbine has proved to be little more useful than placebos. Men should ask their doctors if yohimbine might be right for them.

Another alternative is the vacuum constriction device, a plastic cylinder attached to a pump that draws blood into the flaccid penis. Tight bands then are slipped over the resulting erection to trap the blood inside.

This technique works quite well, but it isn't for everyone. "It really takes away the spontaneity, and it's sort of cumbersome to use," says Dr. Bloom.

Finally, some men opt for penile implants, surgically implanted prostheses that make the penis sufficiently rigid for intercourse. Some implants consist of a flexible, semirigid rod—essentially a permanent erection. Others are inflatable (via a squeeze bulb concealed in the scrotum)

PROFILE IN HEALING

BRUCE MACKENZIE: FINDING A PERMANENT SOLUTION

It took a long time before Bruce MacKenzie of Maryville, Tennessee, suspected that something was wrong. It was true that he and his wife didn't—couldn't—make love, but Bruce thought that had more to do with a failing marriage than with anything wrong with him. "I was chalking it up to being tired, or having too much to drink, or one excuse after another," Bruce remembers.

Then his wife died, and Bruce married his current wife, Eileen. "Of course, I was unable to consummate the marriage," he says. "We agreed that what I needed was tender loving care, and everything would work out all right." But a year later, Bruce still couldn't get an erection. "I went to the family doctor, and he told me it was all in my head. Well, the family doctor can't be wrong, so I just accepted it."

For the next four years, Bruce and Eileen attended counseling and sex therapy groups. Nothing helped. His doctor finally sent him to a urologist, and Bruce learned that the trouble was not in his head. His problem was a direct result of his diabetes, a disease that often causes impotence.

"He gave me two choices," Bruce says. "He said, 'You can opt

and allow the man to pump up an erection any time he wants to have sex. About 25,000 penile implant surgeries are performed each year, and the recipients generally are well pleased.

While doctors today have considerable skill in treating impotence, the most important job begins at home. Being willing to face the problem is the main thing.

for a penile implant, or you can go ahead and not consummate your marriage.' I didn't know anything about option one, but I knew I didn't like option two, so I signed up for option one." The surgery was quick and easy, and it changed his life, Bruce says. After more than a decade, his inflatable implant still is going strong. "It was the best decision I ever made in my life."

Of course, having an "artificial" erection takes some getting used to, he adds. For starters, there's the problem of timing. "You're all ready to go, and you say, 'Wait a minute, I've got to pump it up.'" Another danger is giving technology, not love, star billing. "You've got to be careful that your lovemaking doesn't become so medicinal and mechanical that you're not concentrating on the humanness of it," he says.

Bruce and Eileen were so pleased with their good fortune that they went public. The founders of Impotence World Services and Impotents Anonymous (P.O. Box 5299, Maryville, TN 37802), they now receive thousands of letters a year from men who need help but don't know where to go. "They don't bring it up when they see their doctors, because their pride is hurt," Bruce says. "More than ten million men are suffering from chronic impotence *needlessly*, because impotence is treatable."

INCONTINENCE

C raig is a friendly man, but he absolutely hates sleeping two to a
room. Bunking with buddies is torture, cohabiting a nightmare.
The reason? Craig has a secret he'd just as soon keep to himself.
"I wet my pants. It's that simple," says Craig, of Jacksonville,
Florida. "While I lived alone, it wasn't so bad. I'd put the diaper on
and go to bed, and my dog would jump in beside me—he didn't care! But
it's an awfully embarrassing problem," he adds.

URINE TROUBLE

Craig may feel like he's the only grown man in the world who can't
control himself, but he has plenty of company, says Kathryn L. Burgio,
Ph.D., a behavioral psychologist at the University of Pittsburgh School of
Medicine and the author of *Staying Dry: A Practical Guide to Bladder
Control.* Doctors estimate that more than ten million Americans have urinary incontinence, meaning they can't control their bladder. Older people
especially are more susceptible to accidents. So are young girls, whose
out-of-control giggles sometimes are dampened by sudden and unexpected consequences.

Incontinence can be a serious problem, says Dr. Burgio, who treats
people who are incontinent. "People say to me 'I can't go to church, I can't
go to the wedding, I can't play with my grandchildren.' To avoid embarrassment, they curtail a lot of their physical activities, and they downright
avoid many social situations."

Whether young or old, healthy or sick, most people don't have to live
with urinary incontinence, Dr. Burgio insists. Something is causing the
loss of control. Your job—and your doctor's—is to discover what that
something is. Then you can plug the leak.

SOME POTENTIAL PROBLEMS

When all is well, here's how your bladder works. First it stores the
urine that flows downward from the kidneys. When it starts getting full, it

gives your brain a little nudge: "Please take me to the powder room," it says. If you ignore this gentle request, your bladder will keep getting fuller—and more impatient. Finally it gets desperate. "Listen," snaps your bladder. "If you don't find a bathroom *right now,* you'll never be welcome in this restaurant again!"

If you have what doctors call *urge incontinence,* however, your bladder won't be so accommodating; your urge to go may be quite a bit stronger than your ability to wait. When you get the call, in other words, it's already too late.

Another type of incontinence is called *stress incontinence.* Common in people with weak pelvic floors and caused by changes in abdominal pressure, stress incontinence can occur any time your bladder is jostled—by coughing, laughing or stepping off a curb. "Some people have such weak pelvic floors that every time they cough, they gush," Dr. Burgio says.

Actually, many people with incontinence have both urge and stress incontinence, a mixed breed appropriately termed *mixed incontinence.* But whichever type *you* have, your bothersome bladder can be trained, say doctors. Here's how.

CONTROL THE FLOW

Training your bladder is like training a bouncy (and often forgetful) young boxer: It requires time, patience and lots of understanding. But the odds are in your favor, Dr. Burgio says: About 80 percent of the people who try the following methods will have a noticeable improvement.

Log your bathroom habits. Even before you see your doctor, you should be keeping a scorecard of both hits and misses, Dr. Burgio says. How many times did you use the bathroom? How often did you miss? When you missed, what were you doing? Laughing? Running for the bathroom? Putting your key in the door? Was it a big accident or just a few drops? Knowing your habits will help your doctor choose the treatment that's best for you.

Exercise control. With exercises, naturally. By strengthening your pelvic floor muscles, you can also strengthen your ability *not* to urinate. But before you can exercise these muscles, you have to find them. To do this, clench the muscles around your anus the next time you urinate. Did you slow or even stop the stream? If so, you're squeezing the right muscles. Now it's time for your workout.

The exercise is very simple. All you have to do is clench the muscles . . . count to three . . . relax . . . count to three . . . clench. . . . You should do this 15 times in a row and repeat the cycle at least three times a day. As you build up strength, you will be able to do more—while you're reading, doing the dishes or standing in line at the bank, Dr. Burgio says.

Incontinence is an extremely common problem. Then again, so are the cures. "Some people accept the leakage of urine as a normal part of getting older, but most people can reduce or eliminate it by exercising and using these muscles," Dr. Burgio says.

Control the urge. What's the first thing you do when you get the call? *Panic!* Well, from now on, you're going to show your bladder who's boss. After all, wanting to urinate and having to urinate aren't the same thing, Dr. Burgio says. Your goal is to urinate when you decide to, not when your bladder wants you to.

The next time you get the urge, don't go to the bathroom right away. Don't even think about going, Dr. Burgio says. At first you probably won't last very long—a few minutes, perhaps, or just a few seconds. That's okay. You're training your bladder, and every second counts. The more you practice, the easier it will be for your bladder to wait: 10 minutes today, 1 hour next week, 2 hours next month and so on.

Go before you need to. Particularly for people with urge incontinence, the interval between "I think I have to go" and "Whoops!" can be alarmingly brief. You can prevent emergencies by anticipating them. Go to the bathroom before you get in the car, before you leave the restaurant, before you pick up your tennis racket.

Don't rush. It jiggles the bladder. Besides, people get progressively more desperate the nearer they get to the bathroom. This is because the mind associates going to the bathroom with *going to the bathroom.* If you're already on the brink, Dr. Burgio explains, making that last-minute dash virtually guarantees an accident. Instead, take a mental step backward. Wait for the urgency to subside. When it does, c-a-l-m-l-y proceed to the bathroom. You want to go when you're ready, not when you're desperate.

Squeeze when you sneeze. You can prevent many mishaps simply by tightening your pelvic floor muscles before you sneeze or cough, whack the ball or pick up the groceries.

Don't depend on diapers. There's nothing wrong with insurance, and there may be occasions when you really need that extra protection. But your goal should be to stop incontinence, not accommodate it, Dr. Burgio says.

Finally, don't be discouraged by occasional setbacks, Dr. Burgio advises. If you've been incontinent for years, it will take some time before you're fully in control. "You *can* condition the bladder by changing your habits," she says.

THE BIG GUNS

If, no matter what you try, you can't stay dry, your doctor may start discussing the medical options: drugs, surgery and catheters.

In men, for example, a common cause of incontinence is a prostate gland that grows so large that it interrupts the normal flow of urine. Surgery is a simple solution. When doctors remove the obstruction—it can be done without incisions—they also restore control.

For women with stress incontinence, surgery often is performed to move the urethra (the tube that carries urine from the bladder) into a position that is less vulnerable to changes in abdominal pressure.

When incontinence is caused by weak sphincter muscles—the muscles responsible both for keeping urine in and for letting it out—doctors can tighten things up simply by inserting an artificial sphincter. Or if you have a too-small bladder that's always overflowing, doctors can increase its capacity by augmenting it with muscle taken from your intestine.

Of course, surgery can be dangerous, and it doesn't always work. That's why your doctor may recommend that you try other, less invasive remedies first. If you have urge incontinence, for example, your doctor may recommend drugs such as propantheline, which can increase your control by reducing the bladder's involuntary contractions. If you have stress incontinence, a class of drugs called bladder outlet stimulants can help by causing the sphincter muscle to contract. This helps you retain urine until *you* decide to let it go.

If drugs, exercise and surgery aren't right for you, then you may have to depend on urinary catheters—slender tubes that are inserted through the urethra and into the bladder when you need to urinate. "The idea of putting a tube into one's own body can be intimidating at first," Dr. Burgio writes. "But those who need to learn it are rewarded by acquiring the skills to manage their own bladder."

INFLAMMATORY BOWEL DISEASE

S tan hung up the phone with a bang. "Just my luck," he groaned. "Everyone from work—heck, everyone in town—will be at the game, and I'm stuck at home with this again!" He yanked up his T-shirt and gave the ailing offender, which hung dejectedly over the top of his belt, a resounding slap. As if on cue, an angry growl rumbled to the surface.

Few things could keep Stan down when his beloved Buzzards played at home, but this stubborn little bug, which hit all too often lately, was a devil. It gave him gas, stomach cramps and diarrhea five times a day. That's why he nixed the game. Even with courtside seats, he might not reach the men's room in time. But missing the game—*this* game—was the last straw. "Monday," Stan promised himself, "I'm going to see the doctor."

And it's a good thing he did. It didn't take his doctor long to realize Stan's "little bug" wasn't a stomach flu. After analyzing a stool culture, he knew Stan didn't have an intestinal infection either. Now he was getting suspicious, so he asked Stan to come back the following week for a colonoscopy—a procedure that lets the doctor take a close look at the inside of the intestine. That Monday, Stan showed up at the hospital right on time. The procedure went without a hitch, and a half hour later, the doctor's suspicions were confirmed. Stan had inflammatory bowel disease. "IBD," his doctor called it.

ONE NAME, TWO DISEASES, MANY QUESTIONS

IBD is an intestinal disorder thought to afflict up to two million Americans with pain, cramping and bowel movement irregularities. Because

IBD regularly goes into remission, people like Stan often think they simply have a recalcitrant, if particularly nasty, bug. But there's a big difference between what Stan thought he had and what he really *has*. The flu generally disappears in a week or two. The symptoms of IBD can disappear—but they always come back. In fact, it's lucky for Stan that he wised up and went to see a doctor. Left untreated, IBD is a serious health threat. In extreme cases, it can even be fatal.

There are many diseases that can cause inflammation in the bowel, but when doctors talk about IBD, they're usually referring to Crohn's disease or ulcerative colitis. "Ulcerative colitis only affects the colon, and its primary symptom, in the early stages, is bloody diarrhea," says gastro-enterologist Samuel Meyers, M.D., a clinical professor of medicine at Mount Sinai School of Medicine in New York City. Crohn's disease, on the other hand, can affect any part of the digestive tract. Its primary symptoms are abdominal pain, diarrhea and weight loss.

If Crohn's disease and ulcerative colitis sound similar, well, they are. That's why doctors may refer to them simply as IBD. But *IBD* could also stand for "incredibly baffling disease." That's because doctors don't know how to cure it. They aren't even sure what causes it, although bacterial infections, a flawed immune system and hereditary links all are suspected. One study found that close relatives of people with IBD are ten times more likely to contract the disease than those without a family history of the disease.

IBD IS FOREVER

The only thing that's really predictable about IBD is that it's *unpredictable*. Even though Stan has been plagued by his problems for about a year, he can still work all day on the dock, bowl a few games a month and, until recently, make it to all the Buzzards games. That's because most of the time he *feels* okay—his IBD is under control. Sure, he has diarrhea sometimes, but who doesn't? But when Stan's IBD flares up—usually for a few days every month—he feels bad, really bad. Then the gas, bloating and abdominal cramps hit with a vengeance. The only place he dares go is to the bathroom.

But Stan's reaction to IBD is not necessarily how *you* react to IBD. Everyone experiences IBD differently. For some people like Stan, the symptoms flare only occasionally; for others, the pain can be unrelenting. Some people get constipated; others have diarrhea so often they're afraid to leave the house. If the disease progresses long enough, people can suffer fever, dehydration and malnutrition. And although IBD strikes in dissimilar ways, Dr. Meyers warns, for all sufferers one thing is certain: It *always* comes back.

AN INSIDE LOOK

The walls of a healthy colon are evenly coated with a protective layer called the mucosa. Viewed from the inside, the colon is a nice, healthy shade of pink. "With ulcerative colitis, the tissue is almost red. It's swollen and irritated, as if you rubbed it with sandpaper," Dr. Meyers says. Sometimes only small patches are affected by the disease; sometimes the entire inside of the colon is inflamed. Often it oozes blood—hence the bloody diarrhea.

As you might expect, an inflamed colon, like a skinned knee, can hurt—sometimes a little, sometimes a whole lot. The colon tries to heal itself by exuding fluids to protect the sores. That's what causes the watery diarrhea that often accompanies ulcerative colitis. The inflammation usually is limited to the colon's surface, but sometimes it gnaws right through the colon wall, Dr. Meyers says. If the inflammation goes too far, a colectomy—the surgical removal of the colon—may be required. It's the only "cure" for ulcerative colitis, Dr. Meyers says.

Unlike ulcerative colitis, which occurs only in the colon, Crohn's disease may occur anywhere along the digestive tract, from the mouth to the anus. Most of the time, however, it strikes the colon or the part of the small intestine called the ileum, or both. (Crohn's disease used to be called regional ileitis.) The inflammation of Crohn's disease doesn't stop with the mucosa but typically affects the entire intestinal wall. "In Crohn's disease, there are discrete ulcers surrounded by relatively normal mucosa," Dr. Meyers says. "It's as if you took a melon scooper and scooped out ulcers."

Like ulcerative colitis, Crohn's disease waxes and wanes. Often it leaves thick scars on the bowel wall. This scarring can prevent nutrients from being absorbed, which is why Crohn's disease often is accompanied by weight loss. If the scarring gets too thick, the bowel can actually become obstructed. If this happens, surgery is essential.

Many people with Crohn's disease will eventually require surgery. Doctors will remove a few inches—or a few feet—of the diseased intestine and reattach the healthier ends. But surgery is not a cure for Crohn's disease, Dr. Meyers says. In virtually every case, the disease comes back.

Sounds pretty dismal, doesn't it? But it doesn't have to be. IBD may be for life, but it doesn't have to be a life sentence. There's no reason you have to become a prisoner in your own home, waiting for the pain to go away. With drugs, the proper diet and, in some cases, surgery, the symptoms of IBD can be arrested. In fact, most sufferers can lead entirely normal lives, Dr. Meyers insists. "IBD is *totally* treatable."

INFLAMMATION FIGHTERS

When IBD suddenly flares (this is what happened to Stan the day of the game), your insides can feel as if you swallowed hot lava. Drugs are the best way to squelch the fire, says gastroenterologist Bernard M. Schuman, M.D., a professor of medicine at the Medical College of Georgia at Augusta. Unfortunately, there's no one perfect drug.

One of the drugs most commonly prescribed is sulfasalazine (Azulfidine). Containing both an antibacterial compound and a salicylate (a drug related to the active compound in aspirin), sulfasalazine helps ease painful flare-ups. Taken regularly, it can even help *prevent* flare-ups of ulcerative colitis and some stages of Crohn's disease. But sulfasalazine has its drawbacks: Nausea, headaches and allergic reactions are common side effects.

A related drug, 5-ASA (Rowasa), appears to relieve bowel inflammation *without* side effects. 5-ASA has been most effective when used rectally—in enemas—but there are also oral formulas (Dipentum), Dr. Schuman says. Researchers are trying to improve the oral formulas, he says.

But sulfasalazine and 5-ASA, although relatively safe, don't always work. That's why doctors often turn to the more powerful steroids.

Fast and efficient, steroids are the gold standard when it comes to beating inflammation. But prolonged use can lead to serious side effects, including high blood pressure and osteoporosis. Many doctors prescribe steroids only when less dangerous drugs won't do the trick.

A class of drugs called immunosuppressants can also help relieve the symptoms of IBD. For reasons that aren't yet clear, some people with IBD also have immune system–related diseases, such as arthritis. Doctors speculate that IBD, like rheumatoid arthritis, may be caused by a glitch in the immune system that, in effect, orders the body to attack itself.

However, the potential side effects of the immunosuppressants— pancreatitis, allergic reactions and even cancer—have made some doctors wary of using them.

KEEPING IBD AT BAY

Even though these drugs (and researchers are always looking for new ones) can help relieve the symptoms of IBD quickly, they work only when the disease is active—and you're already in pain. To help prevent the pain from getting started, doctors recommend the following.

Think small at mealtime. Because everyone reacts differently to different foods, it's tricky to recommend a one-food-fits-all diet, Dr. Schuman says. However, there is one rule worth following: Don't overeat. "People will usually do better if they eat frequent, small meals that are easily digested," Dr. Schuman says. In other words, a serving of rice might sit more easily than a Mexican buffet.

Know your fiber facts. Some doctors believe that people who don't eat enough dietary fiber may be at increased risk for IBD. Indeed, in countries where people routinely eat lots of fiber (and relatively little fat), IBD appears to be something of a rarity. But scientists aren't sure if it's the fiber or something else in the diet, or even the environment, that helps prevent IBD.

In fact, fiber can sometimes make IBD worse once symptoms of flare-up begin, Dr. Meyers says. When the symptoms are mild, however, fiber can help slow the flow of diarrhea by absorbing excess water from the gut. And for people whose symptoms lean more toward constipation, a little fiber can help move things along.

Empty the gas tank. Many people with IBD suffer from excessive gas and flatulence, Dr. Schuman says. The best way to prevent a gas attack is to avoid gas-producing foods—beans, for example, and broccoli and cauliflower. If milk and ice cream give you gas, you could be sensitive to lactose. Try avoiding dairy foods when your insides are aching. If you still have excessive gas no matter what you eat, drugs containing simethicone (Maalox is one example) may help, Dr. Schuman says.

Put it to bed. When things get bad, a little rest—make that a little

---

TREATMENT BREAKTHROUGH

HUNTING FOR A BAD GENE

Just about every year, researchers announce that they've discovered the cause of inflammatory bowel disease (IBD). And just about every *other* year, they announce that they were mistaken, says gastroenterologist Samuel Meyers, M.D., a clinical professor of medicine at Mount Sinai School of Medicine in New York City.

"Everybody agrees IBD has a genetic basis, and everybody agrees there's going to be some environmental factor that turns it on—a virus, a bacterium—but the bottom line is we really don't know," says Dr. Meyers.

Understanding the genetic link is crucial, Dr. Meyers says, not only for the person with the disease but also for relatives who might be at risk. If IBD really is hereditary, then there will be, somewhere, a defective gene. The first step is to locate that gene; the second, to correct it. "Theoretically, you can change a gene, and that would be a cure for the disease," he says.

Doctors would also like to know which people with IBD are most at risk for cancer. Currently, doctors can diagnose precancerous con-

bowel rest—can help, doctors say. The less strain you put on your insides, the less crampy they'll be. A diet of broths, purees and easy-to-digest foods help relax the most irritable bowels. Just be sure you don't relax them too much. Many people with IBD simply don't get enough calories, protein, vitamins and minerals. You want to appease your bowels, not sacrifice a healthy diet.

Reach for relief. Keep over-the-counter antidiarrheal medicines on hand for those times when you are inconveniently hit with a bout of diarrhea (like on a day when you have to be in the office). Your doctor may prescribe Imodium or Lomotil—drugs that inhibit bowel contractions and slow the flow of diarrhea. In low doses, these drugs reduce the frequency of bowel movements without turning off the gut entirely, Dr. Schuman says.

TAKE CHARGE OF YOUR LIFE

Anyone can get cramps and diarrhea when they're tense—on tough job interviews, for example, or while waiting for an expensive estimate on the car. But for people with IBD, a few butterflies in the stomach can feel more like a stampede of buffalo. "People with IBD have a lot of anxiety

ditions by looking for cell dysplasia—certain changes in the nucleus of a cell. A new technique, called flow cytometry, would look for danger signs in the body's genetic material. This technique, which still is experimental, could possibly diagnose cancer at the earliest possible moment. "We want to find people who are going to get cancer *before* they get it," Dr. Meyers says.

To treat the pain of IBD, researchers are investigating many drugs—for example, new types of steroids, immunosuppressants and an antimalarial drug called Plaquenil—that may quell the intestinal inflammation of IBD even before it starts. Some of these drugs may be virtually free from side effects, Dr. Meyers says, and safe for long-term use.

In the past, progress in treating IBD was hindered by the public's—and doctors'—reluctance to talk about the bowels, Dr. Meyers says. Today, there's much less embarrassment—and a lot more research. "If you look back from 1970 to now, there have been tremendous advances," Dr. Meyers says. "If the advances continue at that pace, I think there will probably be a cure in the next 20 years."

associated with their disease, and that tends to aggravate the symptoms," Dr. Schuman says.

Stop the stress. The less stress in your life, he says, the less the likelihood of recurrent flare-ups. If you have IBD, he recommends that

---

CUTTING THE CANCER RISK

If there's anything worse than the symptoms of IBD, it's the risk—the colon cancer risk. A risk, experts say, that gets greater with each passing year. After 15 years, up to 13 percent of people with ulcerative colitis may develop cancer; after 25 years, that number jumps to 42 percent—nearly one in two. While these numbers are taken from unusually high-risk populations, they do indicate that people with IBD need to be particularly careful. Here's the preventive health watch recommended by doctors.

Have frequent checkups. Ten years ago, doctors sometimes recommended that people who had had active ulcerative colitis for more than a decade have a proctocolectomy—the surgical removal of the rectum and colon—to eliminate the cancer risk. These days, doctors instead usually recommend yearly (or every other year) colon screenings, says William R. Stern, M.D., a gastroenterologist and associate clinical professor at George Washington University in Washington, D.C. "What we try to do is find changes before they turn into cancer— what we call a premalignant change," he says. "Then we can do surgery before the cancer is developed or when it's still very small."

Watch for changes. Cancer of the colon often develops while IBD is in a quiet stage. When symptoms of cancer—bloody diarrhea, for example—finally do appear, they may be mistaken for a "normal" flare-up of IBD. This means the all-important early diagnosis is delayed. Watch for changes in your symptoms, Dr. Stern says. For example, extra blood in the stools might be a warning sign. Or if you suddenly have diarrhea after years of constipation, you should call your doctor.

Trim the fat. For one thing, high-fat diets are hard to digest—and intestines with IBD just don't need the grief. But there's a more important reason: High-fat diets are associated with an increased risk for cancer, particularly cancer of the colon. And since people with IBD *already* are at risk for cancer, it makes a lot of sense to forgo the fat. "It's just a lot healthier," Dr. Stern says, "and not only for people with IBD."

---

you try to maintain as normal a lifestyle as possible. The more active you are, and the more satisfied you are with your life, the less you'll worry about your discomfort. (For a simple stress-beating program, see "Stress" on page 472.)

Friends can help. For some people, feeling good about themselves isn't all that easy. Some people, he says, tend to suffer in silence. They shy away from talking about their problems. But people *need* to talk. That's why in many cities, people with IBD regularly get together. They form friendships, swap stories and talk about the different ways in which they cope with their symptoms. To learn about IBD support groups in your area, write to the Crohn's and Colitis Foundation of America, 444 Park Avenue South, New York, NY 10016.

Make peace with your insides. For many people, the worst part about IBD is that it rarely disappears altogether. Like bad weather, the pain, cramping and diarrhea always are on the horizon. It's important to be realistic about the disease, Dr. Schuman advises. "Your objective should be to reduce the discomfort to a level you can tolerate, even if that level may not be normal bowel function."

INFLUENZA

On Tuesday, Mr. Hauck stayed home from work with a cough. On Wednesday, Ms. Krampus and Mr. Fiever called in sick. On Thursday, the secretarial staff stayed home, and on Friday, the once-bustling office was all but empty. Only the janitor remained, and he left early after posting a small sign on the front door: *Closed for Flu Season.*

Indeed, empty offices and schoolrooms are familiar sights in winter months as this virulent, highly infectious disease sweeps the country. Every year as many as one in four Americans gets influenza, commonly known as the flu. Among the elderly, the infirm and other high-risk groups, the infection rate may approach one in two.

Some years, influenza strikes worse than others. It's the nature of the beast. In 1918, a supervirulent strain of flu killed about 21 million worldwide. During the winter of 1991–92, a flu epidemic jammed hospitals.

The federal Centers for Disease Control in Atlanta attributes some 15,000 deaths a year to the flu—mostly among the elderly and chronically ill.

If you're in otherwise good health, a brush with the flu is unlikely to have dire consequences. In the short run, however, its fever, chills, coughing and aches can make you feel like you've been hit by a truck.

MASTERS OF DISGUISE

You say you had the flu last year, so you are now immune and can't get it again. Ha! Wishful thinking. The flu virus is a sneaky devil, one that is "constantly changing," says Steven R. Mostow, M.D., chief of medicine at Rose Medical Center and a professor of medicine at the University of Colorado School of Medicine in Denver.

Through a mechanism known as antigenic drift, flu viruses easily change their genetic structures, often many times a year. So even though you'll eventually be immune to this year's flu (if you get infected), you'll still be susceptible to the next strain that comes along. There's a new bug every year, and your immune system just can't recognize them.

So there's really no way you can avoid flu viruses during the flu season. Just about everyone, it seems, is hacking, coughing, sneezing and filling the air with what doctors call aerosolized microdroplets. "Anyone who breathes the mist can contract influenza," says Herbert Patrick, M.D., an assistant professor of medicine and director of the Respiratory Care Department at Thomas Jefferson University Hospital in Philadelphia.

KEEPING THE FLU AWAY

As a first line of defense, you should try to stay away from coughers and sneezers. Next consider rendering the viruses impotent with an annual flu shot. Flu vaccines are made from inactivated (killed) viruses. Killed viruses won't make you sick, but they will stimulate your immune system to make special proteins called antibodies, which will help protect you when you catch a lungful of someone else's bug. Vaccines are effective some 70 to 80 percent of the time. But even when they don't prevent flu, they can help reduce the severity of the symptoms, Dr. Patrick says.

In the past, flu vaccines often were scarce and were recommended (as they still are) for the elderly and for people with asthma, diabetes and other health problems. Today's vaccines are more plentiful, and even healthy people can benefit from preventive medicine, says Dr. Mostow. Some doctors, including Dr. Mostow, are recommending an annual vaccination for *everyone*.

It takes about two weeks after you get the shot for your body to develop full immunity. So don't wait until the flu's already in town before you talk to your doctor. For maximum protection, you should get your shot between October 15 and November 15—*before* the flu season peaks.

FIGHTING BACK

While vaccines are great for prevention, they aren't so good for treatment. In fact, they're useless. A prescription drug called amantadine, however, not only can prevent flu but also can stop it cold once you have it, Dr. Mostow says. "Amantadine is to the flu virus what penicillin is to strep throat," he says.

Amantadine works by preventing flu viruses from replicating. During an actual epidemic, it's often given after immunization but before antibodies have had time to develop. It's also given to people who are allergic to flu vaccines. Used to treat flu, amantadine can reduce by half the duration of the illness, Dr. Mostow says. However, it works best when it's taken soon after symptoms appear. "You don't want to wait two or three days to see how sick you're going to get," he says.

Amantadine can cause insomnia, irritability and other side effects, so it's rarely prescribed for garden-variety flus, Dr. Mostow says. But for people who already are in poor health and for whom a bout with flu can be a serious matter, the drug can be a lifesaver.

TREATMENT BREAKTHROUGH

AN END TO SHOTS?

Since people immunized against flu rarely get sick, the solution to this seasonal misery seems simple: Everyone should get a shot. Unfortunately, it's not so simple. Flu shots must be given every year to be effective, and there are a lot of people who *hate* getting shots.

But good news is on the way. A new vaccine developed at the University of Michigan School of Medicine can be given without a needle. Currently this vaccine is in the final stages of testing before getting government approval.

Unlike the more common needle-injected flu vaccines, which are made from killed viruses, this experimental vaccine is made from live viruses that have been "cold adapted." In other words, they survive not in the lungs but in the relatively chilly nasal passages and upper airways. The location is strategic, because it allows limited growth of the virus without producing any symptoms, while inducing the production of protective antibodies, says Julius Youngner, Sc.D., professor at the University of Pittsburgh School of Medicine.

The trick with live vaccines is that they must first be altered to prevent them from causing disease, says Herbert Patrick, M.D., of Thomas Jefferson University Hospital in Philadelphia. "It's hard to do. It means coming up with a virus that carries all of the right information but none of the virulence."

Live vaccines should offer longer protection than the killed-virus varieties, because they tend to make a stronger impression on the immune system. "I guess you could say that the body's immune system responds better to things that wiggle and move than things that are inactivated," says Dr. Patrick. The new vaccines may also prove to be particularly potent against the most virulent strains of flu.

Best of all (for the shot-shy among us), you don't have to bare your arm for the live-virus vaccine, Dr. Youngner says. "With this, you tip your head back and squeeze a few drops in your nose."

FIGHTING AT HOME

As long as you are in generally good health, a common flu should relent enough that you can go back to your normal activities within four to six days. To ease your aches, try the following.

Humidify the air. The flu will often leave your throat, nasal passages and lungs painfully dry and scratchy. Adding moisture to the air with a vaporizer or moisturizer can help keep your lungs lubed, Dr. Mostow says.

OTC relief. Drugs such as aspirin, ibuprofen and acetaminophen can help cool flu's fever and can help ease your aches and pains as well. Doctors warn, however, that flu-stricken children should *not* be given aspirin, because it can increase their risk for Reye's syndrome, a serious neurological condition. Aspirin substitutes offer the same relief without the risks.

Get your fill of R & R. The *R*s stand for rest and more rest. This infection is sapping your strength. Your body needs to bolster its resources to recover, so plan on taking it easy for a few days (and don't try any really strenuous exercise for at least a few weeks).

If you smoke, stop. Not only does cigarette smoke further irritate your lungs and airways, it also can make you more vulnerable to flu in the first place. And should you have the flu, smoking can make it more difficult for your body to fight off the flu virus and other germs that could potentially cause pneumonia.

Bring on the broth. According to some researchers, chicken soup "is as effective as aspirin at relieving flu symptoms," Dr. Mostow says. "Your grandma was right about that." Chicken soup makes you feel better by helping to clear up congestion. And *all* liquids are helpful when your body is fighting a fever.

IRRITABLE BOWEL SYNDROME

Doctors aren't sure what causes it. They don't always know how to treat it. And they all don't agree what to call it. So it shouldn't be too surprising that they don't know how to cure it.

Irritable bowel syndrome, also known as spastic colon and irritable colon, is the digestive disorder most frequently seen by gastroenterologists. And many say it is also the most puzzling. In fact, some doctors suggest that irritable bowel—or at least the gas, cramping, diarrhea and constipation that often accompany it—affects so many people that it shouldn't be labeled a disease at all. Of course, people who *suffer* from it have a different opinion.

All of this gut-level confusion really isn't surprising, says gastroenterologist Nicholas J. Talley, M.D., an associate professor of medicine at the Mayo Medical School in Rochester, Minnesota. "The digestive system is very complex, and we are only beginning to really understand it very well," he says. "The system has to get the food to the right place, digest it at the right time, get the nutrients into the blood system through the lining of the bowel and then excrete all the stuff it doesn't want. And it has to do all this in a very precise, controlled manner."

CONSISTENTLY INCONSISTENT

It's not uncommon for people with irritable bowel syndrome to have diarrhea—sometimes with little warning—several times a day. Other people stay constipated for weeks at a time. Still others will have constipation one day and diarrhea the next. The one predictable thing about irritable bowel syndrome is that it's unpredictable. As surely as the abdominal cramps and irregular bowel movements are bound to go away, they are just as sure to come back. And when and why they come back is anybody's guess.

The gas pains, however, are different. For some people, they rarely go away. Even though researchers believe that people with irritable bowel syndrome have normal amounts of gas in their intestines, it doesn't *feel* normal at all. It can hurt. Worse, in some cases, it's always threatening to escape. Some people find gas so problematic that they're nervous about mingling in public.

Many people with irritable bowel syndrome never see a doctor, Dr. Talley says. They simply take their diarrhea—or gas, cramping or constipation—in stride. But sometimes irritable bowel syndrome gets too serious to ignore—painful cramps, for example, or diarrhea that just won't stop. This is usually what brings people to the doctor, says Dr. Talley. Symptoms of irritable bowel syndrome can be similar to serious disorders—cancer of the colon, for example, or inflammatory bowel disease. The doctor's first job is to test for such diseases.

When testing has ruled out everything else, the doctor makes the diagnosis: irritable bowel syndrome. It doesn't mean that there's nothing wrong. It means they don't *know* what is wrong. There's no explainable reason why your body should be carrying on like this.

MAKING SENSE OF THIS SYNDROME

Researchers do know that people with irritable bowel syndrome often have intestines that really are—well, irritable. They seem to have unusual electrical activity in their gut that, in some cases, may be related to the colon's tendency to overrespond to stimuli such as food or stress.

This doesn't mean that people with irritable bowel need to have their gut rewired, Dr. Talley says. In fact, doctors aren't sure if abnormal electrical activity, which determines the frequency of muscle contractions, actually causes irritable bowel, or if it's merely present at the same time.

"All it means is that there's something wrong," Dr. Talley says. "But at least we can reassure our irritable bowel patients that it's not all in their heads—it's in their bowels."

Researchers have also found that certain foods can help trigger an attack, says gastroenterologist William R. Stern, M.D., an associate clinical professor at George Washington University in Washington, D.C. The most notorious is milk. Some people with irritable bowel have trouble digesting the lactose found in dairy products, a condition known as lactose intolerance. When they quit eating dairy products, their symptoms often improve. It's possible, Dr. Stern says, to have lactose intolerance *and* irritable bowel syndrome.

Many people are sensitive to sorbitol, a sweetening agent found in sugarless gums and candies, Dr. Stern says. As with dairy foods, sorbitol can cause—or exacerbate—gas, cramps and diarrhea. And high-fat foods, such as hamburgers, french fries and pizzas with everything, are almost certain to make an irritable bowel downright cranky.

But what has become most obvious to doctors is the hold that irritable bowel syndrome can have on your emotions.

MIRROR TO THE EMOTIONS

The bowel, says Rosemarie Scolaro Moser, Ph.D., "is the springboard of the emotions. If you're feeling anxious, you're likely to feel it *there*—especially if you suffer from irritable bowel syndrome."

An irritable bowel can be a painful bowel, says Dr. Moser, staff psychologist at Helene Fuld and St. Francis medical centers in Trenton, New Jersey. Along with it come the fear and trepidation of uncontrollable gas or not being able to get to the rest room fast enough.

Compounding this is the finding that people with irritable bowel syndrome may have a tendency toward anxiety and depression. Experts suggest that some people with irritable bowel syndrome "are often rigid, methodical persons who are conscientious, with obsessive-compulsive tendencies," says Dr. Moser.

Irritable bowel syndrome can be emotionally crippling for those who are susceptible. They may stop going to movies, to parties, to dinner with their friends. In extreme cases, they can even be afraid to leave home, says Dr. Moser.

Learning to cope with the disorder is the best way to deal with it, she says. Here's how.

Identify your button pushers. Before you can cope with stress, you have to recognize it, Dr. Moser says. Try to identify the things or people who consistently press your stress button: rush-hour traffic, too much coffee, an obnoxious co-worker. Then find ways to cope.

Run the other way. One way to deal with stress is to avoid it. Take that horrid Mathilda Gilda—*please!* Every morning, you are upset by her scurrilous office gossip about who's doing what to whom. Don't sit next to her, sit next to another co-worker. *Don't* let Mathilda ruin your morning.

Take charge of your life. Perhaps you don't feel like running from Mathilda anymore and holding back your frustration. Tell her in a non-aggressive way that you prefer not to hear the gossip and would rather talk to her about other topics. A little assertiveness can enable you to express your feelings in a constructive way and ultimately boost your confidence levels—and help relieve your stress.

TURNING OFF THE GAS

It's bad enough that you have diarrhea one day and constipation the next. Then there's the cramping, the bloating, the uncomfortable feeling of fullness you have in between. But perhaps worst of all is the gas.

With irritable bowel, it's usually not one food—beans, for example—that causes the problem. It could be anything from onions, cabbage and bagels to pasta, pretzels and pastries. You can't give up everything!

And you don't have to. The goal is to control *excessive* gas. You can do this by eating some foods, avoiding others and, when necessary, taking over-the-counter flatus fighters. Here's what doctors recommend.

Break the bubbles. Over-the-counter products containing simethicone (Di-Gel, Gas-X) help relieve flatulence by lowering the surface tension of gas bubbles in the intestine. This causes them to break apart and then coalesce into larger bubbles, which are more readily—and more gently—eliminated from the gastrointestinal tract.

Activated charcoal. This product, also sold over the counter, reduces not only the frequency of flatulence but its odor as well. When used occasionally, activated charcoal is entirely nontoxic. Ask your doctor for directions.

Digestive aids. You can buy small packages of a liquid enzyme that may help your body digest some of the sugars—found in beans, peas and other foods—that are known gas producers. Just sprinkle a few drops on your first forkful of food, and eat with confidence!

Milk means trouble. At least for people who are deficient in the enzyme lactase, which the body needs to digest the lactose found in many dairy foods. When people with lactase deficiencies indulge in dairy products, their reward often is a full tank of gas. You might want to give the ax to milk and ice cream. Or buy lactose-free milk. Or use Lactaid, which supplies the missing enzyme.

It helps to know beans. These nutritious legumes are rich in nonabsorbable carbohydrates, notorious for causing intestinal—and occasionally social—discomfort. Soybeans tend to cause the most problems; lentils and limas are safer. All beans will produce less gas when thoroughly cooked. Soaking them overnight and draining and rinsing them before cooking also let out some of the wind.

"If you feel good about yourself, you feel confident," Dr. Moser says. "If you're confident, you're less likely to feel anxiety." And relieving anxiety can only help an irritable bowel.

Picture a river . . . In a British study, 36 people with irritable bowel were told to place their hands on their stomach and imagine a quiet, riverside scene. They imagined that their gastrointestinal tracts were like a slowly flowing river. After four sessions over a period of seven weeks (each session lasted 40 minutes), 20 people said their irritable bowel symptoms improved; 11 of these were virtually symptom-free.

Similar techniques can work for most people, Dr. Moser says. First find a quiet place where you can relax. Concentrate on a soothing mental scene—an ocean sunset, or a spring meadow carpeted with azaleas and topped with flossy white clouds, or whatever visual image works for you. Fill your image with details, she suggests, to make it as real as possible. After 15 minutes of successful imagery, your level of stress should be considerably reduced, Dr. Moser says.

Get on with your life. "Irritable bowel isn't anything dangerous," Dr. Moser says. "It's not a good idea to stop going to the movies, to dinner or to the mall. You basically have to say to yourself 'I'm not going to allow this to restrict my activities or my life.' "

Consider outside help. A psychological counselor can enable you to attack the irrational beliefs in your life that promote stress. He or she can also assist you in learning to be more assertive and learning to relax, says Dr. Moser.

GET YOUR DIET RIGHT

Dealing with your emotions is only half the battle. The other half is your diet.

People with irritable bowel already have cranky insides, Dr. Stern says. Don't make them angrier by packing in rich foods, all-you-can-eat buffets or pizzas at bedtime.

Just as doctors suspect that certain foods can bring on an attack, they also believe that certain foods will help prevent an attack. And they put their biggest hope in fiber.

"We believe that a high-fiber diet, particularly for people with constipation, can be very helpful for controlling the symptoms of irritable bowel," Dr. Talley says. Of course, fiber can help people with diarrhea, too, because it soaks up liquid in the bowel.

Bran is best. "We recommend unprocessed bran for the folks who can hack it," Dr. Talley says. "Take 1 or 2 tablespoons a day. But build up to it slowly." People who eat too much bran without giving their bodies time to adjust may actually experience *more* gas and diarrhea, he warns. (For more tips on how to get fiber into your diet, see "Constipation" on page 125.)

Keep tabs on your diet. Pay attention to how different foods affect you, Dr. Stern suggests. For example, if you spend 3 hours in the john every time you eat an oat bran muffin, it's time to try some rice bran (or corn or wheat bran) instead. If you get cramps when you chew one type of gum, switch brands.

When your bowel is acting up, feed it easy-to-digest meals. Soups and rice dishes always are good. Maintain regular mealtimes and eat moderate servings.

Take an evening constitutional. There's no *scientific* proof that exercise cures irritable bowel syndrome, Dr. Talley says, but many of his patients say that regular exercise helps.

THE OPTIONS OF LAST RESORT

For those times when you can't be inconvenienced by your bowel, doctors say certain over-the-counter drugs can help. Imodium A-D, for example, can help relieve diarrhea. Products containing simethicone or activated charcoal can help with gas.

Doctors save the serious drugs for more severe cases. A class of drugs called antispasmodics, for example, can help relieve cramping by inhibiting the contractions that naturally occur in the lower intestine. Antidepressant drugs can also help alleviate the symptoms of irritable bowel syndrome in very severe cases, because they reduce bowel contractions and help the pain, Dr. Talley says.

GET A GRIP

People with irritable bowel syndrome may spend years searching for a diagnosis, Dr. Talley says. Even when they learn they don't have cancer or inflammatory bowel disease, they still don't know what they *do* have. Without reassurance, and filled with fear, they often get worse. And that frightens them even more.

"We reassure people that there is no organic disease and that this isn't something to be frightened of," Dr. Talley says. "You don't die of irritable bowel—ever. And the fact that it is so common should be of some comfort. You're not alone with these symptoms."

KIDNEY INFECTIONS

Think of your kidneys as your body's own, personal sewage treatment plant (please, humor us). As the cells in your body turn nutrients into energy, they create waste by-products. The kidneys get rid of these by-products, so that your cells don't languish, buried in waste. Your city's public works department only wishes it could a have sewage treatment facility as wonderfully efficient as your kidneys. These two bean-shaped organs, each with over one million tiny filtering units, remove the waste products from the blood, combine them to form urine and send the entire shipment southward toward the bladder, urethra and the great outdoors.

But while this liquid shipment is in transit, danger lurks, especially for women. Bacterial bandits, especially *Escherichia coli,* wait in ambush around the urethral and anal openings. They can invade the urine, multiply, infect the urethra and bladder and then scurry up toward the kidneys. A kidney infection—or nephritis—almost always begins as a lower urinary tract infection. (See "Urinary Tract Infections" on page 523.)

AN EASY DIAGNOSIS

Get a kidney infection, and you'll know it, says kidney specialist Neil Kurtzman, M.D., chairman of the Department of Internal Medicine at Texas Tech University Health Sciences Center and vice president of the National Kidney Foundation. "The pain is excruciating," he says. "It's very sudden and very intense. If I give even the lightest touch to the skin on the back of someone with nephritis, they'll jump off the bed. It's an easy diagnosis."

Despite infection, the kidneys usually keep working, but they'll serve notice they're working under duress, says Dr. Kurtzman. If just one of the kidneys is infected, the pain will be one-sided, spreading down to the groin. The pain comes from the body's immune system cells attacking and killing the bacteria, causing inflammation and fever, sometimes up to 104°F. Along with the fever can come chills, trembling and possibly nausea and vomiting. Since you probably also have urethritis or a bladder infection, you can have pain when urinating—as well as a constant urge to urinate. You may have cloudy or even red-tinted urine. You'll know it isn't the flu.

Women are more susceptible than men to kidney infections. The main reason, Dr. Kurtzman says, "is the anatomical arrangement of their plumbing. They have a very short urethra, which makes it very easy for bacteria to get into the bladder." Despite their anatomical susceptibility, most women still never get kidney infections. "We don't know why some get it and most don't," says Dr. Kurtzman.

NOTHING TO KID ABOUT

Although you'd probably live through a kidney infection without medical care, you shouldn't take chances. Untreated, a kidney infection can cause abscesses and spread to the rest of the body, says Dr. Kurtzman.

Of course, you'll probably be so sick that you wouldn't want to tough it out. The pain is so intense, Dr. Kurtzman says, that people generally opt to go to the doctor. He or she will give you oral antibiotics. You'll feel better in one or two days, but you need to take all the antibiotics (usually about a week's worth) to be sure you've killed off all the bacteria. If you're extremely ill, you may be hospitalized so that you can receive intravenous antibiotics.

Besides being sure to take the full course of antibiotics, you can do a few things to help yourself. Here's what Dr. Kurtzman suggests.

Take painkillers. Aspirin, acetaminophen or ibuprofen can lessen the suffering. Take as needed, but don't take more than the recommended dosage.

Take it easy. Plenty of bed rest will take a load off your kidneys and help them heal faster.

Drink plenty of fluids. Flushing out the kidneys helps to eliminate the infection. "Make sure you get at least 2 quarts of fluids a day," says Dr. Kurtzman.

AVOIDING PROBLEMS

The best way to discourage a potential kidney infection is to make sure you never get a urinary tract infection. By far the most important precaution for women is to be careful of the way they clean after a bowel movement. "Always wipe from front to back, not from back to front," Dr. Kurtzman says. This can help keep the fecal bacteria from invading the urethra.

If you're a man over 50, your best precaution may be an annual prostate exam. As you get older, it's more likely that your prostate will enlarge and keep the bladder from emptying, promoting infection, says Dr. Kurtzman. This enlargement, once diagnosed, can be treated.

LACTOSE INTOLERANCE

Y ou knew there'd be trouble, but you foraged right ahead, devouring a handful of cookies and half a carton of milk. Now you feel rather expansive, kind of like the Goodyear blimp waiting to lift off into the ionosphere.

For some people, consuming dairy products such as milk, ice cream and cottage cheese sets the stage for intestinal woes—bloating, pain, diarrhea and gas.

These people have a condition called lactose intolerance. They have trouble digesting lactose, a milk sugar found in all dairy products in varying amounts and added to many other foods.

DIGESTION CONGESTION

Normally lactose is digested in the small intestine. It's broken down by an enzyme, lact*a*se, found on the cells in the wall of the intestine. In people with lactose intolerance, some or most of the milk sugar is not digested in the small intestine. Instead, it travels to the large intestine, where it is fermented by bacteria.

"The end products of this fermentation process are gases—hydrogen, carbon dioxide and sometimes methane," explains Dennis Savaiano, Ph.D., professor of food science and nutrition at the University of Minnesota–Twin Cities Campus. And in people who have symptoms of lactose intolerance, the process also draws excessive fluid into the bowel, causing watery diarrhea and enough jet propulsion to provide an evening's worth of embarrassment.

Symptoms can start within a half hour of consuming lactose, although they are more likely to occur 2 to 6 hours after downing an offending food.

"You feel symptoms when the lactose reaches your colon," Dr. Savaiano says. "Drinking a glass of milk on an empty stomach will produce symptoms quicker than having a glass of milk with a meal, since solid food absorbs the milk and moves it more slowly through the bowel."

IT'S IN THE GENES

Most people can blame their parents for this problem. It seems to be nearly as hereditary as the color of our skin. If, for instance, you are of Vietnamese heritage, it is certain that milk could make you moan. If you are a black American, your chances are two in three. And if you're a white American, chances are one in five you'll have a problem.

Infants and small children aren't likely to have lactose intolerance, but in most ethnic groups, the ability to digest lactose does begin to drop by age five.

"It's also possible to develop lactose intolerance from sickness that damages the intestinal lining, such as a bad case of infectious diarrhea, intestinal parasites or inflammatory bowel disease," Dr. Savaiano says. Alcoholism, malnutrition, pelvic radiation therapy, even drugs such as antibiotics can cause lactose intolerance.

KNOWING FOR SURE

If you're lactose intolerant, you may know it—or you may not. Some people's reactions may be very mild, says Jay A. Perman, M.D., director of pediatric gastroenterology at Johns Hopkins University School of Medicine in Baltimore. "There's a wide range of possible symptoms, and because lactose is found in an extraordinary variety of foods (such as luncheon meats, cereals and baked goods), many people can't always relate their symptoms to a particular food," he says.

"But there is a very simple way to find out, objectively, once and for all, if you have lactose intolerance," Dr. Perman says. It's a breath hydrogen test, done by a doctor specializing in gastrointestinal disorders.

For this test, you drink a lactose solution on an empty stomach. Then your breath is sampled and analyzed over about 8 hours. (Some doctors have portable breath-collecting kits you can take home.)

"If you are lactose intolerant, the amount of hydrogen in your breath will rise dramatically," Dr. Savaiano says. That's because the gas formed in your colon doesn't all pass as gas; some diffuses through your intestinal wall into your bloodstream and travels to your lungs, where it is expelled. That's what the doctor is measuring when he does this test. (By the way, hydrogen is odorless.)

MAKING MILK A FRIEND

Although you can't prevent lactose intolerence, you can easily treat its bothersome symptoms. Just try these tips.

Put back what's missing. Several over-the-counter products contain lactase, the enzyme missing in your small intestine. Some of these products (such as Lactaid drops) are liquids to be added to a carton of milk. Others (Lactaid caplets, Lactrase capsules) are tablets to take when you eat lactose-containing food. Both work equally well, Dr. Savaiano says. Both include directions on the package about how much to use to eliminate your symptoms. "But you may have to experiment to figure out what works for you," Dr. Savaiano says.

Have yogurt. In yogurt, some of the lactose has been broken down into easily digestible sugars. And yogurt culture comes with its own natural lactase. Look for yogurt brands that say "live cultures" on the label. Avoid those rare yogurts labeled "heat-treated after culturing."

Frozen yogurt brands vary widely in the amount of lactase they contain, so you may want to shop around or ask the manager for nutrition information next time you're at the frozen yogurt parlor.

Make milk part of a meal. Fat and fiber slow the flow of food through the small intestine and allow your system to digest some lactase. So the same glass of milk that gives you problems on an empty stomach may go down easily when consumed with food.

Try chocolate milk. Preliminary research suggests that chocolate milk may be easier to tolerate than white milk. "But no one knows why," Dr. Savaiano says.

Stick to small portions. "Most people do not develop symptoms after drinking a single 8-ounce glass of milk. But many *do* develop symptoms drinking two glasses of milk," Dr. Savaiano says. So go easy on the foods that cause you problems. Eat them in amounts small enough to control or eliminate symptoms.

Know high from low. Milk is the food highest in lactose, with 12 grams per cup. Ice cream has 9 grams per cup, and cottage cheese has 7 to 8 grams per cup. Most hard cheeses are low in lactose, with less than 1 gram per ounce. Other foods that may contain lactose include pancakes, creamy salad dressings, instant foods, instant cocoa mixes, creamed soups, puddings, gravies, powdered eggs, milk chocolate, breads and pastries.

Liquid diet formulas and "instant breakfasts" are milk based and, when reconstituted, can contain up to 22 grams of lactose per 8 ounces, an amount equivalent to almost twice the amount in one glass of milk. So use lactase enzyme drops or tablets if necessary when you're using these products.

Over-the-counter and prescription medications often also contain lactose, although in small enough amounts that only the very sensitive need to be concerned, Dr. Perman says. "To be on a truly lactose-free diet, you have to read labels, because there are hundreds and hundreds of products that contain lactose," he says.

Get your calcium. Much of the calcium in an average diet comes from dairy products. If you're cutting back, you are going to need other sources for this essential nutrient. Good choices include sardines, salmon (with bones), collard greens, mackerel, herring, turnip greens, kale and certain brands of mineral water. You might also want to consult with your doctor about taking calcium supplements.

LARYNGITIS

Oh, you had a great time last night, telling war stories, hooting and hollering and doing your best Luciano Pavarotti imitation. But this morning you woke up with a murderous ache in the back of your throat. When you walked into the kitchen to greet the family, instead of "Good morning!" they heard "Googrrr . . . erg . . . grggoo . . . muhgrrr. . . ."

You've got laryngitis, an inflammation of the larynx, or vocal cords. You've also got the most common symptoms, hoarseness and pain. "Singing badly or yelling and screaming—that kind of thing can inflame the vocal cords," says Barry C. Baron, M.D., associate clinical professor of otolaryngology at the University of California, San Francisco, Medical Center. Other things that can inflame your vocal cords include colds and flu, pollen, dry air, smoke and alcohol.

Regardless of how you get it, laryngitis does not destine you to lead a life of quiet desperation. You don't *lose* your voice to laryngitis—it's more like you *lend* it for a few days. Nevertheless, that's a few days of unnecessary discomfort. Laryngitis is generally preventable.

STOP VOCAL CORD ABUSE!

Keeping your vocal cords in smooth working order doesn't require much effort. All they really need is a little tender loving care—and a sufficient amount of rest and relaxation.

Shhhhhhhhhhhh. You already know that screaming means trouble. But even *talking* can irritate your vocal cords—if you do it incessantly, warns Stephen Mitchell, M.D., chairman of the Speech, Voice and Swallowing Disorders Committee of the American Academy of Otolaryngology–Head and Neck Surgery. If your job entails a lot of speaking, whether you're a teacher, a parent, a salesperson or a motivational speaker, or if you're just a motor-mouth, organize your schedule to give your vocal cords regular breaks.

Stop clearing your throat. Your vocal cords, unlike a lion's, just aren't designed for growling. Besides driving everybody around you crazy, constant throat clearing can cause laryngitis. To break this habit, take sips of water regularly throughout the day, suggests Dr. Mitchell.

Get the drop on postnasal drip. This by-product of a cold or an allergy can irritate your vocal cords, so break up the drip and nasal congestion with an over-the-counter expectorant.

Make sure your home isn't a desert. During the cold winter months, does the heating in your house make the air as dry as burned toast? Indoor heating dries out your vocal cords, and when they get dry, they get irritated. To prevent this, use a properly working and always-clean humidifier, says Dr. Mitchell.

If you smoke, quit. Smoking is a major cause of laryngitis, says Dr. Baron. In fact, puffing on cigarettes month after month can *chronically* inflame the vocal cords. That's why older women who are heavy smokers sometimes have heavy voices.

SOOTHING YOUR SORE VOICE

Suppose you gave your vocal cords just a little more than they could handle, and now they're angry. What can you do?

BEYOND LARYNGITIS

Constant vocal cord abuse can have some alarming consequences beyond simple laryngitis.

SINGER'S NODES. These are small white-gray knots or swellings that grow on the vocal cords. "Your voice can end up being very raspy and hard," says Barry C. Baron, M.D., an otolaryngologist in private practice at the California Pacific Medical Center who treats singers from the San Francisco Opera. "The nodes can stay there permanently, like calluses, unless you train to get rid of them by using your voice differently. Surgery to get rid of them is also an option."

VOCAL POLYPS. These are small, tumorlike growths on the vocal cords that may or may not be malignant. If the polyp is benign, hoarseness may come and go, but a malignant polyp can cause continuous and worsening hoarseness. Cigarette smoking is a big cause of polyps.

CONTACT ULCERS. These are sores on the vocal cords. Along with hoarseness, there may be pain that goes from deep within the neck up to the ear. You may also experience a tickle or urge to clear your throat, a lump in your throat, aching or dryness.

Stop talking, stop dripping, humidify, quit smoking. These are the things you could have done to prevent laryngitis but didn't. If you don't do them now, you may make things worse.

Inhale some steam. Either from a sinkful of hot water with a towel draped over your head or in a nice hot shower. The vapor will moisturize your vocal cords and help them feel better, says Dr. Baron.

Have an afternoon tea. Sipping warm tea may also provide comfort, says Dr. Baron. Sucking lozenges is also good. But gargling with saltwater, an old home remedy for sore throat, may not help your vocal cords much. They're located too deep in the throat.

See a doctor. If you follow the above advice, simple laryngitis will usually cure itself within a few days. If it lasts more than a week, seek a doctor's attention.

LEGIONNAIRES' DISEASE

I t made headlines in 1976, when it affected 221 people and caused 34 deaths during an American Legion convention at a Philadelphia hotel. As perplexed health-care workers scrambled to combat this mysterious ailment that caused high fever, diarrhea, nausea, lung congestion and severe coughing, many wondered if an epidemic was about to sweep the country.

It didn't happen. Instead, Legionnaires' disease—a rare form of pneumonia—slowly faded from public awareness. But it didn't disappear. The federal Centers for Disease Control (CDC) in Atlanta continues to receive reports of about 1,000 cases a year. Fortunately, Legionnaires' is easily treated with antibiotics and is seldom fatal when promptly treated.

Since the Philadelphia outbreak, researchers have linked Legionnaires' to several mysterious epidemics dating back to 1965. They have also identified a platoon of at least 19 types of bacteria that can cause the disease. The bacteria, collectively referred to as legionella bacteria, like water and have been found in lakes and streams and in man-made devices such as hot tubs, ice machines, faucets and hot water heaters.

THIS LEGION DOESN'T MARCH, IT SWIMS

In the past, most outbreaks have been associated with hospitals and hotels. Most likely, that's because some hospitals and hotels keep the hot water at temperatures lower than many people do in their homes. Unfortunately, Legionnaires' bacteria thrive in those lower temperatures, says Victor Yu, M.D., chief of the Infectious Diseases Section of the Veterans Administration Medical Center in Pittsburgh. The bacteria have also been found in homes, however.

"There are a few people who get Legionnaires' disease from contaminated water in their own homes," Dr. Yu says. "How they get it is unclear.

Perhaps they get it by taking a shower and breathing in the aerosols. You *can* get it from a humidifier. A humidifier vaporizes the contaminated water, and you inhale it."

If you do use a humidifier, there are a couple of simple steps you can take to protect yourself.

Clean and disinfect it at least once a week. Bleach and other disinfectants will kill any Legionnaires' bacteria that may be lurking in the humidifier's reservoir. Follow the manufacturer's instructions, Dr. Yu says.

Use sterile water. "If you use tap water contaminated with Legionnaires', the humidifier will send out a mist containing the organism," Dr. Yu says. "Sterile water will eliminate that possibility. Tap water can be sterilized by boiling."

CUTTING THE RISK

Between 2 and 7 percent of all pneumonias are caused by Legionnaires', says Barbara Marston, M.D., an epidemiologist at the CDC. Its symptoms are similar to those of other types of pneumonia and commonly include coughing up phlegm, chest pain, stomach cramps and fever, sometimes in excess of 104°F.

Untreated, Legionnaires' may have up to a 25 percent mortality rate. But proper treatment with the antibiotic drug erythromycin reduces the death rate to about 5 percent, says Richard Kohler, M.D., a professor of medicine specializing in infectious disease at Indiana University School of Medicine in Indianapolis. Two new drugs, clarithromycin and azithromycin, promise to be effective against the disease.

Smokers, heavy drinkers and people who have chronic respiratory diseases such as emphysema and bronchitis are most likely to get the disease. (So quitting smoking and drinking moderately, if at all, will also help reduce your risk.) Organ transplant recipients also are at high risk, because the drugs used to prevent rejection of the transplant by their body also suppress the part of the immune system that would normally fight off Legionnaires', Dr. Marston says.

See a doctor immediately if you do get symptoms of Legionnaires'. "Recovery depends on the overall health of the patient," says Dr. Marston, "but recovery is quite probable."

LUPUS

Three days before her wedding, Angela Richardson wound up in intensive care, looking and feeling like she had been badly beaten. Hives covered her body. Her arms, legs and face were swollen. Her eyes bled. Her joints and muscles ached. Her blood pressure soared. Her doctor didn't even recognize her.

Angela was having her first attack of systemic lupus erythematosus. Her own immune system was beating her up. Had she been afflicted 30 years ago, Angela's life would have been cut short. But today, the life expectancy of someone with lupus is nearly the same as that of someone without the disease. That's how much medicine has advanced on the lupus front, says Dennis Boulware, M.D., associate professor of medicine and chief of rheumatology at the Tulane University Medical Center in New Orleans.

IMMUNITY ON THE RAMPAGE

You want your immune system to do its job of fighting off infection by bacteria and viruses. And when the job is done, you want it to go back to the barracks until needed again. But in lupus, the immune system doesn't quit. "It can't turn itself off," says Dr. Boulware.

Sometimes, as in Angela's case, the disease comes on abruptly; sometimes it's gradual. And as with Angela, most patients with lupus develop it as young adults. Usually it has flare-ups and remissions, although the severity and the symptoms vary greatly from one person to the next. Fever and fatigue are common. About half the afflicted develop a butterfly-shaped facial rash that spreads across the cheeks and nose. Many become extremely sensitive to sunlight. About half get an inflammation of the outer lining of the lungs that makes breathing painful. The symptom doctors worry about most, Dr. Boulware says, is inflammation of the kidneys and the brain.

It's estimated that 16,000 Americans develop lupus each year, adding to the 500,000 who have already been diagnosed. It takes urine and blood studies, x-rays, electrocardiograms and even kidney biopsies to diagnose lupus and discover where it's done its dirty work.

No one knows what causes lupus. "But there's a strong genetic factor. We think people inherit a genetic predisposition for their immune system to turn on but not turn off," says Dr. Boulware. There's about a 1 in 19 chance that parents with lupus will have a child who develops the disease. Unfortunately, if you're born with the genetic predisposition, there's no sure way to avoid lupus. "All you can really do is maintain a healthy lifestyle—good diet, exercise, balance between work and play," says Dr. Boulware.

Lupus strikes women about eight times more frequently than it does men, and blacks much more often than whites. Again, no one knows why.

PROFILE IN HEALING

FRANCES KNUCKLES: "I HAVE LUPUS; LUPUS DOESN'T HAVE ME"

At age 15, Frances Knuckles says, she had her first lupus symptom: serious digestion problems. But another 19 years went by until, in 1983, a rheumatologist finally diagnosed lupus. In those intervening years, she suffered repeated attacks that were misdiagnosed by dozens of doctors.

"The hardest thing was not knowing what I had," Frances says. "I was worried that I was contagious and maybe could kill my husband. One dermatologist told me I was crazy. I told him off and said, 'Don't bother billing me, because I'm not paying.' "

That feisty attitude has made the difference in Frances's life with lupus. Despite spending about ten days out of every year in a hospital—for problems with her intestines, lungs and heart, and the last time, for a liver infection—Frances holds down a full-time job as a bookkeeper and payroll clerk for a tree surgery company in Atascadero, California, where she lives. The job helps her maintain her positive attitude. And prednisone, a steroid medication, helps to control the disease.

Frances gets support from her husband, Bruce, and from the Central Coast Chapter of the American Lupus Society. Frances has Raynaud's phenomenon, the cold-hands ailment that often afflicts people with lupus, so on cold mornings, Bruce starts her car to get the

Among women, female hormones seem to play a role—during flare-ups, women may have irregular menstrual periods or none at all, and flare-ups often dangerously erupt right after pregnancy.

LIVING WELL WITH LUPUS

Despite the devastating effects lupus can have, medical care and self-help techniques let most people adapt in ways that allow them to enjoy life.

Educating yourself will give you a handle on the disease, and the best place to start is with your doctor. It's essential to find a doctor who is highly experienced in treating lupus.

The mainstay medication for lupus is the steroid prednisone. Steroids are the most potent anti-inflammatory drugs we have, "and at one time or

---

heater going, then warms her gloves with a hair dryer. The support group, which she serves as president, offers the companionship of others who really understand.

"We try to look at lupus as just one part of our lives," Frances says. "We also have families, friends, art, jobs, hobbies. We do compare horror stories, but we don't allow gripe sessions, because they go nowhere. In fact, we don't even really talk about the disease itself. We call each other when we're down, or when we're up, we compare notes about treatments."

When Frances gets stressed out—as when an unknowing stranger berates her for parking in the handicapped zone because she doesn't look disabled, despite the fact that she has a permit—"I make myself calm down and chill out," she says. She leaves plenty of time to drive to work, so that traffic is no problem. At work, she has good days when everything goes well and bad days when her heart skips beats and a rash spreads across her face, "but I tough it out," she says.

"When I see the sunset or see the mama deer and her two fawns playing tug-of-war with the Spanish moss hanging from the oak trees in our yard, I'm thankful I'm alive, that I have the beautiful sky above, my family, my friends and my support group," says Frances. "The disease is an inconvenience, not a life sentence. There's so much more to life than lupus. I have lupus; lupus doesn't have me."

another, the vast majority of people with lupus will have to take them," mainly to save their kidneys or brain, says Dr. Boulware. But while steroids can be lifesaving, the side effects of prolonged use can be bad. These include puffiness of the face, acne, weight gain, increase in facial hair, diabetes and liver problems.

Because of these side effects, your doctor won't prescribe steroids unless you absolutely need them. But if you're not on steroids, you'll likely be told to take nonsteroidal anti-inflammatory drugs like ibuprofen and to use topical steroids for the skin rash.

A WINNING STRATEGY

Beyond the medical strategies of your doctor, there is much you can do to make lupus more tolerable.

Shield yourself from the sun. In some people with lupus, the ultraviolet rays of the sun can trigger a flare-up. If you find that you are sun sensitive, always cover up with a sunscreen, long sleeves and pants, a hat and sunglasses before venturing into daylight, says Dr. Boulware.

Avoid alcohol and cigarettes. While it's basic good sense to limit your vices, that goes double for people with lupus, Dr. Boulware says. There are no studies showing alcohol and tobacco can make lupus worse, but logic dictates caution. Lupus often invades the linings of the lungs and heart, organs also targeted by tobacco. And alcohol is an efficient depressant, something no person with lupus needs.

Cut back on caffeine. If you're on medication for lupus, you may already have digestive problems, and caffeine can make these worse, says T. Stephen Balch, M.D., medical director of the Jacquelyn McClure Lupus Treatment Center in Atlanta. In addition, people with lupus may have heart and kidney troubles. Caffeine can increase the heart rate and, since it's a diuretic, can put an unneeded strain on the kidneys.

Beware of colds or flu. Ironically, despite their overactive immune systems, people with lupus are more susceptible to infections of all kinds, Dr. Boulware says. Yet immunizations like flu shots can trigger flare-ups. It's difficult to avoid people with colds or flu, but be sure to get medical attention early if you do become infected.

Load up on fiber. People with lupus often have a mysterious digestive disorder called irritable bowel syndrome (see page 320), causing bloating, constipation or diarrhea, Dr. Balch says. A high-fiber diet may help prevent the problem.

Watch out for protein. If you've got kidney problems because of lupus, too much protein can make matters worse. Check with your doctor about how much protein you should be eating, Dr. Balch says.

Get some exercise. Exercise has been shown to help reduce fatigue and pain in lupus patients. The key here is moderation, Dr. Balch says. Exercise like swimming or walking can improve your conditioning and help you manage lupus better. Talk with your doctor about an exercise program.

Have a life. Family, friends, outside interests, helping others, getting counseling—all of these provide emotional support and may help you keep a healthy outlook, says Dr. Balch.

LYME DISEASE

E very summer, vacationers stream into Lyme, Connecticut, to enjoy the sunshine, beaches and tranquility of this picturesque resort town. But Lyme has a tainted history. Among scientists, medical historians and the national news media, what makes Lyme tick is its *ticks*—more specifically, the tick-borne bacteria, first discovered in Lyme, that cause Lyme disease.

In all fairness to the Lyme Chamber of Commerce, Lyme disease was making people sick long before doctors from Yale and the Connecticut State Health Department arrived in town in 1975 to investigate an outbreak of what appeared to be juvenile rheumatoid arthritis. Lyme disease has been around, at least in Europe, since the 1920s, says William S. Paul, M.D., of Fort Collins, Colorado, an infectious disease expert with the federal Centers for Disease Control in Atlanta. Today it has been reported in 46 states (although it's more common in the Northeast and upper Midwest and along the Pacific coast), so even though the disease first was *identified* in Lyme, it's now a national concern.

OF MICE AND MEN

Lyme disease is caused by the bacteria *Borrelia burgdorferi,* which normally live quite happily (and without causing disease) in white-footed mice. Trouble begins when hungry deer ticks feed first on white mice and then on you. Should *B. burgdorferi* from an infected tick enter your bloodstream, they can make you, unlike the white mouse, very sick indeed.

Most people infected with Lyme disease will develop a rash that gradually radiates outward from the bite site like circles in a pond. You may also have fever, chills, muscle aches and other flulike symptoms. If left untreated, "there's definite risk that it will go on to cause Lyme arthritis or neurological problems such as paralysis of the face, or meningitis, or even heart problems," Dr. Paul says.

Indeed, researchers from Tufts University School of Medicine examined 39 children who had been infected with Lyme disease for ten years and who had not received proper treatment at the onset. The researchers discovered that 12 (31 percent) of the group were still having occasional episodes of joint swelling and pain, the so-called Lyme arthritis.

CREATE A TICK-FREE ZONE

With proper treatment, Lyme disease can be rendered tame, but it's still a lot easier to prevent the disease than to treat it later. To keep ticks at bay:

Get ticked off. If you're in a high-risk area—such as the northeastern United States—be careful of woods and tall grasses from May through October. If you venture out, wear long-sleeved shirts and long pants. Tuck your pants into your socks or boots. For added protection, apply insect repellents containing DEET to your arms, legs and head. You can also spray your clothes with the repellent permethrin, which will help prevent ticks from coming home with you.

Protect your pets. Deer ticks that hitch a ride on Fido's fur may hop

---

TREATMENT BREAKTHROUGH

PURE PROTECTION

If you spend time in the woods in tick-infested regions such as the northeastern United States, there is no absolutely foolproof way to protect yourself from Lyme disease. According to the federal Centers for Disease Control (CDC) in Atlanta, approximately 8,000 cases of Lyme disease are reported every year. Clearly, the danger is real.

One way to reduce the risk, researchers say, would be to create a Lyme disease vaccine. Like the flu vaccines currently in use, this could protect people *before* they get infected, says William S. Paul, M.D., medical epidemiologist for the CDC. But it's a tall order. "The best vaccines we have are for viruses, which are much simpler organisms than bacteria. We need to learn a whole lot more about how the body's immune system responds to Lyme disease before we can develop an effective vaccine," he says.

Still, progress is being made. Researchers from the University of Wisconsin and Wisconsin State Laboratory of Hygiene report developing a vaccine that, at least in one small study, protected hamsters against infection. *All* the hamsters.

But animals are one thing, people are another, says Robert T. Schoen, M.D., of the Lyme Disease Clinic at Yale University School of Medicine. "I think we're still several years away from testing a Lyme disease vaccine on humans."

off to feed on you. If you live in an area known to harbor deer ticks, inspect your pet for ticks and use a repellent before your pet ventures into fields or wooded areas. And during the summer months, keep pets clean with a tick- and flea-killing shampoo. You can also check with your veterinarian for dips and repellent sprays.

Remove ticks ASAP. Deer ticks are extremely small, about the size and color of poppy seeds. The sooner you remove ticks, the better your chances for staying disease-free. It often takes 24 hours before a tick begins to pass on the bacteria. By wearing light-colored clothing, you can spot them and pluck them off before they have a chance to grab hold of you.

Remove them gently. Ticks already embedded are loath to give up a good meal, and removing them can be tricky. Forget such home remedies as coating them with oil or lighting matches to scorch their rear ends, Dr. Paul says. Instead, grasp them with sharp tweezers as close to the skin as possible and gently pull them out. Make sure you pull straight, he adds. "Do not twist—ticks don't screw in or out." It might also be a good idea to save the tick if you're not sure whether it's a deer tick. Your doctor should be able to help you identify what kind of tick bit you. If it is a deer tick, be aware of any symptoms that might develop.

Watch for symptoms. Occasionally, the hallmark rash doesn't appear, and the disease may progress directly to fever, miscellaneous aches, swelling, joint pain or fatigue. If you live in a high-risk area and you suspect Lyme disease, see your doctor right away, Dr. Paul advises.

STOPPING IT COLD

Although Lyme disease still makes people very sick, most doctors agree it can easily be managed. Even in areas where a majority of ticks carry the infectious organisms, fewer than 2 percent of tick bites actually cause disease. Should you get infected, the treatment—and cure—is an office visit away.

"If you get antibiotics at the beginning of the illness, there's about a 95 percent chance you'll be cured of Lyme disease," says Robert T. Schoen, M.D., an associate clinical professor of medicine and co-director of the Lyme Disease Clinic at Yale University School of Medicine. "Even if treatment is delayed until more serious symptoms appear—swollen joints, for example—antibiotics will still knock out the disease in 60 to 70 percent of all cases," he says.

"Frequently it's my job to reassure people that it's not as bad as they think," adds Dr. Schoen. "Yes, Lyme disease has been reported to do serious things. But the average person who has Lyme disease that is detected and treated should have no further problems with it."

MASTITIS

olly couldn't wait to bring her newborn son home from the hospital. She pictured herself breast-feeding Joey in cozy comfort, tenderly caressing his tiny head while gently rocking in the oak rocker.

But Molly's picture-perfect vision of breast-feeding soon developed an ugly blot. After a few weeks, one of her breasts became so tender and swollen, it was hard to tell who wailed louder, Joey or Molly.

Fortunately, a call to her doctor reassured Molly that she was experiencing a mild form of mastitis, an inflammation of the breast that commonly occurs in nursing mothers in the first weeks after birth. Much to her relief, Molly learned that she would not have to give up breast-feeding. In fact, breast-feeding is the prescribed treatment for mastitis.

THE CASE OF THE CLOGGED DUCT

When a nursing mother develops a painful area in her breast and there's no fever, it's usually caused by a plugged milk duct. This occurs when the breast is not emptying as completely as it should. The milk backs up in the ducts, resulting in inflammation.

Take Molly's case, for example. A few weeks after Joey's birth, she returned to work. Up until that time, Joey had nursed on and off all day, which stimulated Molly's breasts to produce lots of milk. When Molly's work schedule abruptly cut back on the nursing schedule, her milk supply exceeded the demand. Her breasts became overly full and, by late afternoon, sore and swollen.

To make matters worse, because her breasts ached, Molly rushed nursing Joey, leaving her breasts only partially drained. Overnight, her right breast became tender, and she stopped nursing from that breast entirely, which was the worst thing she could have done. As a result, milk backed up, a duct clogged, and her sore breast turned scarlet and throbbed like the dickens.

This is a classic example of inflammatory mastitis. "When an abrupt change in the nursing pattern occurs for any reason, it sets the stage for plugged ducts and mastitis," says Karen Ogle, M.D., associate professor of family practice at Michigan State University in Lansing. Also common: Babies who previously nursed all night suddenly become sound sleepers, leaving Mom with breasts filled to the brim.

YOUR BREAST PLAN

What can you do to prevent or treat aching, throbbing breasts?

Lessen your load. "Always nurse at the first feeling of fullness," says Dr. Ogle. Your baby's body should be fully facing the breast during nursing. This helps him to latch on to the nipple properly and to thoroughly empty the ducts of milk. "If you are away from your baby, hand express or pump enough milk to relieve the overfullness," says Dr. Ogle.

Break through the pain. If, like Molly, your breast becomes inflamed, you must continue to nurse to drain it. "Despite the discomfort, now is *not* the time to wean to the bottle," says Dr. Ogle. Stop nursing when you have inflammatory mastitis, and you risk causing an abscess, which will have to be surgically drained.

Once inflammation subsides, however, you can wean by cutting back one feeding at a time. That way, your breasts will gradually slow down milk production.

But for now, while the inflammation persists, try to breast-feed every 1 to 2 hours, followed by gentle hand expression or pumping if necessary to relieve the plugged duct. Begin nursing on the unaffected breast until you feel milk ready to flow from the inflamed breast, then switch sides. Take acetaminophen for pain and drink plenty of fluids.

Apply a little warmth. To encourage the milk flow, apply a warm, wet towel to the sore breast before nursing. You may also help loosen a plugged duct by leaning over a basin of warm water and immersing your breast before nursing.

Free your breasts. Check your bra. It shouldn't be so tight that it constricts milk flow. Also avoid sleeping on your stomach for prolonged periods, which can cause pressure against your breasts.

WHEN TO CALL THE DOCTOR

If, despite following these tips, your breasts remain sore and red for 24 hours or you have a fever, chills or other flulike symptoms, call your doctor. It probably means you've developed infectious mastitis.

Infectious mastitis is caused when a bacterium such as *Staphylococcus aureus* enters the mother's body, perhaps through a cracked nipple, and the organism settles in a milk duct.

In any case, you'll need an antibiotic to clear things up. Stick with the full course of drugs your doctor gives you, so that reinfection doesn't occur.

Once again, continue to breast-feed. "Don't worry about passing the infection on to the baby," says Dr. Ogle. It's the breast tissue that's infected, not the breast milk. The antibiotic that passes into the breast milk is probably fine for your baby, but you should check with your doctor to be sure.

A final Rx: Rest. You need it to build your resistance and to counteract stress, which can hamper the free flow of milk.

MEMORY LOSS

L ouise, it's Maybelle. Did you hear about Grendl Frebbish's daughter? I forget her name. Oh, you know, she's the one who looks like Edward G. Robinson, only she's got her father's Groucho Marx nose. She married that mousetrap salesman over in East Vegeburg—the one who sneaked mice into people's houses the day before he knocked on their doors. Oh, you know her name. Well, she left him for that car dealer who looks like Don Knotts and sold her that 1959 Buick with the big fins but with the backseat and the trunk chopped out to make it into a pickup truck! . . . Yes! Now what is her name? It's right on the tip of my tongue!"

Maybelle complains to her doctor that her memory is failing, but actually, she can remember every important detail of this bit of small-town gossip except Grendl Frebbish's daughter's name (it's Frondella). Actually, she can remember just about every detail of the lives of everybody who lives or who has ever lived in New Hogjowl, Pennsylvania. She's constantly learning new things about them, too. She just has a little trouble recalling bits and pieces of this vital information, especially when under pressure from Louise. She has "tip-of-the-tongue syndrome," known to doctors as benign senescent forgetfulness, or age-associated memory impairment.

PROBABLY NOTHING SERIOUS

Maybelle isn't alone. Half of all people over age 60 have memory problems, but only a few have conditions that can really do damage to their memory, like Alzheimer's disease or the aftereffects of stroke. *"Benign senescent forgetfulness* is a relatively new term that refers to the natural lapses in memory that often come with aging," says behavioral neurologist Frank Benson, M.D., professor of neurology at the University of California, Los Angeles.

After all, your body slows down as you age, so why not your mind? "It happens to all of us," Dr. Benson says. "Look at the difference in the best marathon times between a well-conditioned young runner and a well-conditioned elderly runner," he says. "The older runner's times are darn near twice as long." Memory is just another physical process, he explains, and like all physical processes, it slows down with age.

Memory making begins with learning, moves to storage and then to retrieval. What Maybelle is going through is "not exceptional," Dr. Benson says. "It's pretty well documented that, up until about age 70, people can learn just about as well as younger people, but they're slower at retrieving things they have already learned and less competent at recalling correctly. They need more cues and prompts before they can get going. I'm getting into this age group myself, and I know it exists."

USE IT OR LOSE IT

Still, Dr. Benson notes, your memory is better than you think it is. "A sizable number of people complain that they're forgetful, but when they're tested, they test well," he says. "Maybe not as well as most people, but good enough."

In fact, as you age, "you'll probably lose much more time off the 100-yard dash than you will in your ability to remember things," says neuropsychologist Curt Sandman, Ph.D., co-director of the Memory Disorders Clinic at the University of California, Irvine, Medical School. "We simply don't see devastating losses in memory in older people who aren't sick."

If you've never run a marathon, or even the 100-yard dash, you never will unless you get your rear off the couch, your feet into running shoes and your body in gear. The same goes for your memory, Dr. Benson says. "The old 'use it or lose it' idea may be just as true for mental activity as it is for physical activity. Keeping an active mind is something you should do all your life."

MIND YOUR BODY

Your memory is in your brain, and your brain is in your body. Your brain lives on the same blood and nutrients as the rest of you. To be at its best, it needs the rest of you to be at *its* best.

There's plenty you can do to keep your body in good enough shape to preserve and improve your memory.

Go that extra mile. A brisk, daily 20-minute walk is enough to get your blood pumping all the way up to your head to feed those hungry memory cells, Dr. Sandman says. But you can do more than just aerobics to help your memory, he adds. "We assigned elderly people as foster grandparents to neurologically impaired children. The foster grandparents had to walk several miles a day, they had social interactions they otherwise wouldn't have had, and there were physical demands on them in caring 20 hours a week for another human being." EEGs showed the foster grandparents had higher brain activity, better memory and better sleep, he says.

Follow sound sleeping advice. Be sure to get a good night's sleep, so that you can be alert enough the next day to learn and remember what you want to, say memory experts. Your chances of sleeping well are increased if you don't eat and drink late at night. Sleeping pills don't help much either—they knock you out more than let you sleep, and you can really feel sluggish the next day.

B is for brain food. Your diet plays a big role, too. The B-complex vitamins are especially important, along with the right amounts of protein and carbohydrates. A balanced and varied diet of fresh foods—fruits, vegetables, dairy products, fish, poultry and grains—is an easy way to get everything your brain needs.

One food in particular has been shown to improve memory: a fruit drink sweetened with the simple sugar known as glucose. University of Virginia researchers found that people who drank the glucose drink just before memory tests did much better than those who drank a fruit drink sweetened with sodium saccharin. But check with your doctor before you start guzzling glucose-sweetened lemonade: People with high blood sugar levels (like those caused by diabetes) did poorly on the memory tests. In fact, if your memory is failing, you may want to have your blood sugar checked—that may be your problem.

VARIETY IS THE SPICE OF LIFE

"People who are using their memory and pushing themselves and really maintaining as much interest in what goes on around them as they did when they were kids may well get along better than those who are pretty complacent and going about doing the same things day after day and not challenging their minds," says Dr. Benson. "You've got to learn new things in order to remember them."

Variety is a matter of details, yet the older you get, the less likely you are to pay attention to details, Dr. Sandman says. "What we think happens is that you pay more attention to general principles," he says. "You may ignore the details younger people concentrate on in favor of understanding how the world works. So if you're tested about details that have just happened, you may have ignored them, and you're said to have a bad memory. What really happened is that those details didn't really change the world and so you didn't pay attention to them. It's not really a loss of memory; it's a way of adapting to the world, and we call that wisdom."

In fact, Dr. Sandman notes, many of the older people he tests for memory "don't even care if they do well on these detail tests. They don't think those details are important. They think I'm a nice young guy—I'm 50 years old—and they're just helping me out by trying to be nice and taking my tests."

So what do you do if you're wise but still want to remember details?

Put some spice in your life. "The number one stimulus is variety," Dr. Sandman says. One of his studies challenged Alzheimer's patients and their spouses to do something different each week. Then the couples were given memory tests—not for that special event but for all the little details of their lives that week. "We found that adding spice to their lives improved their memories significantly," says Dr. Sandman.

What kind of spice? "Some of them had romantic lovers' picnics in the park, the kind of thing they hadn't done for 55 years," Dr. Sandman says. Others took short trips. "As they get older, many people tend to become tied very closely to their house," he says. "We encouraged them to take some risks, buy things they had put off buying, indulge in dining out on food they've never tried before. These were all ordinary, simple, enjoyable things that had a jarring effect on their memories."

Stop living in the past. Reminiscing is anything but variety, and it hurts your ability to remember details, Dr. Sandman says. "There's tremendous satisfaction in reminiscing," he says. "I'd ask my patients why they didn't remember a particular event in the past week, and I'd find that they had taken off on this little reminiscing fantasy. It's very seductive. There's no more exotic place to travel than in time. You completely block out the rest of the world. Everything going on around you is quite secondary. But it produces memory loss." Instead, Dr. Sandman advises, "replace the satisfaction of internal trips with external trips."

MEMORY METHODS

Now it's time to give the brain itself a workout. If you've been watching a lot of TV, you'll notice that TV people don't think much of your ability to concentrate for any length of time. Prove them wrong.

Try taking the TV test. "In one study, my patients and I all watched the same TV programs at home," says Dr. Sandman. "Then we all made up tests about the details of the programs. They asked me questions, and I asked them questions. Even though the questions weren't the same, their ability to answer *my* questions improved remarkably, just because they themselves drew up questions to ask me. As a matter of fact, I could answer *their* questions better, too, because I had also drawn up questions to ask them."

All you have to do is watch a program and write down ten questions. Three days later, ask yourself those questions. If done regularly, "it's amazing what this will do for your memory," Dr. Sandman says.

Relax and get emotional. One of the memory problems that causes the most anxiety is the ability to remember names. Well, you can relax. Really. "Just become less anxious about remembering names," Dr. Sandman advises. "Instead, after you're introduced to someone, don't even focus on the name and the face. Instead, focus on interests, on things you have in common with the person. You build an emotional halo around the person."

This means you go deeper than just the superficiality of name. Because you find out more about the person, including things you have in common that you hold dear, this person registers in your emotions. "Emo-

---

WHEN IS IT ALZHEIMER'S, AND WHEN ISN'T IT?

Fear of Alzheimer's disease is common, and it's often the first thing to pop into your mind when you start forgetting things. Yet it's not likely your memory problems are the beginning of Alzheimer's.

The fundamental difference, says neurologist Frank Benson, M.D., is that "people with Alzheimer's don't learn. People with slowing memories can learn." For fast relief from the fear and trepidation of Alzheimer's, take a look at this table, prepared by social worker Lisa Gwyther, director of Duke University's Alzheimer's Family Support Program and assistant professor of psychiatric social work.

ACTIVITY	ALZHEIMER'S	NORMAL MEMORY LOSS
Attending an event	Forgets the whole experience	Forgets parts of experience
Following directions	Gradually unable	Usually able
Taking notes; using reminders	Gradually unable	Usually able
Caring for self	Gradually unable	Usually able

tional memories never die," Dr. Sandman says. Having this emotional focus does two things: You have something to talk about, and that relieves anxiety in a social situation; and it helps you to remember the name.

Go over it again and again. Rehearsal is a tried-and-true method of remembering. College students call it cramming. "If you want to learn and remember something, just rehearse it," Dr. Sandman says. "We had a group of our patients take pictures of each other and write the names on the backs. Then they went over and over the names and, at the same time, used the emotional associations—what these people do for a living, trips they'd taken, how many children they had, anything they felt they could identify with. Now these were people who were having a hard time remembering their spouses' names. After four weeks, they were remembering all the names of the people in the group."

And Dr. Sandman's patients had Alzheimer's disease, so you can imagine how well simpler rehearsals, even without emotional associations, could work for you!

MORE WORDS OF WISDOM

Although memory problems are a normal part of aging, they can sometimes be a symptom of physical or emotional disease. There's a long list of conditions that affect memory, including Alzheimer's disease (see "When Is It Alzheimer's, and When Isn't It?" on the opposite page), depression, fatigue, grief, artery disease, alcoholism and diabetes. So if you notice your memory is starting to slip, discuss it with your doctor.

Of course, you've got to be able to hear and see in order to remember. As you age, the lens of your eye yellows and impairs vision. The power of your ears to hear high-pitched sounds declines. So be sure to have your vision and hearing checked and remedied. And while you're with the doctor, ask if any medications you're taking could be making you forgetful.

If your health is on your side, improving your memory should be simple—exercise your body and mind. There's no reason you shouldn't be able to someday tell your grandchildren, in great detail, how you ran away with Grandpa in his vinyl siding truck while Maybelle was peeking around the corner of the drugstore.

MENIERE'S DISEASE

One of childhood's favorite games is to spin like a top until you get so dizzy you collapse in a heap. Older children like to urge their younger siblings on just to watch them stagger around afterward. Some kids and adults delight in amusement park rides that spin them into a dizzy euphoria.

But for two to five million Americans, dizzy spells come unbidden and unwanted—while they're cleaning house, conducting a business meeting, shopping, entertaining friends or, worst of all, driving. They feel like they're on a merry-go-round, completely disoriented—the sense of unreality only vertigo can create. These people suffer from Meniere's disease, an illness that attacks the inner ear, first robbing them of their balance and then attacking their hearing.

STOP THE WORLD, I WANT TO GET OFF!

Meniere's disease is a mystery. "Whoever finds the cause will probably win a Nobel prize," says Ronald Amedee, M.D., assistant professor of otolaryngology/head and neck surgery at Tulane University in New Orleans. The disease "strikes out of nowhere in totally healthy people," he says. Most are between 35 and 55 years old. "Usually the doctor first finds out about it when a patient calls from the floor of the bedroom or bathroom," says Dr. Amedee.

The attack usually hits one ear. You'll likely notice a loss of hearing in that ear, a sense of fullness or pressure, perhaps tinnitus—ringing in the ear—and the overwhelming dizziness.

The attacks normally last anywhere from a few minutes to as long as 24 hours and can range from mild to severe, says Dr. Amedee. "In the early stages of the disease, you can have two or three attacks per month. Occasionally the attacks can occur more frequently in more aggressive forms of the disease."

Without treatment, Meniere's most likely will eventually burn itself out, and the sufferer will find relief from the incapacitating vertigo. But that burnout "can take as long as 30 to 40 years of misery," says Dr. Amedee. And meanwhile, your hearing in the affected ear can be destroyed. "It's as though the ear were committing suicide," he says.

The destruction occurs because of the intricate links between hearing and balance. "The inner ear is two organs in one," says Dr. Amedee. "It holds the cochlea, the hearing organ, and the labyrinth, the balance organ." In Meniere's, the balance organ goes haywire—and its garbled chemical messages will, without treatment, also eventually destroy the hearing organ.

"Once the disease has burned itself out in one ear, balance is restored, because the other ear compensates," says Dr. Amedee. The other ear also retains hearing. "Those 15 to 20 percent of the people who have Meniere's in both ears have a real problem—although there are still treatment options available," he says.

TREATMENT: A HUGE SUCCESS RATE

Even though the cause of Meniere's is a mystery, doctors have devised highly successful treatments.

First your doctor will likely try the conservative approach. You'll be given motion sickness drugs (antihistamines) to suppress the function of the balance organ, "to give it a rest," says Dr. Amedee. The most popular motion sickness drug is meclizine (Antivert).

Your doctor may also prescribe diuretic drugs, the same ones used to treat high blood pressure, to reduce the pressure caused by the inner ear fluids.

These drugs do have side effects—the antihistamines make you drowsy and, in men, can create bladder problems, while the diuretics may cause weakness or occasionally impotence. But these side effects are tolerable in the face of vertigo. The antihistamines are used only for the short term, while the diuretics are a long-term proposition.

At the same time, the doctor will monitor your blood pressure to make sure it doesn't drop too low, "a very rare occurrence in Meniere's patients," says Dr. Amedee. And you'll go on a low-salt diet—salt makes your body retain fluid, and eating less salt helps the diuretic work and makes lower dosages possible.

"These drugs don't cure Meniere's, but they make the attacks less frequent and less severe, and most important, they help preserve your hearing," Dr. Amedee says. "There's a success rate of 75 to 80 percent— that is, your attacks may be cut to one or two per year at most."

JUDE ARRAS: BACK ON AN EVEN KEEL

Jude Arras was lying under a truck in May 1989, doing his thing as a self-employed welder, when the world suddenly seemed to career out of orbit. "Everything started spinning around me," he says.

The 50-year-old resident of East Carondelet, Illinois, managed to get himself to the hospital, where tests revealed nothing. A week later, an ear, nose and throat specialist told him he had Meniere's disease—verified by a balance test—and put him on Antivert. "A dizzy pill," Jude says.

"I took it for a year, and I slept for a year," he says. Antivert, a motion sickness drug commonly prescribed for vertigo, makes you drowsy—really drowsy. "There was a week or two when I couldn't even get out of bed," he says. "And it didn't do much for the dizzy spells either. They could happen anytime, when I was driving, or working, or just sitting around." The attacks would usually last from 5 to 20 minutes, he says, "but one lasted for a week straight. I had to crawl from my bedroom to the kitchen."

Meniere's often subjects its victims to gossip. "People who know me know I don't drink," Jude says, "but some acquaintances looked down their noses at me." The sense of unreality induced by the dizziness, the anxiety caused by never knowing when an attack would come and the misunderstanding from the ignorant and judgmental combined to send Jude into depression.

He tried a specialist in nearby St. Louis and was given a battery of expensive tests. The result? "The doctor told me to live with it and then relieved my wallet of a few thousand dollars," says Jude.

At the end of that year, Jude read about Tulane University surgeon Ronald Amedee, M.D., and his treatment of Meniere's—inserting a tiny flake of streptomycin in the inner ear to destroy the malfunctioning balance organ while preserving the hearing organ.

In May 1990, Arras had the surgery, had only minor pain and was on the road to recovery.

Today, Jude has no symptoms at all of Meniere's. He's back to regular work and can drive anywhere he wants.

"I went through a year of hell," the soft-spoken man says. "Now life is back on an even keel. It's like being reborn."

SURGERY: WHEN DRUGS FAIL

One out of four or five people, however, won't respond to drug treatment, says Dr. Amedee, sometimes because the disease has progressed too far when they finally see a doctor.

The newest form of surgery, pioneered at Tulane University, has now been performed on hundreds of patients with a success rate of about 90 percent. In a procedure called selective chemical labyrinthectomy, the surgeon makes a small incision behind the ear and applies a flake of streptomycin into the inner ear. Over the next several hours, the drug begins to kill the balance organ. It's an operation for a highly skilled ear surgeon—too much drug, or a miscalculation, can also destroy the hearing organ, says Dr. Amedee. But performed correctly, he says, "the surgery destroys the balance organ and offers the potential to preserve hearing in the affected ear."

In severe cases, a doctor might recommend an even more complicated operation in which the surgeon cuts the nerve leading from the balance organ to the balance center of the brain. "It's a more invasive form of surgery for those patients who have failed to respond to conservative medical treatment," says Dr. Amedee.

TAKING CARE OF YOURSELF

There's no known way to prevent Meniere's disease, and you need a doctor's care to handle it. If you experience any of the symptoms described here, see a doctor immediately—your hearing is at stake.

If you're on drugs for Meniere's disease, "you have to take them daily, as instructed," cautions Dr. Amedee. "Too many people forget or stop taking them because they feel better. The longer you have to take drugs, the harder it is to comply, but compliance is essential to protect your hearing and decrease the potential for severe attacks."

People with Meniere's have an upbeat prognosis, says Dr. Amedee. "In the long run, the vast majority of people do quite well with conservative therapy. They can work, drive, lead very physically active lives. Very few therapies for such disabling diseases can claim that kind of success."

MENINGITIS

Y ou've never before hurt so much. Your forehead is hot enough to roast chestnuts. You've just vomited what seems like your last eight meals. And inside your head, a battalion of cackling gremlins is driving needles into your most sensitive nerve endings. Could it be the flu? Or could it be something worse, like meningitis?

Meningitis, an ugly but fortunately rare disease, often starts off with the same symptoms as the common flu. But along with the fever, nausea and headaches, you might also experience a stiff neck, an oversensitivity to bright light and, occasionally, a deep red or purplish rash.

What these symptoms may mean is that your *meninges,* the membranes that cover your brain and spinal cord, have become infected and inflamed. The cause is usually an invasion by either viruses or bacteria. Sometimes these organisms are carried to the meninges by the bloodstream from another part of the body, such as the lungs. Sometimes a head injury, like a skull fracture, or an infected sinus or ear can open the door to such an invasion.

THE ESSENTIAL DIAGNOSIS

The symptoms of both types of meningitis, viral and bacterial, are the same. But the bacterial kind is much more dangerous—in fact, potentially deadly if not treated quickly. That is why it's important to act on these symptoms immediately by going to your doctor or a hospital emergency room.

There's only one way to tell the two kinds of meningitis apart, says Bradley Perkins, M.D., a specialist in meningitis with the federal Centers for Disease Control (CDC) in Atlanta. That one way is with a spinal tap. Doctors remove a dose of spinal fluid for analysis to tell what kind of organism may be at the source of your woes.

If that organism is a virus, you can breathe a sigh of relief. You'll feel rotten for a while, but you'll probably be well in two to three weeks.

THE VIRAL VARIETY

The kind of meningitis caused by viruses is not only the less dangerous of the two, it's also the more common. These viruses usually spread from person to person and tend to spread quickly among groups, much like a flu. The favorite victims of viral meningitis are children and young adults. "Their immune systems are usually strong enough that they get better without medication," Dr. Perkins says. "Antibiotics don't work against a virus, and antiviral drugs have so many side effects that it's usually not worth giving them."

In other words, if you have viral meningitis, you simply need to tough it out as you would a flu. What can you do to feel better? The same things you'd do if you had the flu.

Stay home and rest. Let your body devote its energy to fighting the infection, Dr. Perkins says. "You won't feel like getting out of bed anyway."

Drink plenty of fluids. Fever dehydrates you. And you've got to keep your elimination system well watered to flush out the debris of the war in progress between your immune system and the virus.

Reach for the bottle. Take aspirin, ibuprofen or acetaminophen as needed for the pain, says Dr. Perkins. But don't give aspirin to anyone under 21 because of the risk of Reye's syndrome, a serious neurological disease.

Darken the room. Your eyes are probably hypersensitive to light, and that can make your headache worse.

Keep eating. It's essential to keep up your strength.

Take an antinausea medication. How can you eat if you're nauseated and throwing up? Try an over-the-counter preparation recommended by your doctor or pharmacist.

Take it easy. Don't go out and run races or dance till dawn right after you've recovered—that's risking a relapse. Again, think of yourself as having had the world's worst flu, and act accordingly. Give yourself time to regain your strength.

THE BACTERIAL BLIGHT

Even though bacterial meningitis is extremely dangerous, it's much less common than it used to be, and if caught early, it is usually highly curable, Dr. Perkins says. Bacterial culprits include very common bacteria like *Streptococcus pneumoniae* and *Hemophilus influenzae* type b (Hib). "Most of us carry these bacteria around, but we don't get sick, because our immune systems keep them in check," says Dr. Perkins. "The people most susceptible are probably those with some kind of immune deficiency or those who have gotten some new strain of bacteria that they haven't developed an immunity to." Babies, the elderly and people traveling through certain nations with epidemic diseases are most at risk.

No matter the specific bacteria, the treatment is the same: hospitalization and intravenous antibiotics. "You should be in the hospital for a minimum of 7 days, and often up to 14 days," Dr. Perkins says. "You'll usually get dramatically better very fast." When you're discharged, you may take oral antibiotics for another couple of weeks. Treatment is essential; without it, bacterial meningitis is fatal at least 70 percent of the time.

Although some forms of meningitis will probably be with us for some time, the kind caused by the bacteria *Hemophilus influenzae* type b may be on the wane. This number one cause of bacterial meningitis in American children is the target of an immunization plan by the CDC. It recommends every child get a first vaccination for *Hemophilus influenzae* type b at two months of age. "We expect a dramatic reduction in Hib meningitis," says Dr. Perkins.

MENOPAUSAL PROBLEMS

Imagine standing beside a roaring bonfire. Your face turns beet red; your chest and arms sizzle with a zillion hot pinpricks. In seconds, your blouse is soaked with sweat, and your hair mats to your brow. You feel uncomfortable and clammy, like you've been shrink-wrapped in plastic.

Now picture yourself standing crimson faced and sopping wet before a meeting room full of people. That's what a hot flash, the most common, uncomfortable and embarrassing symptom of menopause, is like.

A generation ago, there wasn't much a woman having a menopausal hot flash could do. As one woman put it: "With each wave of heat, I felt my body was broadcasting to the world that I was going through the change of life."

Technically, a woman reaches menopause on the date of her last period, usually around age 50, although early signs of menopause can begin four to six years before. Menstruation ceases because the ovaries no longer produce enough of the hormone estrogen to trigger the regular monthly cycle.

When estrogen output grinds to a halt, however, more than the menstrual cycle is affected. Estrogen affects many different tissues and organs throughout your body. So when the hormone flow is stopped, your entire body feels the difference—from your brain down to your bones.

"When estrogen wanes, your body reacts like it's going through a drug withdrawal," says Brian Walsh, M.D., director of the Menopause Clinic at Brigham and Women's Hospital in Boston. The more serious effects involve changes you can't even feel.

LIFE WITHOUT ESTROGEN

Without estrogen to help your bones absorb calcium, you are at increased risk for osteoporosis. And people who have advanced osteoporosis—a disease that involves gradual degeneration of the bones—are more susceptible to bone fracture. Estrogen also helps keep artery-clogging blood fats in check. So a decreased estrogen level may increase your risk of heart disease and stroke.

Most women are all too well aware of other troublesome menopause symptoms. Hot flashes head the list. Three-fourths of all women going through menopause experience these internal heat waves. For many women, they're infrequent and no more intense than a blush after a bawdy joke. Others have severe, sweat-soaking flashes that come in rapid-fire succession. They interfere with daily routines, from driving to conducting meetings, and can jolt you awake again and again throughout the night. These sleep-robbing "night sweats" may be why some women feel wrung out, edgy and muddle-headed during menopause, experts say.

"In a nutshell, a drop in estrogen makes the body's thermostat go haywire," says Dr. Walsh. "The body thinks it's too hot, so blood vessels near the skin's surface dilate, causing the pink flush. Then you sweat to cool off. This gives you the shivers."

Next to hot flashes, vaginal discomfort is the second most vexing menopausal complaint. It's easy to see why.

As estrogen dwindles, the vaginal walls shrink and become thinner, drier and inelastic. This can cause painful friction during sexual intercourse. Blood flow is reduced, so the touch sensation is altered. These symptoms can quickly squelch sexual desire.

Additionally, the vagina becomes more inviting for bacteria, possibly triggering a merry-go-round of vaginal and bladder infections.

Thinned urethral tissues may also increase the frequency of urination. And lax bladder muscles may cause unexpected dribbling when you laugh, sneeze or cough.

A DECADE OF DWINDLING HORMONES

Fortunately, the effects of estrogen withdrawal don't hit all at once (unless you've had a total hysterectomy—in effect, a surgical menopause in which the ovaries are removed).

Normally, a woman's ovaries start gradually slowing down their output of hormones—both estrogen *and* progesterone—in her forties. During this winding-down phase, sometimes called the perimenopause, she may notice subtle "mini-changes." Periods become erratic, for example, or bleeding may get either scantier or, more typically, heavier. As hormones fluctuate, a woman may ride a roller coaster of changing moods. When estrogen peaks, she feels edgy; when progesterone peaks, she feels blue.

Then the other menopausal symptoms emerge, usually hitting in full force within three years after periods stop. Some symptoms subside, others may continue for ten years or more.

Many Ride Out the Symptoms

But here's encouraging news: Many women are able to ride out the waves of menopause until their symptoms subside without undue strain. In fact, even among women who may suffer severe symptoms, few sink into the depths of despair.

Women are developing an upbeat, take-charge attitude about menopause, according to Cynthia Stuenkel, M.D., medical director of the Menopause Clinic at the University of California, San Diego. "They're seeking (and finding) methods that ease them through menopause and help them stay healthy in the years beyond," she says.

Many of those methods are easy-to-use home remedies (more on those later), but by far, the most effective treatment is one that comes from the doctor—hormone replacement therapy (HRT).

Help with HRT

Ever since its introduction in the 1960s, HRT has profoundly improved the quality of life for many women going through menopause.

As its name implies, HRT replaces hormones that the body no longer produces. Today, the standard HRT formula consists of an estrogen pill taken daily for 21 days, followed by a progestin pill, a synthetic version of progesterone, taken for the remaining days of the month. This hormone duo closely mimics the interplay of hormones that a woman naturally experiences during her childbearing years.

Having the option of taking HRT means you don't have to suffer through debilitating symptoms until they finally subside years later. "HRT helps many get on with their lives," says Dr. Stuenkel.

If night sweats are so severe that you're changing sheets like they change guards at Buckingham Palace, for instance, HRT can usually eliminate them in short order, according to Lila E. Nachtigall, M.D., associate professor of obstetrics and gynecology at New York University School of Medicine in New York City and author of *Estrogen: The Facts Can Change Your Life*. Within a week or two, for many women, night sweats will be a memory.

Once hot flashes are extinguished, many women sleep better, feel less edgy and have more energy.

HRT can also help end vaginal symptoms, according to Dr. Nachtigall. Estrogen toughens up painfully thin vaginal tissues and increases lubrication. Tenderness, itchiness and vaginal infections may vanish for as long as you take the hormones.

Restoring vaginal tissues can give a lift to your libido. At the Yale University School of Medicine, researchers found that sexual desire—and sexual activity—increased after three months of estrogen in 90 percent of women who reported a lack of desire.

While the research is inconclusive about HRT's effects on mood, many women find that HRT helps them feel less anxious and irritable.

HRT also helps prevent bone loss and staves off osteoporosis. Estrogen replacement is the main way to effectively stem the unrelenting loss of your bone as you get older, according to Dr. Nachtigall.

When started within a few years of the onset of menopause, estrogen can actually help women recoup lost bone. As for fractures, women who take estrogen may have fewer broken bones than those who do not take it, studies show.

"Very simply, HRT can renew your life," says Dr. Walsh.

Here's more convincing evidence about HRT's lifesaving potential. In a ten-year study of nurses at Harvard Medical School, women who took estrogen cut their risk of heart disease by nearly half. "It appears that estrogen raises the good lipids and decreases the bad lipids," says Dr. Walsh. "This is significant, since heart disease is the number one killer of women over age 50."

CONCERNS ABOUT HRT

Despite all that HRT has going for it, only one-third of the women who receive prescriptions actually take it. The major reason? "Fear of cancer," says Dr. Walsh.

That's understandable. Early versions of HRT contained more potent doses of estrogen and produced five times more endometrial cancer in the women who took it. Excess estrogen causes endometrial (uterine) tissue to grow abnormally.

Today's HRT formulas contain a safer, lower dose of estrogen coupled with progestin, a combination that prevents the buildup of uterine tissue.

But there's still one hard-to-ignore problem: Some preliminary evidence suggests that progestin may contribute to breast cancer. In a much-publicized Swedish study, for example, women using HRT had four times more breast cancer than women who were not using it.

To complicate matters, it appears that progestin reverses to a degree estrogen's heart-healthy effects: It raises the bad lipids.

Even with this uncertainty, doctors believe that if you have severe vaginal dryness or hot flashes, or if you're at high risk for heart disease or osteoporosis (you're thin, fair skinned or have a family history of osteoporosis, or a bone density test reveals dangerously thin bones), the benefits of HRT outweigh any possible risk of breast cancer.

"Women have far greater odds of getting heart disease than breast cancer," says Dr. Walsh.

Until further studies can resolve these perplexing issues, says Dr. Walsh, women should stay up-to-date on HRT information and carefully weigh the benefits and risks with their doctor based on their own medical history and lifestyle.

At this point, HRT may be used with caution by women at risk for breast or uterine cancer or by those with uterine fibroids or liver or gall-bladder disease. If you have high blood pressure, HRT may be okay with close monitoring. All HRT users should have regular breast exams and report any unexplained bleeding to their doctor.

You should, however, expect regular period-type bleeding if you take the combined HRT. Progestin's job of controlling endometrial tissue means the tissue gets sloughed off each month. While these periods may be briefer and lighter and may eventually disappear, they can still be a nuisance, especially when the one plus of menopause is *not* having periods.

Progestin also brings back other unwelcome PMS-like symptoms, such as breast tenderness, headaches and moodiness. Some newer HRT regimens may minimize these side effects.

TAKING CHARGE

"HRT is not a substitute for good prevention habits that can help you stay healthy in the postmenopausal years," says Dr. Stuenkel.

Menopause isn't about popping pills to resolve your problems. "It's about finding ways to take control, so you can make the most of your life as your body changes," says Dr. Stuenkel.

The following nonhormonal self-help techniques have made it possible for many women to take control of troublesome symptoms. You might want to try one or several of these approaches before turning to more potent medication. If you are already using HRT, these methods may boost its effectiveness.

In addition to keeping a fan handy and the room cool, here's how to turn down your thermostat.

Skip the alcohol and coffee. These beverages can make the blood vessels dilate and worsen hot flashes. So can hot and spicy food.

Try vitamin E. If your hot flashes are not devastating, this nutrient could help you have fewer, less intense episodes, according to gynecologist Susan Lark, M.D., director of the PMS and Menopause Self-Help Center in Los Altos, California, and author of *The Menopause Self Help Book*. The recommended dosage is 400 international units (IU) twice a day. If that doesn't do the trick, double the dose. (Check with your doctor first. Vitamin E can be blood thinning.)

Chill out emotionally. In one six-week study of menopausal women, stress was associated with an increase in the frequency, intensity and duration of hot flashes in half of the participants. Try meditation or a soothing tub soak.

Reframe it. You may be able to lessen the intensity of a hot flash by changing how you think about it, says Dr. Lark. One woman associated the sweaty feeling of hot flashes with how she felt after playing tennis. "The hot flashes still came, but I felt less negative about them," she says.

DEALING WITH VAGINAL DRYNESS

To combat the problems caused by a shrinking vagina:

Try artificial lubricants. Vitamin E oil rubbed in vaginal tissues can ease your discomfort, says Dr. Lark. You might also try Replens. This over-the-counter lubricant and moisturizer plumps up the vaginal lining cells with moisture and can actually return shrunken vaginal lining tissue back to normal, studies show. Another plus: Replens creates an acidic environment, which keeps bacteria at bay.

Avoid antihistamines. These drugs dry out mucous membranes in your vagina as well as in your nose.

Engage in regular sex. "Regular orgasm and tender, sensitive love-making can help to relax the pelvic muscles, improve blood flow and keep natural moisture in vaginal tissues," says Dr. Lark.

Practice Kegels. These specially designed exercises improve muscle tone and blood circulation in the pelvic area, says Dr. Lark. To contract the pelvic muscle, use the same motion you would to stop a stream of urine. Do 10 contractions a day—5 fast, plus 5 held for 3 to 5 seconds. Build up to a total of 50 to 100 contractions a day.

SMOOTHING OUT MOOD SWINGS

Luckily, the roller coaster of moods felt during menopause usually levels out within a year. In the meantime, try these soothing remedies.

Sip passionflower tea. This herb, along with others such as chamomile, hops and catnip, has been found to elevate serotonin, which triggers sleep and calmness, according to Dr. Lark.

Walk it out. "Exercise helps discharge excess anxiety-causing adrenaline that many women experience around menopause because of a shift in hormones," says Dr. Lark. Regular exercise may improve your mood by raising endorphins (feel-good hormones that are known to drop during menopause).

Give it a rest. Take an afternoon or midmorning meditation break. Sit quietly with closed eyes. Let your muscles go limp and breathe slowly.

BATTLING BONE LOSS

Experts now say that you need a trio of factors that includes estrogen, exercise (especially weight-bearing exercise like walking) and calcium to build strong bones. But even if you cannot take estrogen for some reason, the other two factors may be enough to slow bone loss if you are not at high risk for osteoporosis.

In a two-year Australian study, researchers found that postmenopausal women who participated in exercise and brisk walking three times

---

HORMONE REPLACEMENT THERAPY: A REVIEW OF THE REGIMENS

The state-of-the-art hormone replacement therapy (HRT) regimen is estrogen in daily doses for 25 to 30 days, accompanied by progestin for the last 10 to 13 days. Sometimes, however, physicians prefer to prescribe the estrogen for only three weeks, with one week off—plus, of course, overlapping days of progestin.

Unfortunately, that's when monthly bleeding begins. At this point, two-thirds of HRT users stop their medication because of this period-like bleeding.

The good news is that it's possible to sidestep bleeding and other side effects by customizing your HRT formula. Here are your choices.

DAILY LOW-DOSE PROGESTINS. A low dose (2.5 milligrams) of progestin given every day produces bleeding only for about six months. There's no final word yet on how this regimen affects bones or blood fats.

THE PATCH. A medicated adhesive is attached to your abdomen, where it releases estradiol, a pure form of estrogen thought to be less cancer causing. Estradiol bypasses the liver and is best for women who can't take HRT orally but who have severe hot flashes and vaginal problems. Early studies indicate the patch may protect the bones and heart.

VAGINAL ESTROGEN CREAM. It increases lubrication and relieves dryness and itching. Effects may be noticed in less than a week. You can use cream on and off and resume treatment when symptoms return. Estrogen is absorbed by the bloodstream but has fewer risks than when taken orally. You may need an occasional progestin pill.

---

weekly and also took 1,000 milligrams of calcium daily showed a significant slowdown of bone loss.

You can also fortify your bones by avoiding the calcium bandits such as excess coffee and salt. (For more bone-saving tips, see "Osteoporosis" on page 392.)

There are also several strategies to help protect your heart that you should incorporate into your life, whether you take HRT or not.

"Stopping smoking, eating a high-fiber, low-fat diet, getting regular aerobic exercise and practicing stress management are all proven, non-hormonal ways to prevent heart disease," says Dr. Lark. "The sooner you start using these preventive strategies, the more likely you'll remain disease-free in the years beyond menopause."

MENSTRUAL PROBLEMS

As generations of women can attest, the menstrual cycle can run like a clock—a bad clock. Periods can begin late one month or end early another. Or they can begin late and end early the same month. One month blood flow can be heavy, the next month, light. The signs that it's coming can come on like clockwork month after month. Then suddenly it hits with no hint at all—usually when you're someplace like the company picnic, where the line to the ladies' room is 30 women long.

Although unpredictable and inconvenient, most menstrual cycle "irregularities" are nothing more than that. Early, late, heavy, light—rarely are these problems cause for concern (although you should tell your doctor about them when you go for your yearly checkup). When your period stops altogether for no known reason, however, it's a sign of something wrong. You should see your doctor right away.

AMENORRHEA

If you haven't had a menstrual period for three months or longer and can eliminate the usual suspects (pregnancy and menopause), you have a condition called amenorrhea. "Stress, depression and anxiety are all known to create this condition," says Sadja Greenwood, M.D., assistant clinical professor of gynecology at the University of California, San Francisco. So are crash dieting, sudden weight gain and some prescription drugs. Athletes with too little body fat who exercise too much are also susceptible.

There are also physical problems that can push your hormones out of balance and your periods out of sync. Ovarian cysts, for example, can throw a big wrench into your body's works. You should see your doctor to find out the cause.

Suddenly going without your period may seem like a blessing in disguise, but really, it is just the opposite. Amenorrhea means that your ovaries are no longer putting out an egg every month. You may also have less estrogen secretions than normal, which can put your health at serious risk, warns Dr. Greenwood. Estrogen is a female hormone that shields the body from bone loss and, to some degree, heart disease.

Even more serious is the increased risk for uterine cancer among women who regularly miss their periods, Dr. Greenwood says. Even if you "normally" menstruate only once or twice a year, your doctor may give you supplemental hormones every few months to "trigger" a period and thus lessen the cancer risk.

PLANNING YOUR PERIODS

Supplemental hormones may be the simplest, most efficient way to regulate your cycle. But for many women, changes in weight, lifestyle and exercise habits can help make their periods more punctual.

Step off the fast track. "I'm definitely pro-exercise, but the people who exercise the most can have the most difficulty with their periods," Dr. Greenwood says. "Moderation is the most important thing. Forget what other people say you should do or what the fashion models look like. Do what feels right for you."

Add a few pounds. Go ahead and cheer—it's not often you get advice like this! Doctors aren't sure why, but women who lose too much weight or who have too little body fat—as is often the case with runners and other athletes—tend to miss their periods. If you're not an athlete but you've been practicing a strict diet, Dr. Greenwood says, try relaxing a bit to help regulate your cycle.

Take a break. A mental break, that is. If stress is causing your periods to take a break, then getting rid of the stress will bring them back, says Dr. Greenwood. (See "Stress" on page 472 for ways to help alleviate stress.)

CRAMPS

If you're a woman between the ages of 13 and 50, there's an eight in ten chance that you have an intimate acquaintance with cramps. These monthly miseries, doctors say, are the number one reason women take time off from work and school. Worse, cramps often are accompanied by nausea, headaches, back pain and diarrhea.

To refer to the whole package, doctors use the term *dysmenorrhea*—Greek for "difficult monthly flow."

"It's not completely understood why some people have cramps more than others," says Dr. Greenwood. "But all the things that doctors used to think were psychosomatic—the cramps, nausea and diarrhea—do seem to have physical components."

Even though menstrual pain rarely indicates serious problems, Dr. Greenwood says, there are exceptions. If your flow suddenly increases, or your cramps become worse, or intercourse is painful, you should see your doctor.

THE CONTRACTION CONNECTION

Doctors aren't sure what causes most cramps, but a class of hormones called prostaglandins seems to be the star in this monthly play. Produced by the uterine lining (the endometrium), prostaglandins actually make the uterus contract when it's time for your period. These contractions do two things: They expel the endometrium from the uterus, and they give you cramps.

Doctors have found that women with the worst cramps—and the strongest uterine contractions—also have the most prostaglandins. This can be a problem, because prostaglandins also stimulate the intestines, which can cause menstrual nausea and diarrhea. They also are the hormones responsible for sending pain messages to the brain, Dr. Greenwood says. Consequently, women with plenty of prostaglandins can have plenty of pain.

Generally, cramps are most severe among adolescents who have just started menstruating, Dr. Greenwood suggests, possibly because the uterus isn't yet accustomed to these monthly contractions. In most cases, cramps become less severe as women get older. They're also relieved by childbirth.

YOUR ANTICRAMP STRATEGY

Nobody's going to recommend pregnancy as a "cure" for cramps. There are other remedies that take less than nine months to work!

Break out the aspirin. Or the acetaminophen, ibuprofen or any of the prescription nonsteroidal anti-inflammatory drugs, such as Motrin, Naprosyn and Indocin. These drugs inhibit the production of prostaglandins, Dr. Greenwood says, and often are the first choice for relieving painful cramps.

Whisper in your partner's ear. Sex researchers William Masters, M.D., and Virginia Johnson have found that orgasm can help reduce both cramping and backache. "At the time of orgasm, the uterus does contract, and that seems to help some people," says Dr. Greenwood.

Have a workout. Doctors agree that mild to moderate exercise, especially aerobic exercise like swimming or bicycling, is one of the best ways to relieve cramps.

YOUR SECONDARY STRATEGY

If nothing above seems to help, your doctor may prescribe oral contraceptives, which have been found to alleviate menstrual symptoms in some women. And that should do the trick. Not only can oral contraceptives relieve cramping, says Dr. Greenwood, but they can reduce other menstrual symptoms—acne, for example, and breast tenderness—as well.

MISCELLANEOUS PROBLEMS

Even women otherwise blessed with regular, trouble-free periods will sometimes notice changes in their cycles. One month may bring spotting, for example, or heavy bleeding. Most of such changes are caused by transitory shifts in your body's chemistry, and everything should soon return to normal. But such changes also can indicate potential problems—a uterine tumor, sexually transmitted infection or a malfunctioning thyroid gland. These possible conditions need to be examined before your doctor can give you a clean bill of health.

Spotting, the appearance of small amounts of blood between periods, is one of the most common bleeding problems women take to their gynecologist. And no wonder: It's tough to feel secure when your period becomes an all-month event.

Unless spotting is accompanied by a lot of blood, it probably isn't serious but should be checked by your doctor anyway, Dr. Greenwood says. Unless any abnormalities show up, your doctor may give you oral contraceptives to help regulate your cycle. If you don't want to take contraceptives, then progesterone pills (taken for a few days each month) can help.

Heavy bleeding, a condition called menorrhagia, can be more serious. Because a little blood goes a long way, it may be difficult to tell when you're bleeding "too much." But most women, during their period, lose about 4 tablespoons of blood. If you think you're losing more than that, or if your periods last longer than seven days, see your doctor.

"A common cause of heavy bleeding is the development of uterine fibroids [a benign overgrowth of the uterine muscle]," says Dr. Greenwood. "But it could be a number of things, including lack of ovulation. When women aren't ovulating and they have a lot of estrogen, that can ultimately lead to uterine cancer. That's what we really worry about with heavy bleeding."

Another problem sometimes associated with heavy bleeding is iron-deficiency anemia. In fact, doctors recommend that all women, particularly those with heavy periods, eat plenty of iron-rich foods such as raisins, prunes, deep green, leafy vegetables and dried or fresh beans. Dr. Greenwood suggests that you also talk to your physician about iron supplements.

MONONUCLEOSIS

A ha! So you've been smooching and fogging up the car windows again! And now for a week you've had a sore throat, fever, swollen glands, headache and wobbly knees. Whatever could it be? Oh, let's see, could it be . . . *(ominous drum roll)* kissing disease?

That's what mononucleosis is often called, but kissing is only one of many ways this infection spreads. The villain here in most cases is really the Epstein-Barr virus (EBV), a type of herpes virus nearly as common and as widespread as the cold bug. About half of all kids and practically every adult carries it. (In most persons, the virus lives in a dormant state in certain white blood cells without causing any illness. It is sporadically present in the saliva.)

Yet mono is far from epidemic. "Ninety-five percent of the world's population is infected with EBV, but most never know it, because they've never had obvious mononucleosis," says infectious diseases specialist Peter Axelrod, M.D., assistant professor of medicine at Temple University School of Medicine in Philadelphia. Even among those who do get sick from EBV, the symptoms are usually so mild that most people will think they have a cold or flu.

TEEN FEVER

Just like a cold or flu, mono may be spread by coughing, sneezing, sharing eating and drinking utensils and, of course, kissing. "But because it's not nearly as contagious as a cold or flu, and because most people's immune systems can effectively limit or eliminate symptoms, you don't usually see more than one person in a family getting mononucleosis," says Dr. Axelrod.

Those most likely to experience full-blown symptoms are teenagers, particularly those whose first encounter with the virus occurs at adolescence. "There may be a fundamental difference in the way teens' immune systems react to EBV, but it's not really understood," says Dr. Axelrod. Roughly 1 in every 150 teens suffers full-blown mono, most commonly between ages 15 and 16 for girls and between 18 and 21 for boys.

"The typical teenager who gets mono can be out of commission anywhere from two weeks to three months, but it's really variable," says Dr. Axelrod. The disease brings fever (often over 102°F), sore throat, swollen glands and an enlarged spleen. The few middle-aged people who get it are much more likely to also have an enlarged liver and jaundice, and they often do not have a sore throat or swollen lymph glands. Everybody with mono is likely to feel extremely fatigued.

Once you've gotten over the worst of the illness, one or more of the symptoms may return during the following year. "These relapses show that even though your immune system has controlled the virus, it isn't controlling it completely," says Dr. Axelrod. The most common symptom to reappear is tiredness, he says, and that intermittent tiredness can last up to a year.

The good news is that once your immune system learns to fully control the virus, you can never get mono again—not even if you attend a double-feature drive-in movie with your infected sweetheart!

MOBILIZING AGAINST MONO

Can you avoid contracting the mono virus? Not easily, says Dr. Axelrod. "You can usually avoid flu by not going near anyone who has it, but mono is different. Nearly everybody carries the virus, and most carriers have no symptoms. I suppose if you lived in a bubble and never touched anybody and had all your food sterilized, you'd never get EBV or mono. But if you're a human being who lives on earth, there's nothing you can do to prevent it," he says.

So rather than trying to isolate yourself from the mono virus—you can't—learn what you can do to neutralize the little devil. You may want to see your doctor to make sure that what you have is mono and not something else—the symptoms can mimic a host of diseases. But other than making a diagnosis, there is very little your doctor can do, besides recommending the following.

Rest. You won't feel like doing much else anyway. "Don't count on working your normal hours or going to school," says Dr. Axelrod. "It's better to restrict your activities. Treat your tiredness by getting extra sleep and rest."

Take acetaminophen. That's Tylenol or Anacin-3, or the generic equivalent. It will lower your fever and help relieve aches and pains and sore throat. Aspirin will do the same thing, but no one under age 21 should take aspirin because of the risk of Reye's syndrome, a serious neurological disease.

Drink plenty of fluids. Drinking water or fruit juice will help rehydrate and cool your feverish body, and it may help your sore throat. Lozenges can offer additional help for your aching throat.

Watch football. That is, don't play it. Stay away from all contact sports for at least a month *after* you feel better, Dr. Axelrod says. This is because an enlarged spleen is common in mono, and a blow to your abdominal area can rupture the spleen—and that could be deadly.

Take your time. It's best not to rush back into a full schedule right after you feel better, says Dr. Axelrod. Take time to relax and give your body a chance to get the virus under complete control.

MOTION SICKNESS

I f there is anyone who should be concerned about motion sickness, it is Diane Van Dien. Owner of the International Sailing School in Punta Gorda, Florida, Diane can't afford to get woozy—not when there are greenhorns on deck nervously awaiting orders.

"I've sailed for 30 years, and I've just recently started having problems with motion sickness," she says. "For example, I was helping deliver a large sailboat from Punta Gorda up to Clearwater when I began to feel funny, like I had a headache coming on. My stomach got a little upset, too—it was a terrible feeling!"

A PROBLEM OF PERCEPTION

You don't have to be a sailor on the high seas to get the "I'm turning green" blues. Some people get sick when they ride in cars, buses or airplanes. Some get sick in elevators. Others get sick at carnivals, where the merry-go-rounds make their stomachs go 'round. "Although some of us are more vulnerable than others, if you have the right sort of stimulus, just about everyone will become motion sick," says Edwin M. Monsell, M.D., Ph.D., head of the Division of Otology and Neurotology (ear and ear-nerve medicine) at Henry Ford Hospital in Detroit. And as with Diane, motion sickness can occur even after a lifetime of smooth sailing.

Actually, it's not only motion that makes you sick but also your *perception* of motion. Here's what happens. Inside your inner ear, there are five balance sensors, which, along with your eyes and your brain, help you to keep your balance. But when your eyes and inner ears perceive different things, you can get a bit off-balance. When you read in the car, for example, your eyes are fixed on the page; they say you're sitting still. Your sensitive inner ears, on the other hand, know very well that you're cruising. The ensuing argument may cause motion sickness.

MOTION POTIONS

Since a bout with motion sickness can make the most longed-for journey seem entirely too long, those who are sensitive may prefer to ward off trouble before it begins, Dr. Monsell says. In fact, it may be easier to prevent motion sickness with drugs than to relieve it once you're already down.

You've probably taken antihistamines to relieve occasional cold or allergy symptoms. These drugs do more than clear stuffed-up noses. Certain kinds of antihistamines, taken before a trip, can help beat motion sickness. Perhaps the best known is dimenhydrinate (Dramamine). This over-the-counter drug works by preventing chemical signals from traveling from your inner ear to that part of the brain called, appropriately, the vomiting center.

Remember, however, that these antihistamines are more effective at preventing motion sickness than at relieving it, Dr. Monsell says. If you take them when you're already queasy, it may be too late. Take your pills a half hour to an hour before departing, following the dosage instructions on the bottle, he says.

More powerful than the antihistamines, a drug called scopolamine also works by inhibiting chemical signals from traveling through the central nervous system. But scopolamine has too many potential side effects to be taken in pill form. Instead, it is commonly affixed to a prescription adhesive skin patch, which you stick behind your ear when you travel. The patch steadily releases small amounts of the drug for up to several days. This helps maintain steady—and safe—levels of scopolamine in your bloodstream.

But scopolamine, like the antihistamines, depresses the central nervous system and can cause drowsiness, a dry mouth or blurred vision, Dr. Monsell says. "Don't take any motion sickness drug if you're driving," he warns.

CALMING THE QUEASIES

Oops. You forgot to take your medicine. Or maybe motion sickness took you by surprise. What can you do about it? Here are some tips to help you calm the queasies.

Close the book. Reading in the car is one of the most common causes of motion sickness, Dr. Monsell says. Even people with otherwise steady stomachs may find the combination of reading and riding too much to handle. If your head starts to swim, pack away the book until you reach solid ground.

Focus on the scenery. When you concentrate on objects outside the vehicle, you're forcing your eyes to *see* the same motion that your inner ears *feel*. Once your senses are in agreement, your stomach should start calming down, Dr. Monsell says.

Put the kids up front. Because their nervous systems aren't fully developed, kids are more susceptible to motion sickness. What's more, they often occupy the rear seat, from which their field of vision is substantially curtailed. On long trips, this can push their sensitive stomachs over the edge, Dr. Monsell says. To help little Johnny keep his lunch down, a seat near the windshield can help. Of course, make sure little Johnny wears his seat belt!

Keep your distance. Through the power of suggestion, nausea can be contagious. When one deckhand gets sick, there's a fair chance that others will, too. Don't try to help a fellow sufferer. There's not much you can do, and *your* stomach may be the next to go.

Stay busy. You may have noticed that it's usually passengers, not drivers, who get motion sick. Researchers at Pennsylvania State University have found that people who keep their minds busy (by solving mental problems) are less likely to get sick than those who passively go along for the ride. So if you're getting queasy, try to stay busy. Take the wheel for a few hours. Count license plates. Sing a few songs.

Find the steady seats. Whether you're sailing to Greece or flying from Topeka to Dallas, minimize your discomfort by grabbing the most stable seats. On airplanes, the seats over the wings are the most stable. When sailing, the place to be is amidships (for you landlubbers, that means in the middle of the ship).

Hold still. If you're already sick, of course, you probably don't feel like doing anything more vigorous than leaning over the rail. In fact, this

---

ACUPRESSURE TO THE RESCUE?

Some travel shops sell elastic wristbands that will press a hard plastic button against the inside of your wrist. According to acupressurists, pressure at this point—the so-called P6 position—can help relieve the nausea caused by motion sickness. But do the bands really work?

In one study at England's Institute of Naval Medicine, blindfolded volunteers were strapped into rotating chairs, where they were whirled and whirled about. No, the acupressure wristbands didn't prevent them from getting sick to the point of wanting to vomit. The researchers admit, however, that this challenge was particularly "severe"—and that the bands might work for some people under less turbulent conditions.

is good medicine. By keeping yourself still, you're giving your inner ear time to stabilize, Dr. Monsell says. If space permits, lie down and hold your head very still. In time, the world—including your stomach—should stop spinning.

Pack a lunch. Studies have shown that people who eat before traveling get sick less often than those who depart with their tanks on empty. However, Dr. Monsell adds, greasy things that sit in the stomach for a long time and are hard to digest can make matters worse. Instead, eat a light meal of protein and easy-to-digest carbohydrates—a plate of pasta, for example, or a slice of bread. You can also pack snack foods such as crackers to nosh while you travel. "My secret is peanut butter and jelly sandwiches," says the sea-going Diane Van Dien. "They calm my stomach down right away."

Leave the alcohol at home. It can change the way your brain and inner ears sense motion, adding to the tendency to have motion sickness, Dr. Monsell says. When you're traveling by air, you should avoid carbonated beverages as well. "With the changes in pressure, all those little gas bubbles can give some people stomach problems," he adds.

Get some fresh air. When you're already queasy, unpleasant odors—and particularly the smell of tobacco smoke—can turn your stomach upside down. Turn it right-side up again by cranking down the car windows or taking a soothing walk on deck.

Pack some ginger. Long a folk remedy for upset stomachs, powdered gingerroot has been recommended for motion sickness as well. In one study, volunteers were given either 100 milligrams of Dramamine or two capsules (940 milligrams) of ginger. Then they were seated in a motorized revolving chair and told to stop the chair when they began feeling nauseated. The people taking ginger lasted 57 percent longer than those taking Dramamine.

According to Varro E. Tyler, Ph.D., professor of pharmacognosy (the study of the medical uses of plants) at Purdue University, travelers may get relief by taking two 500-milligram capsules of ginger before embarking on their journeys. Or if you prefer tea, try mixing 1/4 teaspoon of powdered ginger in a cup of hot water and drinking it down. Repeat every 4 hours as needed.

DISEASE
FREE

MUSCLE PAIN

N o pain, no gain," the bulging bodybuilder with the Cro-Magnon brow always says. "No brain," responds anyone who has ever been greeted on a new day with a stiff salutation from aching muscles.

A certain amount of muscle aches, strains, soreness and stiffness almost is inevitable. "If you increase activity, there's little to do to stop the tissue response," says Terry Malone, Ed.D., executive director of sports medicine, associate professor of physical therapy and assistant professor of surgery at Duke University.

With proper precautions, your twinges should be mild enough to remind you that you had a good, healthy workout, not bad enough to keep you from wanting to do it again. That's why it's helpful to know just what's happening to your muscles when you exert yourself—and why it's important not to *over*exert yourself.

THE SORE SCORE

Common muscle soreness typically has two causes. There's the immediate discomfort of heavy, extensive physical effort, which fades soon after the exertion. And then there are the sneakier aches of delayed muscle soreness, which appear from one to three days after the activity.

Delayed soreness happens any time you do something to which your body is not accustomed or when you use muscles you normally don't work, Dr. Malone says.

When you're challenging your muscles, "you're stimulating nerve endings, tearing muscle fibers and accumulating waste products like lactic acid," says Richard Bachrach, D.O., president and medical director of the Center for Sports and Osteopathic Medicine in New York City. "You're also slightly bruising the muscles, and they bleed inside."

As gruesome as this sounds, it's a perfectly natural process that muscles undergo as they grow stronger. But you don't want to go too far.

To prevent excessive soreness and possible injures, follow these precautions.

Grow accustomed to your pace. Curiously, once those tiny tears heal, the muscle becomes stronger and more capable of meeting the particular demand that originally caused them. "People build up a tolerance, and they do so rather quickly," Dr. Malone says. The work no longer produces pain—as long as you perform it regularly.

The best way to protect yourself against the stealthy soreness of spring-cleaning or a weekend of room painting or the volleyball game at

---

DISMOUNTING THE CHARLEY HORSE

It can awaken you in the dead of night with biting pain, or it can knock you off your feet with a sucker punch in broad daylight. Commonly known as a charley horse, this muscle cramp in the thigh or leg can crack you with a crippling cringe of pain as the muscle involuntarily flexes and refuses to relax.

Nothing can prevent them, but they can be treated easily, leaving the ache a fleeting, if somewhat agonizing, memory.

"Cramps are usually the result of an imbalance of potassium or sodium in the body, resulting from a loss of water," according to Terry Malone, Ed.D., executive director of sports medicine, associate professor of physical therapy and assistant professor of surgery at Duke University.

A cramp can also be caused by a blow to the muscle or can be the body's defense mechanism to a blow—the bruised muscle contracts to prevent its use, sort of like a bug rolling itself up into a little ball to protect itself.

When a cramp hits, "drink fluid immediately," Dr. Malone says. At the same time, you have to stretch the cramped muscle by contracting its antagonist, the muscle responsible for movement in the opposite direction. If, for example, you've got a charley horse in the calf, you must pull the foot up to a 90-degree angle with the leg. That helps stretch the calf. If you have a cramp in the biceps on the front of the arm, Dr. Malone says, you straighten your elbow using the triceps muscle on the back of your arm.

After you've stretched out the cramped muscle, massage the area to stimulate blood flow.

---

the annual family picnic is to stay in shape. "Get yourself on a good, positive exercise program that strengthens the muscles," advises Dr. Bachrach. "Exercise is a great manager of all sorts of pain. Aerobically conditioned people don't suffer from aches and pains as much as unfit people."

Get strong. A regular weight-training regimen not only makes your body more durable for everyday and not-so-everyday activities, it also strengthens the muscle/tendon connection, helping to prevent strains, according to Dr. Malone.

Take time to stretch. By making you more supple, stretching and warming up help prevent common soreness and more severe injuries. And the increase in body temperature that accompanies the stretching and warm-up makes muscles and tendons more flexible and elastic. "Muscles, ligaments and tendons that are warmed up are less likely to tear," says John Skowron, a licensed physical therapist and director of Raleigh Community Sports Medicine and Physical Therapy in Raleigh, North Carolina.

Stretch gently through the muscle's full range of motion. Hold your stretches for 10 to 15 seconds. But don't bounce into the stretch. Forceful, "ballistic" movements contract the muscle with undue stress. "That's undesirable," says Dr. Malone.

PRICE IS RIGHT

The relatively minor aches of overtaxed muscles will dissipate on their own after a day or two, and experts say you don't really need to treat them. But for severe soreness from overuse and for muscle yanks, cranks, strains and pulls, doctors advise *PRICE,* a mnemonic string on the finger that stands for *P*rotect, *R*est, *I*ce, *C*ompress and *E*levate.

Protect and relatively rest the muscle. You don't have to remain completely bedridden until the soreness abates, Dr. Malone says, "but you should refrain from certain actions that'll use the muscle."

Put the icing on the ache. Ice reduces inflammation and swelling, numbing the skin and reducing and preventing secondary muscle spasms that would prolong the pain. "It contracts blood vessels at first," Dr. Bachrach says. After the cold is removed, a rebound surge of blood rushes to the sore area as the vessels dilate. "The cold makes the body think it needs to send more blood there, which helps to heal the damaged tissue," he says.

To chill the area, don't bother with an ice bag or gel packs. "Use a bag of frozen peas," Dr. Malone says. "It'll conform exactly to the area, and you can safely apply the cold without it being too cold. Gel packs might get too cold."

Ice your muscle pain for 10 to 15 minutes, until the skin begins to feel numb, Skowron suggests, and repeat the quick chill every couple of hours. After each treatment, move the muscle through its full range of motion.

Ease into the squeeze. The muscle should be compressed with an elastic bandage while it recovers, according to Dr. Malone. The wrap should not be too tight, just firm enough to provide some support.

Raise it when you rest. You probably won't need to be strung up in traction while your muscle pain heals, but you should be elevated slightly while you sleep. If the problem's in your legs, placing several books under the foot of the bed will provide all the elevation you need, Dr. Malone says. "Don't prop up the limb on pillows," he says. "It's uncomfortable to do, and a lot of people don't sleep on their backs."

The massage is the medium. Sore muscles often are knead-y . . . they need a good rubdown. A massage squeezes blood into the muscles, Skowron says, and causes them to relax. It also stimulates nerve endings.

Have your massage therapist use firm pressure, but not too hard—it shouldn't hurt, Skowron says. The muscle should be worked for 10 to 15 minutes.

Don't baby your bruise. "Don't immobilize a strained muscle," Dr. Malone says. "You have to allow its safe use." Protect it, rest it, ice it, compress it, and elevate it, but also work it, moving the joint to which the muscle is attached through its full range of motion to prevent stiffness. Initially, just move it on its own, but eventually add some resistance, with dumbbells or ankle weights, to strengthen the muscle and tendon.

HEAT . . . IF YOU INSIST

While it undoubtedly feels good, heat offers an illusory sense of healing, and it actually can aggravate inflammation and swelling as well as delay recovery, according to Dr. Bachrach. "People have more problems accommodating to ice than heat," Skowron adds, "but you should never use heat on an acute muscle injury, such as a pull or a strain, especially one in an arm or a leg."

For mild aches from overuse or overexertion, Skowron says, heat at least feels good and provides some temporary pain relief during the heat treatment.

Moist heat, dry heat, lotions, electric blankets, infrared lamps—they're all the same to the body. "They're all superficial, and they will not heat up the damaged muscle below the surface of the skin," Skowron says. Moist heat subjectively seems to feel better than dry heat, but no evidence exists to prove it works any more effectively, he says.

The active ingredient in some of the sports ointments, says Dr. Malone, is capsaicin, the same stuff in hot sauces and chili peppers that scorches your mouth.

All those muscle creams provide a burning sensation that works as a counterirritant, according to Dr. Malone. "It brings a feeling of warmth, particularly superficially, but it doesn't go lower into the muscle," he says.

If you want to use heat, warm the sore area for 15 to 20 minutes. "Any prolonged periods of time may cause more discomfort," Skowron says. "And don't fall asleep with an electric heating pad on. You could wake up medium well-done, with blistering burns. We do see that occasionally."

NASAL POLYPS

The next time you look in the mirror, admire your nose. Why? Because apart from its good looks, your nose is a sophisticated tool. Not only does it trap particles and pollutants from incoming air, it adjusts the temperature and moisture of the air as well. Your nose is also the window to two of your senses. It's what enables you to smell a rose or to fully enjoy a tasty meal.

If you have nasal polyps, however, the entire system can break down, says Jeffrey P. Kirsch, M.D., an otolaryngologist/head and neck surgeon at Tulane University Medical Center in New Orleans. Nasal polyps are small, noncancerous growths within the nose or sinuses. "Some people may have 50 or 100 polyps," says Dr. Kirsch. "They come in clusters, like grapes."

STILL A MYSTERY

This doesn't mean that things resembling the California Raisins will soon be protruding from your nostrils. Nasal polyps usually grow too deep in the nose for you to see or touch them, Dr. Kirsch says. In fact, you can have polyps for years and not even know it.

Trouble begins when they grow large enough to block one or both of your nasal cavities. When that happens, your sense of smell can go haywire. Nose breathing becomes difficult, and you may notice a distressing post-nasal drip—a consequence of having a surplus of mucus-producing nasal tissue. In addition, polyps can contribute to a breathing disorder called obstructive sleep apnea, which not only can disturb your sleep but also may even contribute to your risk for high blood pressure or an enlarged heart.

Although nasal polyps were first described some 3,000 years ago, doctors still aren't sure what causes them. They do know that one in three people with polyps also has allergies or allergic-type symptoms. People with asthma, aspirin sensitivities and cystic fibrosis often get polyps, and men get them twice as often as women.

When you take your stuffed-up nose to your doctor, he may recommend a procedure called nasal endoscopy—an examination with a pencil-size instrument called a fiber-optic endoscope—to see what's wrong. Since nasal polyps can resemble some types of cancer, he may take a tissue sample as well. When polyps are small and your symptoms slight, your doctor may counsel patience. If the polyps are more advanced, however, you have several options: drugs, surgery or a combination of the two.

EASY TO TREAT, HARD TO BEAT

"The initial treatment of choice usually is nasal steroids," Dr. Kirsch says. Prescription drugs such as betamethasone, sprayed in the nose, sometimes will quickly shrink nasal polyps, allowing normal or near-normal airflow through the nasal passages. "We may give oral steroids to get the ball rolling and then switch to nasal sprays," he adds.

However, nasal polyps will often resume their growth once the drugs are discontinued. Consequently, many people will use nasal steroids several times a day, often for years. Unlike oral steroids, research has shown that long-term use of steroid nasal sprays is quite safe in most patients, says Dr. Kirsch.

When steroids don't do the trick, surgery may be recommended, he adds. Most of the time, the procedure is quite simple. Under either local or general anesthesia, the surgeon snags the polyps with tiny snares and forceps. Once the polyps are removed and the nasal lining tissue has healed, a marked improvement in symptoms may be seen. The procedure usually takes between 1 and 3 hours and is generally very safe.

There is a catch, however. While polyps are easily removed, they frequently grow back, Dr. Kirsch says. Researchers at Brown University/Rhode Island Hospital in Providence studied 167 people with nasal polyps, 143 of whom had polypectomies. Of these, 57 required a second operation, and 11 eventually required six or more operations! "The recurrence rate is very high, and some people require surgery every few years," Dr. Kirsch says. "In general, we usually start with a trial of medication. If that doesn't work, then surgery can be considered."

NECK PAIN

A spoon jams in the garbage disposal—what a pain in the neck. The guy in the office down the hall interrupts you with idle chitchat—what a pain in the neck. And all sorts of arrangements have to be made for that dinner party this weekend. That's a whole succession of pains in the neck.

From the car to the kids to garbage-can lids, anything can be a pain in the neck. But why is an ache in that skeletal bridge between head and body such an apt metaphor for all of life's woes?

The neck is "one of the most sensitive areas of the body," says Jerel Glassman, D.O., staff physician and education coordinator at St. Mary's Spine Center at St. Mary's Hospital in San Francisco. "A lot of things can go wrong with the neck. It is a busy area, in which major nerves, arteries and vessels must channel through a narrow opening—a real 'bottleneck.'" In addition, what we often call "neck pain" may have its origin in nearby joints and muscles. "The body is a mosaic of interrelated parts, and the neck sits atop this structure in a most vulnerable position," Dr. Glassman says.

What causes the top of this "mosaic" to start to crack? Most often, it's a case of owner abuse.

STRAIGHT TALK

When it comes to neck pain prevention, your posture—when standing, walking and at work—is the place to start, Dr. Glassman says.

Give your walk a lift. Your head should not be thrust forward, and your chest and back should be straight. From crown to tailbone, "there should be no accentuations in any of the natural curves of your head, neck and back," Dr. Glassman says. "Think of yourself as tall and rising through gravity, almost as if you have a string attached to the top of your head that lifts you."

Keep it moving. The particular and peculiar demands of your job can have a profound effect on the welfare of your neck. "A lot of problems have to do with bad work positioning," says licensed physical therapist John Skowron, director of Raleigh Community Sports Medicine and Physical Therapy in Raleigh, North Carolina.

The preventive prescription is often simple: "Move around. Get up and down. Take breaks," Dr. Glassman says. If you sit in front of a computer for hours a day, give your neck a wake-up call by putting an alarm clock near your desk, set to go off at intervals of a half hour or 45 minutes, he suggests. Stand, stretch and do a slow neck roll or two. "You're built for motion," Dr. Glassman says, "and any time you restrict motion, you're going to have trouble."

Watch how you yak. Cradling the telephone receiver between your ear and shoulder is outright neck abuse, says Dr. Glassman. Use your hands—that's how *hand*sets were meant to be used! If you're on the phone a lot, use a headset.

PILLOW TALK

Sometimes we create problems for our necks not during the day but at night! Perhaps instead of counting sheep tonight, you should count the number of pillows you've been sleeping on.

Stop the stack attack. "Don't sleep on an excessive number of pillows unless you've been told to do so by a doctor," Dr. Glassman says. A high stack forces the neck into an unnaturally flexed position for an extended time. Your pillow should be no thicker than the distance between your shoulder and your ear, just enough to keep the neck cushioned and straight.

Roll it up. Special pillows designed for head and neck support are fine, Skowron says, but you may find similar benefits without the additional cost if you simply roll up a hand towel and place it under your neck.

Get on your side. Sleep position can also play a role in creating or preventing neck pain. Dozing on your stomach with your head turned to the side is a sure ticket to crinks the next day. While sleeping on your back is all right, lying on your side with your knees slightly bent is easiest on the skeleton, says Dr. Glassman.

Go with the foam. Mattresses matter, too. "If people sleep on very firm mattresses, they'll often wake up stiff," Dr. Glassman says. He recommends mattress pads made of between 4 and 5 inches of medium-firm foam.

POWER OVER PAIN

The stronger and more flexible your neck and shoulder muscles, the more resistant you'll be to common aches and pains. And the same exercises performed to bolster your neck against pain may also work out the kinks if or when they do occur.

Work it through the range. Tilt your head to one side, trying to touch your ear to your shoulder, Skowron says. Slowly roll your head down to your chest and around to the other shoulder. Repeat several times.

Put your chin in and head up. Lie on your back, tuck your chin toward your chest, and raise your head with your neck muscles. Hold for a few seconds, lower your head, then repeat five to ten times, says Dr. Glassman.

Put your hands behind your head. While seated or standing, place your hands behind your head, with your fingers intertwined. Push your

---

WHIPLASH: WHEN YOUR NECK'S A WRECK

When is a pain in the neck *really* a pain in the neck? When it's whiplash.

Whiplash is "a woefully undertreated and mismanaged condition," says Jerel Glassman, D.O., a staff physician and education coordinator at St. Mary's Spine Center in San Francisco. A violent, vigorous forward and backward throw of the neck is what causes it. And this complex condition may involve injury to the neck, head, spine or other areas.

But whiplash's potential damage isn't limited to the musculoskeletal system. Your brain could also suffer. "It gets a jar, too," Dr. Glassman says.

Whiplash usually occurs in auto accidents, so the best thing you can do to minimize injury is to drive carefully and to make sure the headrests on your car seats are adjusted properly, says physical therapist John Skowron, director of Raleigh Community Sports Medicine and Physical Therapy in Raleigh, North Carolina. "Properly adjusted" means that the middle of your headrest is comfortably supporting the middle of the back of your head. That will keep your head from flying in the event of an accident.

If you do have an accident and you experience any neck pain, back pain or nausea—either immediately afterward or within the next day or two—see your doctor.

Treatment depends on the severity of whiplash. In mild cases, ice compresses on the neck, along with some aspirin or ibuprofen, may be enough to cure the crunch. In serious cases, you may need more intensive medical treatment, ranging from several days' bed rest to wearing a temporary neck brace to receiving physical therapy.

head into your palms against the resistance of your arms. Hold for several seconds and relax. Next gently pull your head forward, tucking your chin against your chest. Repeat the series three times. Next lace your fingers behind your head below the base of the skull. Slowly roll your head back over your hands. Repeat three times.

Do a decisive shrug. Shrug your shoulders up toward your ears while keeping your arms straight. Start off with no weights; then, provided you're not currently in pain, try it with light dumbbells—say, 3 to 5 pounds. Do 12 to 15 repetitions.

ICE AND HEAT TREATMENTS

While a little bit of prevention could go a long way toward eliminating problems, you still may someday yank, crank, misuse or overuse something in your neck.

For otherwise normal pains in the neck, give them the cold shoulder. Physicians and physical therapists agree that ice is almost always best for rips and tears, pulls and strains in your neck and shoulders.

Ice up and stretch. Ice offers a natural if somewhat chilly anesthesia and helps to reduce inflammation and swelling. It also helps stimulate blood flow, as the body tries to heat up the cold area. Wrap up some crushed ice cubes in a towel, or grab a bag of frozen peas, and apply to your neck for 10 to 15 minutes at a time, Dr. Glassman says. Afterward, stretch the neck and shoulder muscles with some slow neck rolls.

Get hot under the collar. Some people are just too sensitive to tolerate ice on their necks. For them, and for those of us who have lingering neck pain even after a day or two of icing, it may be time to turn up the heat. Heat your sore neck and shoulders for about 15 to 20 minutes, Skowron suggests. Use whatever is handy—a sports cream, hot compress or warm shower. "You'll usually know after one or two applications if the heat is helping," Skowron says. He also suggests trying both heat and cold, then choosing the most effective.

RED FLAGS AROUND THE NECK

Often neck pain can be taken care of at home with the above treatments, but if the pain or stiffness persists for a week, or if it's accompanied by other symptoms, a more severe problem may exist.

"If the pain migrates down your shoulders and into your arms, or if your arms and hands become numb and you find yourself dropping things, see the doctor," Skowron says. Neck pain can come from serious conditions such as tumors and injured spinal disks—but rest assured, these are rare.

OSTEOPOROSIS

The patient was only in his sixties, but the radiologist examining his x-rays saw an unhappy sight. Instead of the white shapes that a healthy 60-year-old man's bones cast on film, this patient's bones cast dark shadows. The bones were so porous that many of the x-rays passed right through them. The diagnosis: osteoporosis.

Clearly, the man was in bad shape, but his doctor's diagnosis didn't faze him. After all, Nes-Ptah, who once worked at the Temple of Amun in ancient Egypt, has been dead some 3,000 years. Now he resides in Boston's Museum of Fine Arts, where radiologist Myron Marx, M.D., made his house call.

BAD TO THE BONE

Unfortunately, osteoporosis, a condition in which bones lose minerals and become progressively weaker, is still with us. It affects some 25 million Americans, most of them women. But now research is revealing some of the weapons—diet, hormones and exercise, to name a few—we can use against the disease.

Drugs are one way to slow or reverse bone loss. "There may be modest gains in bone with a number of treatments like diphosphenates, calcitonin and sodium fluoride," says B. Lawrence Riggs, M.D., president of the National Osteoporosis Foundation and professor of medical research at Mayo Medical School in Rochester, Minnesota. (They're most commonly prescribed for people who have full-blown osteoporosis.) And estrogen replacement therapy has been shown to be the most effective way to prevent bone loss during the years around menopause.

Better yet, there are steps most people can take to slow and stop bone loss and even to achieve modest gains in bone density—to stop osteoporosis before it starts. If Nes-Ptah were alive today, his poor old bones might be in a lot better shape!

A Combined Effort

There are no shortcuts to better bone health, scientists say. "You want the whole environment for bones to be as positive as possible," explains Gail Dalsky, Ph.D., director of the Exercise Research Laboratory at the University of Connecticut Health Center's Osteoporosis Center in Farmington. "You need good nutrition, including calcium, healthy hormone levels and several different kinds of exercise."

The importance of a multilevel approach was dramatically illustrated in a study conducted by the Human Nutrition Research Center at Tufts University in Boston. Scientists there found that both exercise and calcium helped plug up different spots on the skeleton. While calcium boosted bone at the femoral neck (a section of the thighbone), exercise helped prevent bone loss at the spine. "In areas where exercise worked, calcium had no effect, and in places where calcium helped, exercise had no effect," says study coauthor Miriam E. Nelson, Ph.D.

The study involved 36 postmenopausal women. Half walked for 50 minutes three times a week for one year, while the rest remained sedentary. The walkers saw a small, 0.5 percent increase in their bone mass in the spine, while the sedentary women saw a 7 percent drop in the same spot.

At the same time, half the women in each group received a milk-based supplement containing 831 milligrams of calcium. The rest had a similar drink with only 41 milligrams of the mineral. The women who drank the high-calcium formula enjoyed a bone density leap of 2 percent in their thighbones, while the low-calcium drinkers suffered a 1.1 percent drop. The study was short term, so it's difficult to say what would happen to the women's bones over longer periods of time.

"The 7 percent drop in bone at the spine in the sedentary women in only one year is remarkable," says Dr. Nelson. "The fact that exercise appeared to stabilize that adds weight to the idea that you need both exercise and dairy products to maintain bone health."

Dieting Right

High calcium intake today helps prevent fractures tomorrow. That's why experts recommend that most women consume at least 1,000 milligrams of calcium daily. Women past menopause who are not on estrogen replacement therapy should get 1,500 milligrams daily.

Sounds easy, but the shocking fact is that most women don't get anything near those levels—even women who are trying to eat right. University of California, San Diego, biology professor Paul Saltman, Ph.D., recently completed a study in which he tracked the food intake of 137 postmenopausal women in the San Diego area. "These were all women who said they were taking good care of themselves," says Dr. Saltman. "But the fact was, over two years, their calcium intake from food averaged only about 560 milligrams a day."

Why is calcium so hard to get? One reason is that many people shun dairy products, the best source. What's more, even people who eat the same foods won't absorb equal amounts of calcium. "Some women absorb only 15 percent of the calcium in their foods, while others absorb three times as much," says Robert Heaney, M.D., chairman of the U.S. Office of Technology Assessment's scientific advisory panel on osteoporosis. The differences may be genetic, he says, and while people can't do much about their genes, they can eat calcium-rich foods to make up for possible absorption problems.

Just as people aren't alike in the calcium they absorb, foods aren't alike in the calcium they offer. Very few nondairy foods are as calcium-loaded as dairy products. What's more, in some calcium-rich foods, the

BEST AND WORST CALCIUM SOURCES

You already know milk is a great source of calcium. But did you know that almonds can also tip the scale in your favor? So can sardines. But forget meat . . . with one possible exception. "I've been told that alligator meat is high in calcium," says Robert Heaney, M.D., chairman of the U.S. Office of Technology Assessment's scientific advisory panel on osteoporosis. "But we haven't tested it—yet!"

But even though meat flunks the calcium test, it's a rich source of manganese, zinc and copper—all vital to bone health. "We can easily show that when growing animals don't get enough of these three minerals, they develop bone abnormalities," says Dr. Heaney.

Dairy products are by far the richest in calcium, and that calcium also is easily absorbed by the body. Depend on dairy to achieve your recommended calcium intake. Some examples:
- Yogurt (from skim milk): 8 ounces, 452 milligrams
- Skim milk: 1 cup, 302 milligrams
- Buttermilk: 1 cup, 285 milligrams
- Skim milk mozzarella cheese: 1 ounce, 183 milligrams
  Fish with edible bones are good sources of calcium. (Sardines can also be high in fat.) Some examples:
- Sardines: 7 pieces, 321 milligrams
- Salmon, pink, canned, with bones: 3 ounces, 181 milligrams

calcium isn't available to the body. For example, cooked spinach weighs in with a hearty-sounding 122 milligrams of calcium for every 1/2 cup serving. The hitch: It's also loaded with a chemical compound called oxalate that makes the calcium unavailable to the body.

Experts recommend calcium supplements for women who don't eat dairy products. But don't exceed 2,500 milligrams a day, since too much calcium can contribute to kidney stones. (See "Best and Worst Calcium Sources" below.)

THE ABCS—OF D

One more key ingredient in the recipe for strong bones is vitamin D. The nutrient is available from both foods and sunlight—your skin manufactures it when exposed to the sun's ultraviolet light. But getting adequate amounts of vitamin D can be a problem for faithful users of sunscreen.

Sunscreens are used to protect the skin from the damaging effects of

---

Greens and beans are moderately high in calcium, and that calcium is available to the body. Unfortunately, you'd have to eat mounds of them to meet the daily calcium level—1,000 milligrams—that experts recommend. Depend on them as supplementary calcium sources. Some examples:

- Bok choy: 1/2 cup shredded, cooked, 79 milligrams
- Mustard greens: 1/2 cup, chopped, cooked, 52 milligrams
- Kale: 1/2 cup, chopped, cooked, 47 milligrams
- Pinto beans: 1/2 cup, cooked, 45 milligrams
- Kidney beans: 1/2 cup, cooked, 39 milligrams
- Broccoli: 1/2 cup, chopped, cooked, 36 milligrams

Like greens, nuts and dried fruits are good supplementary sources of calcium, but you'd have to cover your plate with them to meet daily requirements. Also, nuts are high in fat, and dried foods are loaded with calories. Some examples:

- Figs, dried: 5 pieces, 135 milligrams
- Almonds, toasted, unblanched: 1 ounce, 80 milligrams
- Hazelnuts: 1 ounce (16 nuts), 55 milligrams
- Brazil nuts: 1 ounce (6 nuts), 50 milligrams
- Prunes, dried: 5 pieces, 21 milligrams

Some odds and ends: Spinach is high in oxalic acid, which makes its calcium unavailable to the body; meats have insignificant calcium content.

sunlight. Unfortunately, they also prevent one of the most beneficial effects of sunlight—the production of vitamin D in the skin. And without vitamin D, bones won't harden, says Michael Holick, Ph.D., M.D., director of the vitamin D laboratory and professor of medicine at Boston University School of Medicine.

Dr. Holick believes it's very important that children and young adults apply a sunscreen before going outdoors for prolonged periods of time. They're outside every day, so it's unlikely sunscreen use will lead to vitamin

---

MEDICATIONS TO MONITOR

There are several medications that can weaken bone, especially if they're taken for a long time.

"Recently it's become clear that people who take too much thyroid medication by pill can lose bone," says B. Lawrence Riggs, M.D., president of the National Osteoporosis Foundation. According to a study of 26 premenopausal women, for example, those receiving long-term treatment with L-thyroxine showed decreased density in certain bones. "Endocrinologists now feel that the dose of thyroid medication prescribed ten years ago or earlier was too much. Many women are still taking these old dosages, and the result can be bone loss."

Talk to your doctor. For women, taking more than 150 micrograms of L-thyroxine may be excessive, says Dr. Riggs. A blood test can help your doctor determine the proper dose.

Drugs such as cortisone, hydrocortisone and prednisone, prescribed for conditions ranging from rheumatic disorders to respiratory disease, can also cause problems. Ask your doctor if other drugs might be better for you.

Antiseizure medications such as phenytoin (Dilantin) and phenobarbital can create a vitamin D deficiency. (Vitamin D is vital to healthy bones.) Your doctor should check vitamin D levels every two to three years and may recommend supplementation.

A diuretic often prescribed for people with hypertension and kidney problems, furosemide (Lasix) can lead to excessive calcium loss through the urine. As an alternative, physicians can consider diuretics in the thiazide class that help preserve calcium in the kidneys.

In rare cases, heparin, a blood thinner used against stroke and clotting, can cause bone problems if it is taken intravenously for a long time. (It is more often administered under the skin, where it is less likely to cause problems.)

D deficiency. But the elderly don't make as much vitamin D in their skin as children and young adults. If they always wear a sunscreen, they may not develop enough vitamin D for good bone health.

What to do? Milk is fortified with vitamin D, and just 2 cups provide the recommended dietary allowance of 200 international units (IU) of vitamin D. People who can tolerate some sun can go outside without sunscreen for 5 to 10 minutes, in morning or late afternoon, three times a week. If they're out longer than that, they can apply sunscreen, thus enjoying the beneficial effects of sunlight while preventing potential damage. For those who can't take any sun or milk, Dr. Holick recommends a multivitamin supplement with 200 to 400 IU of vitamin D.

But while some vitamin D is good, more isn't necessarily better; excessive doses of vitamin D can weaken bones and can cause toxicity.

BEWARE OF (SOME) BEVERAGES

Beer was a staple food in ancient Egypt, but we can only speculate as to whether it contributed to Nes-Ptah's osteoporosis. Doctors today know that the worst beverages for the bones are the alcoholic kind. Taken in excess, alcohol can interfere directly with the body's ability to absorb and use calcium.

And there's another kind of brew that has long been suspected as an accessory to osteoporosis: caffeinated coffee. The case against coffee is a murky one, with contradictory answers to the questions of whether it weakens bone and how much coffee you need to drink to see that effect.

In a recent study, coffee consumption was found to increase the risk of hip fracture in middle-aged women. When compared with women who drank less than 1½ cups of coffee per day, women who consumed more than 6 cups per day nearly tripled their risk.

In an earlier study, New England researchers analyzed data on coffee and tea consumption and hip fractures among 3,170 men and women aged 50 to 84. (The data were collected for the Framingham Heart Study.) Compared with people who drank 1 or fewer cups of coffee per day, those who drank 1½ to 2 cups daily had a very small and insignificant increase in risk. But the risk of people who drank 2½ cups or more a day was 69 percent higher than nondrinkers and single-cup drinkers. Tea drinkers could drink twice the number of cups to reach the same risk level.

The researchers looked for a relationship between high coffee consumption and low milk consumption to see if that accounted for the increased risk. It didn't.

Douglas Kiel, M.D., the lead researcher on the study and an assistant professor of medicine at Brown University in Providence, Rhode Island, notes that even with an increased risk of 69 percent, the total overall risk of hip fracture is still very small. He adds that much more research into the coffee connection is needed. Scientists don't know exactly how caffeine might affect the skeleton. Some speculate that caffeine harms bone directly, while others postulate that it may lower calcium levels in the bones.

"I wouldn't want people to give up their favorite beverage based on this one study," concludes Dr. Kiel. "But it does argue for moderation. Try to keep it at two cups. Cutting back is a painless and potentially helpful practice." More suggestions: Add milk to the coffee you do drink as an

---

TREATMENT BREAKTHROUGH

DESIGNING A PILL TO BUILD BONE

Living bone is constantly changing. At millions of places throughout the skeleton, bone tissue is simultaneously breaking down and building up again, a process of regeneration called bone remodeling. But when you have osteoporosis, bone disappears faster than it can be replaced. Eventually, doctors hope, there will be special drugs that will help the body create new bone—without the side effects of drugs currently in use, says Robert Lang, M.D., medical director of Osteoporosis Diagnostic and Treatment Centers in New Haven and Bridgeport, Connecticut.

For example, estrogen, a female hormone that rapidly diminishes after menopause, is essential for preventing bone loss. However, estrogen replacement therapy, which sometimes is needed to keep bones strong, can contribute to blood clots and some types of cancer. In the future, Dr. Lang says, researchers will be looking for new drugs "that have the beneficial effects of estrogen without the side effects." Actually, prototypes already exist for these "anti-estrogens"—estrogen-like drugs that stimulate bone growth *without* stimulating side effects. "Today, we're making designer molecules and designer antibodies, and the same will be true of hormones," he says.

Another area of research focuses on a class of proteins called growth factors, which naturally, in the absence of osteoporosis, stimulate bone growth. "A growth factor has been identified that stimulates the osteoblasts," Dr. Lang says. Osteoblasts are special bone cells that are essential to the bone-building process. Now that researchers know what they're looking for, they hope to synthesize in the laboratory "designer" drugs that will help build bone when the body won't.

extra source of calcium. And if you're choosing between a cup of coffee and a cup of milk, do your bones a favor and pick the milk.

BONE UP WITH EXERCISE

"The evidence that exercise is beneficial to bone is overwhelming," says Sydney Lou Bonnick, M.D., director of osteoporosis services at the Cooper Clinic in Dallas. "You can maintain or even increase your bone mass through appropriate types of exercise."

Exercise puts "beneficial stress" on the skeleton, stimulating bones to thicken. Researchers postulate that three kinds of exercise are best for the skeleton: weight bearing, impact loading and resistance training.

Weight bearing means just that: carrying body weight on the bones. Walking is a good example—better is walking with a loaded backpack. "Research does show that women who do weight-bearing exercise have stronger bones than those who don't," says Dr. Dalsky.

Add impact-loading exercise for better results. An example of impact loading is jumping up and down. The skeleton carries not just body weight but the force from the movement, called compressive force. That's why brisk walking is better than strolling. "It's weight bearing in either case," says Dr. Bonnick, "but when you go faster, your feet strike the ground with greater force."

The hottest news among exercise physiologists: Strong muscles lead to strong bones. Research shows that resistance training (in which muscles resist an opposing force, as in lifting weights) actually builds bone density where the muscles attach. "If you compare all athletes for bone density—the runners, football players, soccer players, swimmers, weight lifters—the winners are surprising," says Dr. Bonnick. "They're the weight lifters."

Fortunately, you needn't heft 500 pounds above your head for top-notch bones. The Nautilus, Universal and other exercise machines at your health club can build muscle and bone, as can free weights and stretch bands.

Resistance training for bone is a new area of study, and so far the bone gains are small, but scientists are hopeful. "When people do these exercises for six months to one year, which is as long as most studies have gone, research demonstrates a 3 or 4 percent increase in bone mass," notes Dr. Bonnick. "That's not very much, but over a longer period of time, over a lifetime, the increase could be much greater. Then we are talking about significantly increasing bone strength."

Incidentally, people who can't do vigorous exercise because of arthritis, balance problems or other disabilities shouldn't give up. Almost any kind of activity is better than none, says Dr. Dalsky. "If people are limited physically, even gentle exercises like swimming and walking can help the bones."

Also give a little extra thought and sweat to building the hipbone. Back and hip machines at a health club can help. So can walking, stair climbing, running, aerobic dance—anything, in short, that keeps you on your feet, Dr. Dalsky says.

Since different exercises build different parts of the skeleton, it's best to cover your bases—and your bones—by doing many exercises, not just one. "We're just starting to understand which sites of the skeleton exercise builds," says Dr. Dalsky. "We still don't know what an ideal exercise program for bone would look like. In the meantime, for both bone health and overall fitness, my advice is to do a program that combines aerobic weight-bearing exercise with some strength training."

Finally, a warning from the exercise physiologists we consulted: Women who exercise may still need estrogen at menopause to prevent dramatic bone loss. "Most of us in the exercise and bone field say that at menopause, exercise does not replace the need for estrogen," says research physiologist Barbara Drinkwater, Ph.D., at the Pacific Medical Center in Seattle. "Even master athletes should consider estrogen to block the rapid bone loss that comes with menopause."

OVERWEIGHT

U p and down, up and down. You lose weight, you gain it back—and then some. Or you give it your best shot and don't see a slimmer, trimmer new you. You seem to be eternally twirling on the end of a diet string held by purveyors of all sorts of weight-loss elixirs and out-and-out quick-fix fads.

Feel frustrated? Helpless? Condemned to a life of love handles or saddlebags? You are not alone. Between 90 and 95 percent—that's right, 90 to 95 percent—of people treated for being overweight fail to keep it off.

Why bother, then, if you're doomed to fail? Because you *can,* in fact, achieve a lower, healthier weight. How? By exercising and learning to eat low-fat meals, says G. Kenneth Goodrick, Ph.D., an assistant professor of medicine at Baylor College of Medicine in Houston.

And just how long do you have to eat low-fat food and exercise before the flab comes off and stays off? "From now until death," he says.

A CORPULENT CORPSE

It's a frightening prospect, and we don't mean to scare you, but death could come quicker if you're overweight, for obesity is a bona fide disease. Every candy bar, every gallon of ice cream, every french fry and every fatty slab of red meat should carry a warning from the surgeon general that their use is associated with an increased chance of heart disease.

Fat increases blood pressure, lowers the level of high-density lipoproteins (HDL, the "good" cholesterol) in the bloodstream and heightens the chance of developing diabetes, according to JoAnn Manson, M.D., assistant professor of medicine at Harvard Medical School and an associate physician at Brigham and Women's Hospital in Boston. "All increase the risk of heart disease, coronary artery disease and stroke," she says. "They're major risk factors."

For reasons not completely understood, fat concentrated in the abdomen and upper body is more dangerous than fat pooled in the hips, Dr. Manson says. A quick gauge of how much at risk you are of developing heart disease is the waist/hip ratio. Divide the circumference of your waist by the circumference of your hips at their widest point. Women are at greater risk if their ratio is more than 0.80, and men, if their ratio is 0.95 or above.

To some extent, whether you become fat and where you deposit the flab are determined genetically. "But it's not destiny that you're going to be fat or have these health complications," Dr. Manson says. The formula is simple. People gain weight when they consume more calories than they expend. Successful, permanent weight loss demands a lifelong monitoring of what you eat and what you do to burn those calories. And the only way to balance that scale is to make everlasting changes in diet and exercise.

THE DIET OF A LIFETIME

Any weight-loss expert will tell you: Crash diets and fad diets don't work. Severe calorie restriction or unnatural reliance on certain foods while avoiding all others may work initially, but not in the long run, says Dr. Goodrick. A diet that treats food as the enemy is simply not realistic.

"With food as your foe, the idea of eating becomes anxiety provoking, and you have even less control," says Dr. Goodrick. In addition, crash diets actually set up the body to crave high-fat foods. "It's no wonder to me," Dr. Goodrick sighs, "that 90 percent of overweight dieters relapse."

If you want to shed your excess pounds and keep them off, incorporate these principles into your lifestyle.

Cut the fat. One of the most important causes of obesity is dietary fat, which not only has more calories per forkful than either protein or carbohydrates but also may be more likely to be stored as fat in the body.

Trim fat from the meats you eat, and use only low-fat dairy products, desserts and salad dressings. Low-fat eaters naturally eat fewer calories, Dr. Goodrick says. "When you eat high-fat foods, you tend to eat more calories," he says. And you may become more lethargic. "People eating high-fat diets sleep more," he says. "They're sluggish. Their red blood cells tend to sludge together and don't transport oxygen as well."

Ease into the eating change. Don't make abrupt, drastic alterations in food choices or calorie intake. "The trick is to switch to low-fat eating gradually," Dr. Goodrick says. "If you do that, you can lose excess weight without feeling deprived."

A body drastically deprived of sustenance thinks it's starving. "We're programmed to conserve calories," Dr. Goodrick says. If you starve your-

RACHEL IRIZARRY: PICTURING THE FUTURE

Beneath the pounds of fat that padded Rachel Socas Irizarry's frame lay the stunning face and svelte figure of a model.

By the time she was 17 years old in 1982, Rachel tipped the scale at 307 pounds. "I had severe high blood pressure in the 200/100 range and an enlarged heart," she remembers. Not a promising health profile for one so young.

But she was determined to lose weight, and she started by eating salads and walking. Within eight years, she was standing, 5 feet 11 inches tall and 153 pounds, before photographers and television cameras as a part-time model.

"I never thought I'd get as far as I did," she says with some degree of disbelief. "But I did."

Rachel first developed a mental image of what she wanted to look like. "You need to visualize yourself and the body type you'd like," she says, "or picture yourself doing some hobby you can't do now because of the weight. Use that as an incentive to get started. I chose modeling, as it was something I always wanted to do."

She then altered her eating patterns by eliminating fat. "You have to change your eating habits, not just diet," she says. "Once you make the adjustment, it becomes a permanent part of your lifestyle. I used to always put butter and sour cream on my baked potato. Now I wouldn't even think of it. I automatically just eat it plain."

Once the pounds began to drop, weight loss became its own incentive. "All the positive feedback I received was so inspiring," she remembers. "You see the changes in the mirror, and you want to continue."

Exercise helped Rachel lose the fat and keep it off, and her Orlando, Florida, home now resembles a small gymnasium, complete with a treadmill, stair-climbing machine, stationary bicycle, mini-trampoline, dumbbells and stacks of workout videos. She walks the treadmill for 30 minutes five days a week and uses the other devices often.

"If I can do it, anyone can," she says. "You need to choose a goal you really desire. You have to do it for yourself. No one else."

And what of her rampant high blood pressure? She was able to control it completely through losing the weight, giving herself a health profile that matches her figure.

self, your metabolism slows to a crawl, and your body begins to store—as fat—whatever it does consume.

Know your nutrition. Read and learn about healthier food choices, so that you can eat wisely at home and when away. Take the skin off chicken. Broil or bake; don't deep-fry. Drink skim milk. Eat low-fat frozen yogurt instead of ice cream. Buy tuna packed in water, not oil.

"Alternative menu planning is easy," says Patrick M. O'Neil, Ph.D., clinical psychologist and director of the Weight Management Center at the Medical University of South Carolina in Charleston. "It has been estimated that people routinely eat only about ten different meals, and they rotate among them. And they have even less variety in their breakfasts. When you think of it that way, making long-term changes is pretty manageable." And when adequately armed with a knowledge of fat facts, you can eat low fat when you're not preparing the meals or when you're dining out.

Mind your menu math. You certainly don't have to count every calorie, Dr. O'Neil says, but you should be aware of certain nutritional rules of thumb. "A pound of body fat contains roughly 3,500 calories," he says. "To gain a pound of body fat, you need to eat 3,500 more calories than you burn. To lose a pound, you have to do the opposite."

Overall, fat should comprise no more than 20 to 30 percent of the calories you consume. Protein should make up another 15 percent, with the remainder coming from carbohydrates, preferably complex carbohydrates from grains and vegetables, Dr. Goodrick says.

Gaining and losing clearly is easier than you might think when you break it down into 100-calorie increments—the equivalent of a can of light beer or two-thirds of a regular 12-ounce soft drink. "One hundred calories a day is roughly 10 pounds a year," Dr. O'Neil says. "On a daily basis, if you eat 100 calories more than you burn, expect to gain 10 pounds in a year. Ten pounds is not that much, but 10 pounds a year for ten years is 100 pounds."

Now turn that formula on its head and consider cutting just 100 calories a day. "That seems more doable," Dr. O'Neil says. "Extrapolate it to a year or more, and you can see where you're really making a difference in weight loss."

FITNESS FIGHTS FATNESS

In stripping off the weight and keeping it off, exercise "is very significant, especially in the long run," Dr. O'Neil says. "It's even more critical in maintenance than in weight loss itself." These calorie-burning exercise basics should become routine parts of your life!

Muscle up your metabolism. Your metabolic rate—how many calories you expend while at rest—is determined by the amount of lean muscle in your body. "Strength training is good," Dr. Goodrick says, "because it increases lean tissue, and you won't lose the muscle you otherwise would lose from decreasing calorie consumption."

And don't worry if you see the needle on the scale rising a pound or two after you begin a strength-training regimen. "With muscle gain, you

THE YO-YO IS A NO-NO

You've seen the ads. You've heard the spiels. You've probably tried them. And you probably feel somewhat gullible now that you realize what you always suspected in the back of your mind: Liquid diets and easy-off weight-loss gimmicks can't work, because they're too good to be true.

But you're not just a bit poorer in finances; you're a bit poorer in health, for yo-yo dieting is downright dangerous. "Weight cycling appears to be even more harmful than maintaining an elevated weight with no loss," according to JoAnn Manson, M.D., assistant professor of medicine at Harvard Medical School and an associate physician at Brigham and Women's Hospital in Boston.

The reasons aren't clear, she says, but it appears that yo-yo dieting is associated with higher fat deposits in the abdomen and upper body. Once you've lost and then regained fat, it tends to accumulate in the torso. And upper-body fat, as opposed to fat on the hips and legs, is a strong predictor of stroke and heart disease.

In addition, Dr. Manson says, "it's extremely stressful to the system physiologically and emotionally to constantly diet and regain."

Liquid meal substitutes are appropriate only in certain situations that are carefully supervised by physicians. "They're a way to help the more overweight person lose a significant amount of weight pretty quickly," says Patrick M. O'Neil, Ph.D., a clinical psychologist and director of the Weight Management Center at the Medical University of South Carolina in Charleston. Liquid meal supplements are recommended only when part of a comprehensive program to help you make long-term lifestyle changes, he says.

The liquid nostrums are completely unrealistic, weight-loss experts say, because people do need to eat, and they need to exercise to maintain any lower weight they achieve. "If you're expecting the powder alone to keep the weight off, then you're barking up the wrong tree," says Dr. Manson.

actually have an increase in weight," Dr. Manson says, "because muscle weighs more than fat."

Prepare for the long haul. Take a walk—on the mild side at first, but weight-loss experts emphasize that each exercise session should last longer than 30 minutes for maximum benefit. "During the first half hour, you're just burning glycogen stores in the body," Dr. Goodrick says. "You don't burn excess fat until you've been exercising beyond a half hour." The psychological high sparked by the body's production of mood-elevating endorphins also doesn't kick in during exercise routines shorter than 30 minutes.

TREATMENT BREAKTHROUGH

FAT AND THE FUTURE

Obesity researchers have been no more successful than their patients in finding a cure for weight gain. And other than modifications in instilling good exercise and eating habits, it doesn't seem as though the future holds any hope for any techno-toner or cyber-slimmer that will melt off the pounds.

"In a Westernized, industrial environment such as the United States, it seems as if we're almost predisposed to gain weight," says Patrick M. O'Neil, Ph.D., a clinical psychologist and director of the Weight Management Center at the Medical University of South Carolina in Charleston. "There's ready access to lots of high-fat food, high-calorie food, and there's usually no great deal of physical exertion required."

The required breakthrough must be a behavioral one, according to G. Kenneth Goodrick, Ph.D., an assistant professor in the Department of Medicine at Baylor College of Medicine in Houston. People have to overcome bad habits about inactivity and indulgent eating.

"We're set up as a society where it's easy to get high-fat food and difficult to exercise," he says. "If we as a nation are serious, we have to educate children in school about the dangers of obesity and the need for healthy eating and exercising." Physical education classes should be mandatory for 45 minutes a day for all kids from kindergarten through twelfth grade, he maintains, "and it should be taught so they'll enjoy it."

The food industry should play a continuing role by offering more nonfat alternatives, he suggests, and government can help by offering safe walking and jogging paths in parks.

Brisk walking is a fine way to begin a new fitness lifestyle. Ease yourself into hour-long hikes three or four times a week, Dr. Goodrick says.

Like your workout. Just as you should avoid short-term dieting binges, you should also shy away from excessively strenuous or exceedingly demanding workouts that no one realistically could maintain. Select an exercise program that you can see yourself doing for the rest of your life, Dr. O'Neil says. That's because you *will* be doing it for the rest of your life.

THE NEW YOU

Once you're on a weight-loss roll, the results themselves should provide ample encouragement to stick to your new eating and exercising regimens. "You'll see it on the scale, you'll hear the compliments as people notice the change. You'll feel different," Dr. O'Neil says. But it's at this point that some people may let down their guard. "It's easy to make dietary and exercise changes when you're seeing the results so quickly," he says. "The real difficulty starts when the rate of weight loss slows down, and you and others don't notice as much change. The compliments wane, and you start to take your new size for granted."

This is when people often think they can revert to old habits, says Dr. O'Neil. They can't. "These are eating and exercise patterns that you have to stay with forever," he says.

While the temptation is great to indulge and let down your guard, weight-loss pros have some suggestions for permanent behavior modification.

Take it easy. "One of the most important challenges is that obesity is a chronic problem that needs a long-term solution," Dr. O'Neil says. "Everybody wants a quick fix; it's human nature." Weight loss won't come easy, and it won't come fast. Expect to lose only about 1/2 to 1 pound of fat a week.

Make it easy. "You don't get extra credit for difficulty," Dr. O'Neil says. "Don't get into a sackcloth-and-ashes mind-set of severe calorie restriction and exhaustive exercise. You won't be able to continue that for long."

Weigh every day. "You have to do it whether you want to or not," Dr. O'Neil says. "It's one of the few things we're pretty nonnegotiable about. You've got to weigh yourself every day for the rest of your life." Keep a daily log of your performance on the scale. The idea is not to make you a slave to your scale. You'll learn that today's weight doesn't necessarily reflect what you did yesterday, but you'll be able to see whether your overall trend is in the right direction.

Plan for setbacks. "Draw a line a few pounds above your maintenance weight—3 to 5 pounds, not 30 or 50," Dr. O'Neil says, "then plan what to do if your weight ever goes above." You might want to consider drinking one fewer beer or cola a night or skipping that buttery bag of popcorn at the movies. Continue this recovery plan until your weight is safely below the line.

Check the charts with a grain of salt. Those old standard height/weight charts are somewhat outdated and unrealistic, physicians say, and they shouldn't be used to plan your ultimate weight-loss goal. "If you weigh 200 pounds and the chart says you should weigh 120 pounds, shoot for 160 pounds," says Dr. Goodrick. Don't heighten expectations only to perhaps have them plummet. "Seek a weight halfway between where you are now and where you should be on the charts," he advises.

PARKINSON'S DISEASE

W henever 34-year-old registered nurse Diane Carlin took a break from her hospital routine of taking temperatures, giving shots, testing blood pressure and writing down medical information, she noticed her right arm would shake. As time passed, other problems cropped up: She couldn't keep up her normally fast pace, and she even started to feel a little clumsy. Her fingers couldn't grip coins in her change purse, she was having a hard time brushing her teeth, and her handwriting was getting small and hard to read—worse, even, than a doctor's. She got so depressed, she had to turn to medication for relief.

Extensive medical testing eliminated all possible causes but one: Parkinson's disease. But she was "too young" for that. Unfortunately, as it turned out, she wasn't.

The diagnosis was a long time coming, and when Diane got the word, she cried. "To this day I'm not sure whether I was crying because I had Parkinson's," she says, "or crying with relief, because I finally knew what it was." As you'll see, she's taken that diagnosis and run with it.

ANOTHER MYSTERY OF THE BRAIN

Diane's case is unusual only in that she was so young. Each year 50,000 Americans get the same diagnosis. An estimated 1.5 million now have it. If you're over 50, there's a 1 in 500 chance that you'll get Parkinson's; if you're over 60, your chances go up to 1 in 100. You're also slightly more at risk if you're a man. But it's neither inherited nor contagious.

Parkinson's symptoms begin slowly, usually affecting one side of the body. The most notorious symptom is tremor of the hands, feet and head. Rigidity is another prominent symptom. A person with Parkinson's gradually loses the ability to move his muscles at will. The muscles become stiff, and movements slow down. As the muscles tighten up, the face may lose its expressiveness, posture becomes stooped, and the hands and feet, deformed. As the disease progresses, a person with Parkinson's may have a hard time walking, turning over in bed, dressing, bathing and talking. He may also lose his balance and fall. His voice becomes a high-pitched monotone, he drools and is constipated. His mental processes eventually slow down; he can become depressed and suffer spells of sweating and feelings of heat or cold.

Yet through all this there is no pain, and Parkinson's itself is not life-threatening. The mind usually remains alert and active, imprisoned in a body that just won't cooperate.

In some ways, Parkinson's resembles Alzheimer's disease: It attacks the brain, no one knows the cause or cure, and it always gets worse the longer you have it. Like Alzheimer's, it's greatly feared. But unlike Alzheimer's, there are very effective drugs and even some self-help measures that can, for years, hold the worst of Parkinson's at bay.

THE DOPAMINE CONNECTION

Although the cause of the disease isn't known, the cause of the symptoms is very well known. In the area of the brain just above where the spinal cord leaves the skull—the part of the brain that controls movement—you have about 500,000 brain cells that make dopamine, a chemical neurotransmitter that relays messages between cells. To work, dopamine must always be in delicate balance with acetylcholine, another neurotransmitter.

For some reason, in Parkinson's, the cells that make dopamine and supply it to the brain begin to die. Yet it's not until at least 80 percent of the cells are dead that the first symptoms of Parkinson's appear. Too little dopamine means too much acetylcholine, causing you to lose control over your movements.

What's killing the dopamine cells? No one knows. But dopamine's role is so central to Parkinson's that most research has zeroed in on this chemical, whether for divining the cause, devising treatments or discovering a cure.

THE DRUGS OF CHOICE

Levodopa (L-Dopa) is the main drug used to fight the symptoms of Parkinson's. The brain uses the drug to synthesize dopamine and to make up for some of the loss of the brain's own dopamine. Its benefits can be dramatic, and people who take it can quickly resume an almost normal life.

MANY MORE ACTIVE YEARS

It's like something out of *Brave New World:* transplanting the dopamine-producing cells from the brains of miscarried or aborted eight- to nine-week-old fetuses into the brains of people with Parkinson's. The transplanted cells start producing dopamine, and the people regain many of their neurological functions.

No one knows if fetal implants will reverse the symptoms of Parkinson's. Yet such implants are one of the most intriguing and futuristic lines of Parkinson's research. "Unpublished information from England and Sweden is looking reasonably good," says gerontologist Franz Hefti, Ph.D. "But it involves only 10 to 20 patients."

For researchers, Parkinson's is a baffling disease. "We're not coming up with a single cause and a single cure," Dr. Hefti says. "It's more likely that we'll face a situation like that of cancer or diabetes or heart disease—we'll probably find that Parkinson's has multiple causes, and some of these causes will have cures, but others will not."

What could these causes turn out to be? "I think that 20 years from now, we'll find that a genetic predisposition is one likely cause," he says. "And maybe some environmental exposure to chemicals, but not necessarily man-made chemicals—they could be natural chemicals."

How about diagnosing Parkinson's early, before so many dopamine cells have been destroyed that symptoms appear? "I don't think there will be a simple test that will tell who will and who won't get Parkinson's," Dr. Hefti says. He does think, however, that tests such as brain-imaging techniques—where doctors will be able to look at the brain and actually count dopamine cells—will be feasible for people thought to be at risk, like those with a possible genetic predisposition.

"In 20 years, I think we'll have very successful treatments for symptoms, including improved drugs that replace dopamine with fewer side effects," Dr. Hefti says. "They'll also be effective longer, allowing those with the disease to be more active longer. On top of that, we'll have one or maybe several ways to slow down the progression of the disease by implanting cells, whether they're fetal dopamine cells or brain cell growth factors. I don't think this is going to cure it, but it's better than no progress at all."

But this potent drug also has drawbacks. Side effects can be severe—but worse, L-Dopa eventually stops working. The longer you take it, the more you experience the "on-and-off syndrome"—periods of time during the day when the medication works fine and you can move easily, followed abruptly by periods when it doesn't work at all, despite the fact that you're taking the proper dose.

L-Dopa's side effects include visual hallucinations, confusion and sudden jerking movements.

"L-Dopa is still the most effective treatment we know," says Franz Hefti, Ph.D., professor of gerontology at the University of Southern California and a research scholar of the National Parkinson Foundation. "It works very well at the beginning of treatment and continues for a number of years. But the longer people take it, the less well it works, and they need higher and higher doses. The side effects increase, and we end up with burned-out people."

Because of L-Dopa's side effects and limitations, doctors now don't prescribe it for mild symptoms, saving it for more advanced stages of the disease. But, says Dr. Hefti, there are other drugs to help Parkinson's sufferers that work in different ways and that can also help reduce dependency on L-Dopa.

One such drug is deprenyl. It can help preserve the brain's own dopamine. Some studies have shown that people taking deprenyl may be able to cut their dosages of L-Dopa by 10 to 30 percent.

A Nutritional Possibility

One exciting development in Parkinson's research offers hope in vitamin therapy. In one small study at Columbia University, 17 patients in the early stages of the disease were given high doses of vitamins C and E. Compared with other patients, the group on vitamins was able to function 2½ years longer without drug treatment for advanced Parkinson's!

How might vitamins C and E affect a mysterious nervous-system disease like Parkinson's? They, like L-Dopa and deprenyl, are antioxidants, substances that scoop up free radicals and neutralize them.

But just like other drugs, high doses of vitamins should not be taken without a doctor's supervision. Besides, the results of this small study still need to be verified. You should talk to your doctor.

Self-Help: The Parkinson's Workout

Since Parkinson's attacks movement, keeping your muscles as flexible as possible can go a long way in helping to fight the debilitating effects of the disease, say experts. That makes exercise, physical therapy and occupational therapy the most important nondrug treatments for Parkinson's.

Stay active. Whatever it is you decide to do, decide to do it every day, says Terry Moon-Sperling of Rehab Works of California, Inc., an occupational therapist and a board member of the National Parkinson Foundation's California chapter. "We tell our clients never to sit for longer than an hour at a time," Moon-Sperling says. "The longer you sit or remain immobile, the harder it is to get moving again."

But this doesn't mean you have to become a triathlete. When you're having one of your "off" periods, "just relax and make that your quiet time," Moon-Sperling advises. When you're having your "on" periods, you have to exercise moderately. Conserve your energy. Overactivity or overexercising could end up increasing your "off" time.

Exercise means gentle aerobics, like walking, riding an exercise bicycle or using a rowing machine. This will help you maintain your range of motion, improve your coordination and boost your speed of movement. It's best to exercise in frequent, short intervals—say, two or three times a day for 5 to 10 minutes each session, she says. And be sure to discuss your exercise schedule with your doctor before you start.

Reach for a helping hand. There are two main forms of exercise—active, like aerobics, and passive. Passive exercise is when a physical therapist—or a family member who has studied a book or videotape or has taken a class on physical or occupational therapy—stretches your trunk, neck, arms and legs. This keeps the muscles from shortening due to rigidity. If you have any joint problems, it's probably best if you have a therapist work on you, Moon-Sperling says.

Find the easy way out of the chair. You have trouble getting out of a chair, let alone walking. What do you do? "Don't struggle to do something," Moon-Sperling advises. "Stop and start all over again. People with Parkinson's have problems with planning their movements. They sometimes have to talk themselves through it. It's mind over matter. You have to integrate your mind and body, because you've lost the automatic connections. And it helps to work in a rhythm."

For example, your chair has you trapped. Rock back and forth rhythmically three or four times, and use your momentum to help you get up. It's best to sit only in firm chairs that are higher off the floor; the same goes for beds, so put your bed and chair on blocks.

Take one giant step forward. For a person with Parkinson's, walking often is more like shuffling. One way to overcome this is to learn to exaggerate your movements. This doesn't mean you'll be taking giant steps—instead, you'll turn your shuffle into normal steps, Moon-Sperling says. And when you walk, walk to music in your head, something with a nice, steady rhythm. Because it's likely you have trouble keeping your balance, don't be shy about using a cane or walker—it beats falling.

Say you have to step over a threshold, but your feet feel like they're trapped in cement. You stand there willing your feet to move, and they won't. "Instead, tell yourself to lift your *knee* up, and your foot will follow," Moon-Sperling says. Your body is playing tricks on you, and you sort of have to play tricks back, fooling it into doing what you want.

Dress and sleep with ease. Getting dressed can be a slow, awkward process. Again, musical rhythm can help—maybe a slow, light, graceful waltz. See an occupational therapist for new strategies for dressing, Moon-Sperling advises. You can learn simple things, like making sure you slide the most affected arm and leg into your clothes first.

There's no such thing as a Parkinson's person tossing and turning in bed—such movement is impossible. But Moon-Sperling has a simple solution to finding a more comfortable sleeping position—satin sheets. "They make it real easy to slide around," she says. "It's amazing how well they work."

Turn to the special effects. There's a lot of inexpensive equipment that can help normalize daily life for people with Parkinson's, Moon-Sperling says: shoes with elastic shoelaces already tied or with Velcro fasteners, eating utensils that keep your food on a steady course from plate to mouth, special pens that are easy to grip (an occupational therapist can train you to write bigger and better).

There's a motto Moon-Sperling likes to pass on to her clients, who may sometimes feel embarrassed by the clumsiness Parkinson's causes: "It doesn't matter *how* you do it as long as you *can* do it."

How One Brave Person Copes

To a person with Parkinson's, every minute is a reminder of the loss of control—a heavy burden to bear. But Diane Carlin is living proof it can be borne. Caring for someone with Parkinson's can also be tough—as with Alzheimer's disease, you're not always sure when to help and when *not* to help. That's why both the victim and caregiver must talk and ask and listen. The more you know about Parkinson's, the better for both of you. Understanding her disease has helped Diane come to terms with her limitations. It has also given her courage.

"Ever since the diagnosis, my philosophy has been that I can choose to live each day *living* with disease or I can choose to live each day *dying* with this disease," Diane says. "I have chosen to live with it and do something about it. And what I'm doing is fighting it, for myself and for everyone else who has it."

And so she *communicates*. She doesn't let her family overprotect her or, on the other hand, deny that she has Parkinson's—she both reassures them and helps them face the reality she has to face.

When Diane visits her doctor, she goes equipped with a list of questions about her symptoms, the drugs she has to take, her therapy—she wants as much control over her treatment as possible. She rides her bicycle, knowing someday she'll have to replace that exercise with something else—a key word, *replace,* not *give up.*

One major replacement in her life was to volunteer at the National Parkinson Foundation when she could no longer be a nurse. Another replacement was even more personal: Her 23-year marriage collapsed under the stress Parkinson's can create, but she later met and married a man with Parkinson's who had called her asking for help.

"Adapting to new symptoms and increasing impairments is not always easy," Diane says, "but living a quality life is very much worth the struggle."

PELVIC INFLAMMATORY DISEASE

Each year, thousands of women discover that they can't get pregnant—all because their fallopian tubes have been blocked by an often silent infection called pelvic inflammatory disease (PID).

The cause? Almost always it's a sexually transmitted disease, and often that disease is chlamydia, says Lisa Hirsch, M.D., assistant professor of obstetrics and gynecology and director of outpatient OBGYN services at the University of California, Irvine, Medical Center. Strictly speaking, when the same germs that cause sexually transmitted diseases in the vagina work their way up the cervix into the fallopian tubes, that's PID. Often, however, infections (even non–sexually transmitted ones) in the uterus, ovaries and cervix are also called PID.

In some cases, symptoms can be so mild that a woman is fooled into thinking they're just part of being a woman. In other cases, PID can bring pelvic pain, abscesses in the tubes and ovaries and pain during intercourse. It can also lead to ectopic (tubal) pregnancy, a condition that's potentially life-threatening to the mother and always fatal to the fetus. The most common complication, however, is sterility. Of the one million American women who will have an episode of PID this year, 12 percent will become infertile as a result of that one episode. A second episode will sterilize 25 percent of the victims, and a third raises the rate to 50 percent.

But you can lower your risk of contracting PID. In fact, this is one disease that is almost entirely preventable.

A PROTECTION PLAN

Preventing PID is relatively simple, but both you and your doctor have to be conscientious and aware, says Beverly A. Sansone, M.D., assistant clinical professor of obstetrics and gynecology at the University of California, Irvine, Medical Center and medical director of Planned Parenthood of Orange and San Bernardino counties. Dr. Sansone suggests how to avoid PID.

Practice safe sex. Preventing PID starts with preventing sexually transmitted diseases. That begins with smart sex. Yes, yes, using a condom can be tedious until you learn to include it as an integral part of sex. But it can help prevent sexually transmitted diseases, so it's a small price to pay to retain your fertility, says Dr. Sansone. The safest sex, of course, is to be had in a mutually monogamous relationship. Women who have multiple sexual partners have more than 4 1/2 times the risk of getting PID compared with those in monogamous relationships.

Avoid intercourse if infected with a sexually transmitted disease. You don't want to spread a sexually transmitted disease to a loved one—nor do you want to give yourself PID. Intercourse can spread infectious germs upward to where they can cause PID. "We think that sometimes the bacteria hitch rides on the backs of sperm, which are carried up into the fallopian tubes," says Dr. Sansone. There's more to lovemaking than intercourse, and you don't need to refrain from affection.

Get checked immediately. The earlier PID is discovered and treated, the greater your chances of limiting harmful effects. "Doctors have to have a high index of suspicion to be able to detect PID," says Dr. Sansone. Although they're getting better, overall, "they still have to get more interested," she says. If you have reason to suspect PID and your doctor doesn't seem too concerned, find another doctor—a gynecologist is probably your best bet.

IF YOU HAVE IT

Doctors are finding PID to be the cause of so much infertility that they're beginning to treat it more seriously. "In the past," Dr. Sansone says, "we started treatment only when there was fever and considerable pain. Now, if you have mild pain, especially during intercourse, a slight discharge and a slight tenderness in the pelvic area, we'll treat you for PID."

Treatment is aggressive. The doctor will take cultures, but he won't wait for the results before putting you on antibiotics. "If it's your first time with PID and your symptoms are severe, you'll often be hospitalized, because the doctor won't know how long you've had it or how much damage has already been done," says Dr. Sansone. If your symptoms are mild, you'll be treated as an outpatient, get an antibiotic shot for possible gonorrhea, take broad-spectrum oral antibiotics for other possible causes and return after two or three days for a follow-up.

"Antibiotics work so fast and make you feel better so soon that in three days the doctor will know if they're working," Dr. Sansone says. "If you don't start getting better right away, you'll probably be hospitalized for even more aggressive treatment." It takes ten days to clean up chlamydia—so you have to take all your pills, even if you feel fine after only three days.

If the disease has damaged the fallopian tubes to the point of making normal pregnancy impossible, doctors sometimes recommend in vitro fertilization for women who still want to have children.

TAKING ACTION

Aside from taking your antibiotics, there are a few other things you can do to help yourself.

Make sure your partner gets checked, too. You and your partner, even if monogamous now, could have picked up infections before you began your relationship and could be passing them back and forth between the two of you. It makes no sense for you to get treated for PID if your partner is going to reinfect you. He should get checked for infection and be treated if necessary.

Take painkillers. Ibuprofen (Advil, Motrin), aspirin or acetaminophen (Tylenol) can relieve the pain and tenderness of PID.

Avoid sex. It may be too painful anyway, and you don't want to risk continuing reinfection from germs that haven't yet been killed by antibiotics or that come from an untreated sex partner.

Rest, eat well, drink plenty of fluids. "Treat yourself as if you had the flu," Dr. Sansone says. "Rest, fluids and food help your immune system help the antibiotics work. Much of the outcome depends on your own immunity."

Keep track of your temperature. "If it goes over 101°F, call your doctor," says Dr. Sansone.

When you knock out the sexually transmitted disease, you knock out PID, but your problems may not be over. "If PID has been brewing a long time, you may already have complications," says Dr. Sansone. "You may have defeated the infection, but you can still have adhesions or blocked tubes."

If you have been trying to get pregnant and still can't, even after curing PID, doctors may insert a laparoscope—a tiny telescope on a long, thin tube threaded through your navel—to get a close-up view of damage. Surgery can often remedy adhesions and reopen tubes closed by infection.

PHLEBITIS

You'd probably think that any disease with a name like *phlebitis,* which involves inflamed veins, would likely be mighty serious. Actually, it's usually not.

Phlebitis generally occurs on the surface veins of the leg. It's not hard to diagnose. There's usually redness and a hard swelling along the affected vein. And oh, yes, it hurts.

Who gets phlebitis? The top candidates are people with varicose veins, those raised and twisted lines of blue just beneath the skin of the legs. Often it's an injury in one of these protruding veins that causes the vein to inflame.

So the best way to prevent phlebitis is to treat your varicose veins kindly and gently. That means staying active, elevating your legs whenever you can, wearing compression stockings and doing all of the other good things suggested in "Varicose Veins" on page 527.

QUICK CARE

Should you develop phlebitis, rest assured that it will probably cure itself within a week or so. But you should check with your doctor to be sure veins deep in the legs aren't affected. If you develop a fever, see your physician right away. In the meantime, here are a few simple steps to help speed your recovery.

Keep moving around. Long periods of standing or sitting keep pressure on the blocked vein. Perhaps the best favor you can do for your phlebitis is to get active. "Don't stay in bed all day. Continue your normal activities. *Move* around," says Michael Silane, M.D., clinical associate professor of surgery at Cornell Medical School and associate attending surgeon at New York Hospital–Cornell Medical Center. If your normal schedule includes a lot of sitting or standing in one place, intentionally getting up and walking at least several times a day for the duration of the inflammation could make a huge difference, he says.

Raise your leg. While you're watching television or reading, lie down and put up your leg, says Dr. Silane. This will help the blood flow. After the phlebitis is gone, raising your leg should become a lifelong habit to help control varicose veins.

Apply heat. A heating pad or warm towel applied for 15 minutes can soothe the painful area around the clogged vein, says Dr. Silane.

Take a painkiller. Aspirin or ibuprofen may relieve much of the pain and reduce the inflammation. Take your pills or capsules as needed, following the directions on the bottle, says Dr. Silane.

Try some zinc. Zinc oxide ointment, available over the counter at your pharmacy, may help relieve any itching you have. Just smear this onto the area that itches.

DEEP TROUBLE

Although most superficial phlebitis is not dangerous, it has a cousin that is: deep venous thrombosis, sometimes referred to as deep thrombophlebitis. Deep venous thrombosis is usually caused by a blood clot in one of the veins deep within the leg. The big danger is that such a blood clot may break free and travel to the lungs. And that can be fatal, says Francis Kazmier, M.D., head of the Section on Vascular Medicine at the Ochsner Clinic in New Orleans.

Ironically, unlike superficial phlebitis, deep venous thrombosis often causes no redness or lumps. If it causes any symptoms at all, those symptoms may include pain and swelling in the leg, with some blue discoloration. Another irony is that if you develop deep venous thrombosis, you need to be hospitalized—but you may already be in a hospital! That's because the most common cause of deep venous thrombosis is extended inactivity, says Dr. Kazmier. Aside from those bound to hospital beds, others susceptible to developing deep venous thrombosis include those who take oral contraceptives, overweight people who sit for long stretches of time and pregnant women.

Doctors who suspect deep venous thrombosis often rely on ultrasound, a highly accurate and painless test, to make a firm diagnosis. If detected, they also treat it aggressively. You'll get large intravenous doses of a blood-thinning medication. After you're discharged, you'll take an oral blood-thinning drug, such as Coumadin, for a period of weeks to sometimes months, depending on your condition.

Contrary to what you may think, the blood-thinning medications don't dissolve the clot. They keep new clots from forming while your own body dissolves the clot.

PNEUMONIA

Richard Levine of Albuquerque eats well, sleeps well and looks like a weight lifter—the rewards for spending thousands of hard, hot days making bricks at one of the largest adobe-brick manufacturing plants in the Southwest. But despite nearly 60 years of robust good health, Richard has two weak points: his lungs.

"The first time I had pneumonia, I was a student at Berkeley in 1968," Richard remembers. "My chest hurt like crazy, and I couldn't breathe—it was terrible. When I went to the doctor, he listened to my lungs and slapped me into bed in the hospital for a week. I just couldn't move." Richard's second bout with pneumonia—and another week in the hospital—came ten years later. After the third time, he was fed up. He finally took his doctor's advice and stopped smoking. "You know, I haven't had pneumonia since," he says.

IT GETS YOU WHEN YOU'RE DOWN

Actually, it's not cigarettes that cause pneumonia but viruses and bacteria that move into your lungs and bronchi, causing infection, inflammation and congestion. Ironically, the germs that often cause pneumonia—*Streptococcus pneumoniae,* for example—normally live in your throat and airways, and they even dip into your lungs without causing trouble. It's usually when your guard is down—after years of smoking and drinking, for example, or when you've been sick with another illness—that your lungs become vulnerable to these everyday bugs, says Steven W. Stogner, M.D., a fellow in the Division of Pulmonary and Critical Care Medicine at Louisiana State University School of Medicine at Shreveport. "Any illness, especially that of the lung, can predispose you to pneumonia caused by an organism that would not otherwise be virulent," he says.

When it's mild, pneumonia can be mistaken for a cold, Dr. Stogner says. In more serious cases, it can put you to bed for days with wracking coughs, burning fever and teeth-chattering, bone-rattling chills. In fact, pneumonia ranks sixth among death-causing diseases, killing more than 40,000 Americans every year. This is because pneumonia often strikes people whose systems are already weakened by other underlying health problems, like heart disease, asthma or emphysema. "If you think you have pneumonia, you need to see a doctor," Dr. Stogner warns. "People can die from pneumonia."

Since pneumonia tends to strike when your natural resistance isn't up to snuff, the best way to prevent it simply is to stay in tip-top shape.

KEEPING IT AT BAY

Of course, no one is healthy all of the time, and it's impossible to avoid entirely the multitudes of pneumonia-causing germs (a few of which are nasty enough to get you even if you're in the best of health). But you can keep your defenses in fighting form and greatly reduce your chances of getting pneumonia. For starters:

Encourage coughs. "One of the risk factors for pneumonia is being unable to properly clear secretions from the airways," Dr. Stogner says. People who smoke or who have frequent colds or other respiratory tract infections will often harbor large amounts of mucus in their lungs and airways, he explains. Bacteria *love* phlegm. And the more bacteria you have in your airways, the greater your chances for getting pneumonia. In other words, those productive coughs—those that bring up phlegm— really are *protective* coughs.

Keep your distance. Some pneumonias are contagious while others are not, but catching a lungful of anyone else's germs is pushing your luck. If you're in the sickroom with someone with the disease, try to keep a few feet between you and whatever it is they're blowing, sneezing or coughing. Frequently washing your hands is added insurance, Dr. Stogner adds.

Snuff the cigarettes. Cigarette smoke essentially paralyzes the hair-like projections in your airways, called cilia, that help expel mucus and other secretions. If the cilia aren't working, the mucus—and hordes of bacteria—stay inside.

TREATMENTS OF CHOICE

If you have a stubborn cold or flulike symptoms and congestion in the lungs that does not get better after a few days, you could have pneumonia, and you should promptly see your doctor, Dr. Stogner says. A course of antibiotics may be all that is needed to clear it up. If your pneumonia is caused by a virus, your doctor may prescribe a virucide such as amantadine or acyclovir.

These drugs may provide quick relief from symptoms, but the infection generally lasts longer than the symptoms. Unfortunately, many people feel so much better that they assume they're cured and quit taking the drugs. "Your doctor prescribes the *exact* amount of antibiotics he wants you to take," Dr. Stogner says. If you give the germs a reprieve by stopping your medication prematurely, he warns, they may very well rally and make you sicker than before.

While pneumonia can sometimes be treated at home, some people are hospitalized for more intensive care. In the hospital, you might be given oxygen to give your inflamed lungs a little help. Or if you're having trouble cleaning the phlegm because of an ineffective cough, your doctor may insert a flexible tube into your trachea (windpipe)—a procedure called nasotracheal suction—to clear things out.

Pleurisy, an inflammation of the lining of the lung, is a common complication of pneumonia that makes coughing, even breathing, terribly painful. Your doctor might give you codeine or other drugs to ease the pain. You might even get an intracostal nerve block—an injection that dulls the nerves near the rib cage.

After you get out of the hospital, you'll still have to take things slowly for a few weeks. Your lungs have taken a terrible pounding. They need some rest.

GIVE YOURSELF SOME TLC

To give your healing a helping hand, Dr. Stogner recommends the following.

Fill up on fluids. Pneumonia's hot fevers will dry you out like the desert sun. You need to drink plenty of fluids—about six to eight glasses a day—to avoid dehydration.

Thin your phlegm. You already know how important it is to clear mucus from your lungs and airways. But because pneumonia often is accompanied by pleurisy, the slightest cough can be terribly painful. One possible solution to discuss with your doctor is to take over-the-counter drugs called expectorants. Essentially, these make your coughs more productive with less effort, Dr. Stogner says.

Lie on your side. By supporting, or splinting, your rib cage, this position should make coughing and breathing somewhat less painful.

Take some aspirin. Not only can aspirin help relieve your aches and pains, it will help cool your fever as well. Check with your physician about whether you should use aspirin or a substitute such as acetaminophen.

Get plenty of rest. Your lungs have been through the wringer, and they need time to recover, Dr. Stogner says. This isn't the time to overexert yourself. A gradual increase in daily activities is suggested.

After you've concluded this long, painful, breathless journey, naturally you'll never want to get pneumonia again. In fact, your doctor may recommend you take something to make sure that you don't.

A SHOT OF PREVENTION

If you're at high risk for contracting pneumonia—that is, you are elderly, you have chronic lung disease, diabetes or *any* debilitating disease or you are in close contact with anyone who has pneumonia—you should ask your doctor about a pneumonia vaccine. "For certain types of pneumonia, the vaccines are very good," Dr. Stogner says.

But pneumonia is sufficiently rare in healthy persons, and easy enough to treat when it does occur, that doctors don't routinely give the vaccinations to everyone.

Because of modern antibiotics and antiviral drugs, pneumonia isn't the marauding scourge it once was. If left untreated, however, it can certainly be a very dangerous disease; people die from it every year. But most pneumonias are tamed easily with drugs. Even Richard Levine, who twice stayed in the hospital, treated his third attack at home with antibiotics. Don't panic if you think you have pneumonia, Dr. Stogner says. But don't wait to call your doctor either. Early diagnosis and treatment are of paramount importance.

PREMENSTRUAL SYNDROME

G ail started the morning by knocking her bowl of Oaties off the table and onto her new silk blouse. "Would you look at that," she muttered, as milk dripped from the table and the cat sauntered over for a little taste. But as she swung her legs out of harm's way, a splinter snagged the back of her stocking. "Oh, blast!" Gail exploded, as the run streaked from her ankle to her thigh. "I *told* him to sand that stupid chair!" She twisted around to inspect the damage. That's when she stepped on the cat's tail. The cat yowled, Gail's heel snapped off, and her designer glasses flipped off her nose and splashed into the sink. "Oh-h-h," she moaned, as she burst into tears. "This is worst day of my entire life!"

THOSE MONTHLY BLUES

Actually, Gail was exaggerating. She feels just as horrible for a few days *every* month. So do the millions of American women who regularly suffer symptoms of PMS—premenstrual syndrome. Doctors agree that PMS, for many women, is only a minor nuisance, a brief shower on an otherwise lovely day. For others, however, PMS can be an emotional and physical hurricane that tears into their life for a week to ten days before their period, turning everything inside out and upside down.

PMS appears to be triggered by the cyclical changes in a woman's hormones, says Gay M. Guzinski, M.D., chief of the Division of Benign Gynecology at the University of Maryland School of Medicine in Baltimore.

Even though doctors have linked more than 150 symptoms—these range from weight gain and breast tenderness to insomnia and full-blown depression—with PMS, little is known about the causes of this disorder. It occurs most often in women in their thirties (often following childbirth), and it seems to get worse with advancing age. The severity of PMS may change from month to month, and it usually gets worse during times of stress.

In the past, women with PMS were more likely to receive cheap shots ("It's like I always say, Blanche, a woman can't be president when every month . . .") than sound medical advice. Today, PMS is recognized—and treated—as a very real disorder.

THE PREMENSTRUAL BLUES

Many women have monthly symptoms, but for women with disabling premenstrual problems, Dr. Guzinski says, it's common to feel depressed, anxious, angry or out of control. Like Gail, you might wake up feeling as nervous as a cat on a screen door. Breast tenderness is very common— some women pad their bras with cotton to take away the ache. Others retain so much water before their period that they feel like the dancing hippos in Disney's *Fantasia*. Finally, there are those out-of-control, not-to-be-denied cravings for cake, candy, ice cream and chocolate.

As we'll see in a bit, indulging food cravings isn't necessarily a bad thing—as long as you crave healthy foods. Grazing on junk food, on the other hand, can quickly boost your dress size. For many women, the combination of extra pounds and changing hormone levels pushes their self-esteem right through the floor.

"Before their periods, some women feel ugly and don't want anyone to see them," says Candace S. Brown, Pharm.D., assistant professor of clinical pharmacy and psychiatry at the University of Tennessee at Memphis. "Some women get so depressed that they isolate themselves from others, stay confined to the bedroom, don't answer the phone or may miss days from work. Still smaller numbers of women may have thoughts of suicide or fear they may harm others, such as their children."

PMS is rarely this serious, adds Dr. Guzinski, because even though many women experience one or more premenstrual symptoms, relatively few—certainly less than 10 percent—have the full-blown, disabling symptoms of PMS.

THE RIGHT FOODS

In the past, doctors advised women with PMS to steer clear of bread, potatoes and other complex carbohydrates. These foods, they said, would increase fatigue, lethargy and other symptoms. Today, doctors know better. Complex carbohydrates can boost the brain's supply of serotonin, a chemical in the body that may be in short supply in women with PMS.

In a study at the Massachusetts Institute of Technology, women with and without PMS were invited to eat whatever they wanted in the laboratory dining room. Researchers counted the calories they consumed. They

---

PROFILE IN HEALING

JOYCE VENIS: SHE KNEW SHE WASN'T CRAZY

It took Joyce A. Venis 11 years, 22 doctors and thousands of dollars to prove she wasn't crazy. Even then, when a specialist explained that she had premenstrual syndrome, "my family doctor told me I was still crazy," Joyce remembers. "That's one of the biggest frustrations about PMS—the not being believed."

But Joyce, a psychiatric nurse in Princeton, New Jersey, who has had PMS since the birth of her first child more than 20 years ago, knew something had to be wrong. "Before I'd get my period, my body size would change so drastically my clothes wouldn't fit. My fingers would swell so much that writing was very difficult. I couldn't think straight—and as a nurse who has to be alert, that was very difficult," she says.

Joyce's first reaction, after being diagnosed as having PMS, was relief—she *knew* she wasn't crazy! But her second reaction, she admits, was horror: "I was told no sugar, no salt, no alcohol and no caffeine. Now that was depressing! As a PMS-er, I craved salt and sugar—I felt like my life was over. But I adapted," Joyce adds, "and now I'm the best I've ever been."

Joyce still has PMS, of course, but through trial and error, she has discovered ways to control it. Take, for example, her cravings for sweets: Rather than slamming down bag after bag of dime-store chocolates, she practices what she calls "controlled cheating." Before her period, Joyce buys the best chocolates she can afford. Because they are too expensive to gobble, she explains, she eats less. She also feels like she's getting a little treat—at a time of the month she needs it most!

Joyce also tries to schedule burdensome chores and errands either after or well before her period. This helps keep the premenstrual stress to a minimum. "You want to be prepared," Joyce says. "If you're prepared, you can control the symptoms instead of them controlling you."

found that women with PMS, during the premenstrual phase, tended to gobble up about 275 extra calories with every meal. The women without PMS, on the other hand, ate the same amounts before their periods as after. In other words, women with PMS don't just *think* they're eating more. They really are.

In a related study, the researchers asked women how they felt before and after eating carbohydrate-rich meals. Before eating, many of the women felt angry, tense and depressed. Afterward, they felt calmer, more alert and vigorous.

What these studies suggest is that it's natural for women with PMS to eat more carbohydrates as they approach their menstrual periods. What's more, adding carbohydrates to the diet may actually be an unconscious form of self-treatment.

But eating the *wrong* carbohydrates can worsen your moods as well as your waistline, says Dr. Guzinski.

Susan Lark, M.D., director of the PMS and Menopause Self-Help Center in Los Altos, California, and author of *Premenstrual Syndrome Self-Help Book,* has designed The Women's Diet—a diet she says women should eat every day, not just before their periods. This diet recommends avoiding sweets (candy, cookies, cakes and soft drinks), shunning fried and fatty foods, limiting protein and eating an abundance of complex carbohydrates—cereals, pasta, fruits, vegetables, whole-grain breads and so on. A sensible diet, Dr. Guzinski agrees, can help reduce, if not eliminate, many of the physical and emotional changes that come before your period.

SOOTHING SELF-HELP THERAPIES

There isn't a cure for PMS, Dr. Brown says. There are, however, many ways to mollify the monthlies. For example:

Get a workout. Aerobic exercise—such as brisk walking or swimming—not only relieves the stress that invariably accompanies PMS but also can boost levels of your body's natural painkillers, called endorphins, says Dr. Guzinski.

Forgo the coffee. There's trouble brewing in that shiny percolator, Dr. Brown warns. "Caffeine makes you more jittery, and if you're *already* jittery and anxious, that's the last thing you want. Other caffeinated beverages such as colas and some teas should be avoided."

Plan ahead. Try not to schedule three interviews, four parties and five root canal operations for the week before your period, advises Joyce A. Venis, R.N., a psychiatric nurse who specializes in PMS (and a PMS sufferer) in Princeton, New Jersey. "Get things done in advance, so you don't have to burn the candle at both ends when you're pre-mens," she says.

Take some quiet time. According to a Harvard study, quietly meditating for a half hour each day can help relieve some symptoms of PMS.

In the study, 46 women were divided into three groups. Women in the first group practiced a form of mental relaxation for 15 to 20 minutes twice every day. Women in the second group spent an equal amount of time reading. Women in the third group went about their daily lives and, like the other women, were asked to chart their symptoms.

After three months, women in the relaxation group had a 58 percent reduction in symptoms, compared with 27.2 percent for the readers and 17 percent for those who made no changes in their lives.

MEDICAL RELIEF

There are several prescription and over-the-counter remedies for some symptoms of PMS.

Try ibuprofen. Used as directed on the label, this nonprescription medication (Advil, Midol and Nuprin) is a safe, inexpensive way to help relieve premenstrual symptoms such as palpitations, headaches, diarrhea, nausea and cramps, Dr. Guzinski says.

Calm it with calcium. In one study, 60 women with PMS who were given calcium supplements (1,000 milligrams a day) experienced less pain, water retention and depression. Ask your doctor if calcium supplements might help with your symptoms.

Be on the safe side. Some researchers believe that small doses of vitamin B_6 (50 milligrams a day) may help relieve PMS-related depression and irritability. You should be aware, however, that B_6 is toxic in large doses (more than 500 to 800 milligrams a day) and can cause a tingling in the hands and feet called peripheral neuropathy, Dr. Brown says. Higher doses of vitamin B_6 should be undertaken with the supervision of your doctor.

WHEN ALL ELSE FAILS

Prescription drugs may also help. For example, some women take diuretics to reduce bloating. A drug called bromocriptine (Parlodel) can help relieve breast tenderness. Finally, some doctors prescribe anti-anxiety medications (buspirone, alprazolam) and antidepressants (fluoxetine, nortriptyline) to ease anxiety, irritability and depression caused by PMS.

If you suspect you have PMS, don't hesitate to get medical attention, says Dr. Brown. For many women, the prescription won't be for medicine but for some much-needed quiet time. "PMS will always get worse when other things in your life are in a bad state," she says. So above all, take it easy for a few days.

PROSTATE PROBLEMS

In a man's younger years, the prostate, a small gland at the base of his bladder, quietly churns out the semen that fuels his sex life. As he ages, however, the prostate sometimes assumes another duty: causing trouble. It can get sore, tender and inflamed. Like a summer zucchini, it can grow large and cumbersome. Finally, it's one of the leading sites of cancer in American men.

But relatively few men are prostrate because of their prostate. Most prostate problems can be assuaged with rest, antibiotics or, most commonly, surgery. Some doctors suggest that extra sex can help. Ah, *now* you're interested!

WHEN BIGGER ISN'T BETTER

Every night, millions of American men, with tired eyes and a brimming bladder, leave the comfort of their bed to seek relief. But to their sorrow, their relief is short-lived: No sooner do they settle back to sleep than their bladder, like an inexhaustible well, is full again.

These uncomfortable fellows belong to what is perhaps the least exclusive club in the world: The Fraternal Order of Men with Enlarged Prostate Glands. Just about every man over 50 has an enlarged prostate, a condition doctors call benign prostatic hyperplasia. Many men with this condition feel the need to urinate often, sometimes every hour. Many will have painful urination, a diminished urinary stream or a feeling that their bladder never is empty.

Here's what happens. As urine leaves your bladder, it first passes through a channel in the prostate gland called the prostatic urethra. If the prostate gland becomes enlarged, it begins to block the prostatic urethra and, consequently, the flow of urine. That's why men with enlarged prostates often have weak urinary streams. What's more, the bladder has to work extra hard to push urine through the narrowed urethra, the tube that carries urine from the bladder through the penis. Eventually the bladder gets tired and finds it more restful to stay full than to try to empty.

Many older men can hold tremendous amounts of urine because the bladder's stretch receptors have become less sensitive, says Steven R. Gambert, M.D., professor of medicine and gerontology and associate dean for academic programs at New York Medical College in Valhalla. "These men often will get an upper urinary tract disorder, which can occur if urine goes back up into the kidneys. That can cause all sorts of problems, including kidney failure," says Dr. Gambert.

PLUMBING REPAIR

Some men can have an enlarged prostate for decades with no problems whatsoever. If the normal flow of urine gets significantly impaired, however, it may be time to open things up, says Mark S. Soloway, M.D., a professor of urology and chief of urologic oncology at the University of Tennessee at Memphis and attending physician at Baptist Memorial Hospital, Memphis. Basically, you have two options: drugs, or surgery.

A class of prescription drugs called alpha blockers—for example, Minipress and Dibenzyline—can help relax the smooth muscle that surrounds the prostate, thus allowing the overgrowth to move outward from the prostatic urethra. Once the urethra is clear, urine can once again flow freely. But these drugs don't actually *shrink* the tissue, Dr. Soloway says. They offer temporary relief, not a cure.

Surgery, on the other hand, can cure an enlarged prostate simply by removing renegade tissue. "Many men, of course, would like to avoid an operation, but surgery is tried and true," Dr. Soloway says. In fact, approximately 350,000 surgeries for this condition are performed every year, and it's one of the most common operations performed on men 65 and older.

Surgical incisions rarely are required, Dr. Soloway says. Instead, most surgeons prefer a technique called transurethral resection of the prostate, in which prostatic tissue is removed by inserting tiny instruments into the penis, through the urethra and up into the prostate. The surgery is quite simple, Dr. Soloway says, and "about 80 percent of the people who have it are dramatically improved."

GETTING THE BUGS OUT

For most of his 70 years, Walter Leika of Colonia, New Jersey, slept just fine. That changed in 1985, when he picked up a dose of bacterial prostatitis—an infection in his prostate gland. Of course, Walter didn't know he had prostatitis. He just knew he was always waking up to go to the bathroom. Then six years later, his big toe got infected. "I went to the doctor, he gave me antibiotics, and I started going to the bathroom once a night again."

Bacterial prostatitis, while easily treated, is quite rare, says Dr. Soloway. It occurs when bacteria from the colon get into the urethra. Once in the urethra, bacteria can take a leisurely swim upstream until they reach the prostate gland. There they make themselves at home by making *you* miserable. The prostate gland may get infected and painfully inflamed. Like Walter, some men will need to urinate every few hours. Others will have painful urination, perhaps accompanied by fever, chills or low back pain.

A few aspirin and a relaxing bath can make you feel better, but what you really need are antibiotics, Dr. Soloway says. In most cases, antibiotics will clear up the infection in just a few days.

PROSTATE SURGERY: A MAN'S BIGGEST FEAR

The same man who might run into a raging fire to rescue a kitten will buckle at the knees should his doctor mention prostate surgery. It's not merely his life that's being discussed but—gulp!—his sex life.

Guys, you can calm down, says Steven R. Gambert, M.D., a professor of medicine and gerontology and associate dean for academic programs at New York Medical College in Valhalla. If you had erections before surgeons worked on your prostate, there's a good chance you'll have them afterward. If you had orgasms . . . well, you might notice some interesting changes.

Most men who have surgery for benign prostatic hyperplasia will have retrograde ejaculations, Dr. Gambert says. This means your semen, instead of coming out of the end of your penis during orgasm, will go backward into the bladder. This isn't a painful sensation, nor will it necessarily change the quality of your orgasms, but the *idea* of ejaculating backward does take some getting used to, he says.

Much more serious—and more threatening to a man's sexual functioning—is the radical prostatectomy. This is the removal of the entire prostate gland, a procedure sometimes required for men with advanced prostatic cancer. "In the old days, many of the nerve fibers that control erections might have been cut, and that would lead to impotence," Dr. Gambert says. Today, surgeons can often spare the nerves, thus sparing erections. It may, however, take six months to a year after the surgery before a man feels like his old self again.

Not so easily treated (and perhaps much more common) is *nonbacterial* prostatitis, Dr. Soloway says. It produces some of the same symptoms as its bacterial cousin, but what causes it remains a mystery. "Most men who have discomfort in the area of the prostate have a sort of nonspecific congestion, and it's unclear entirely what's going on," Dr. Soloway says.

A SEX RX?

Stephen N. Rous, M.D., author of *The Prostate Book,* suggests a very specific remedy for nonbacterial prostatitis: more sex. Because the prostate produces much of the fluid that comprises a man's ejaculate, any decrease in sexual frequency will allow semen to accumulate to potentially painful levels, Dr. Rous reasons.

Certainly there are plenty of men out there who will follow Dr. Rous's advice to the letter! But some doctors aren't convinced that a prostatitis Rx should be spelled s-e-x.

Some doctors suggest that the term *nonbacterial prostatitis* is incorrect—that the disorder might be caused by bacteria that medical tests can't yet detect. In fact, many doctors treat bacterial and nonbacterial prostatitis exactly the same—with antibiotics. "Many men with nonbacterial prostatitis will get well, but that may be independent of the antibiotics—they might have gotten well anyway," Dr. Soloway says.

THE CANCER TRAP

Are you ready for the bad news? Then here goes: If you live long enough, there is a good chance you'll get cancer of the prostate gland. Doctors estimate that perhaps 30 percent of American men 50 years and older may already have prostatic cancer. Among men who live into their nineties, that number may shoot to 80 percent. But don't panic! The statistics for prostate cancer may sound scary, but they really aren't as bad as they seem. Here's why.

Most of these cancers won't catch up with you. Many more men will die *with* prostate cancer than *from* it, says Dr. Rous. This is because prostate cancer usually grows very slowly.

But cancer of the prostate *can* be deadly. In fact, it's the third largest cause of cancer deaths in men, Dr. Soloway says. He advises all men over 40 to have yearly rectal examinations to screen for early signs of trouble. Catch prostate cancer in time, and you could save yourself from being a statistic.

TRIM THE RISK

Better yet, you may be able to prevent prostate cancer in the first place. One way to do this is at the dinner table.

Trim the fat. Researchers have found that men who skimp on high-fat foods such as eggs, meat and cheese may substantially reduce their risks for prostate cancer. In one study, researchers in Utah investigated the diets of 358 men with cancer of the prostate. Eating high-fat foods, the researchers concluded, "was the strongest risk factor" for developing prostate cancer.

Add some fiber to your diet. Some researchers believe that foods high in dietary fiber—for example, beans, dried fruit and whole-wheat breads—can further lower the prostate cancer risk. In one study, investigators examined the diets of thousands of men. Those who ate the most fiber had the lower risks for prostate cancer.

Stay active. According to a Harvard study, men who stay active all their lives may have only half the risk of prostate cancer compared with those who are inactive. In the study, researchers examined the exercise habits of 17,719 men. Among men over 70 years old who were highly active, the risk for getting prostate cancer was 53 percent of the risk of inactive men. Researchers suggest that exercise, by decreasing testosterone levels, may decrease the risk for prostate cancer as well.

There are many dietary and lifestyle factors—including exercise, losing weight and eating certain vegetables—that may help lower your risk for *all* cancers. For more tips on things to do—and things to avoid—see "Cancer" on page 78.

PSORIASIS

P soriasis sufferers, take heart—and not the proverbial heartbreak. While it's true that the disorder's behavior is capricious and unpredictable, you may not have to suffer this interminable, sometimes itchy, unsightly skin condition any longer. The frequency and severity of psoriasis flare-ups can be lessened, doctors tell us. First you have to learn to recognize and minimize the "triggering factors." And in the event of a flare-up, talk with your doctor about how you might benefit from one of the latest medical treatments.

While you may have to experiment a bit, "everybody can be helped, depending on how much time and effort they're willing to put into it," says Cynthia Guzzo, M.D., director of the University of Pennsylvania's Psoriasis Clinic in Philadelphia.

Psoriasis is skin growth gone awry. Normally, skin cells mature and shed in 28 to 30 days, making way for new cells. In psoriasis, new skin cells develop seven times faster than normal. Poorly developed, psoriatic skin cells can't shed fast enough to keep pace with the rapid growth. Instead, they pile up, forming raised, scaly plaques. The layers closest to the body surface appear red, because the affected area is inflamed. As the dead cells are pushed farther from the skin surface, they form silvery white scales over the plaques. Generally, these scaly, red telltale signs of psoriasis show up on the elbows, knees, scalp and lower back, but other parts of the body can be involved.

SNUFF OUT THE SPARK

Experts are still looking for the actual cause of psoriasis. They know it's not contagious and think there may be a genetic link. In one out of three cases, the disorder can be traced through the family, though it sometimes skips a generation.

But having the tendency simply sets the stage for a flare-up. People with the disorder can go through periods during which their skin looks normal. That's because psoriasis itself is like a bomb—something must trigger its fuse to set off an explosion. Unfortunately, that something could be just about anything. Experts have pinpointed some key triggers, among them the climate, damage to the skin (from dryness, a scratch, sunburn or chafing, for example) and a reaction to certain drugs and infections (such as strep throat). Recently, a clear link has been made between stress and psoriasis.

To prevent psoriasis attacks and minimize their severity, try to heed the following advice.

Moisturize. Skin that's prone to psoriasis tends to be dry. Lubricating is particularly important during the winter months, a time when psoriasis tends to flare up because of the dry, cold air.

Avoid bathing with perfumed and deodorant soaps, which can be drying. A 5- to 10-minute bath in comfortably warm water with a superfatted cleansing bar is your best bet. Just be sure to rinse well; soapsuds residue can be irritating and drying. Then while your skin is still damp, seal in the moisture with petrolatum, lanolin or any good over-the-counter moisturizer. Perfumed or tinted brands are okay if you're not allergic to them. (Psoriasis and skin allergies don't necessarily go hand in hand.) Running a humidifier, especially during drier weather, is also recommended.

Avoid prolonged sun exposure. Sunburn, like other skin irritations, can worsen a psoriasis outbreak. "Most people know their skin type and can tell how much they can get before they start to burn," says Christopher E. M. Griffiths, M.D., an assistant professor of dermatology at the University of Michigan Medical School, Ann Arbor. Still, he recommends you consult a dermatologist to determine a safe length of exposure and the appropriate sunscreen, which should be used all over.

Limit your alcohol intake. There appears to be something to the alcohol/psoriasis connection. In a recently published Finnish study, doctors noted a higher level of alcohol consumption among patients with severe psoriasis. Among a control group of 285 patients with other skin problems (such as dermatitis and acne), alcohol consumption was much lower. What's more, one in three of the psoriasis patients reported that drinking seemed to worsen their condition, whereas only one in nine of the controls reported such a connection with their skin problem.

Doctors aren't sure whether it's the alcohol or the stress (which leads some people to drink) that exacerbates psoriasis symptoms, or whether the worsening symptoms prompt many to turn to the bottle.

Other research suggests that alcohol increases the activity of a certain kind of white blood cell in psoriasis patients but not in people who don't have the disease. This increase was most evident in patients who said that drinking made their psoriasis worse. The researchers theorized a connection between the alcohol-induced activity of white blood cells and worsening of the patients' psoriasis.

Don't get irritated (literally). Psoriasis often flares up in areas traumatized by a scratch, bump or abrasion. While it's not always possible to protect your body from such assaults, you can avoid snug-fitting or elasticized clothing. Bra straps and tight waistbands rubbing on the skin are often culprits in a localized flare-up, Dr. Griffiths says.

Look after your overall physical state. "The skin is like any other organ of the body—it's going to be influenced by a good, balanced diet and adequate exercise," says David L. Cram, M.D., a clinical professor of dermatology at the University of California, San Francisco.

Beware of certain medications. A few drugs have been identified as occasionally causing psoriasis flare-ups. These include antimalarials; propranolol hydrochloride and other beta-blocker medications used to control high blood pressure; lithium; the heart medication quinidine gluconate; and topical (rub-on) steroids (when used for prolonged periods). Talk with your doctor or pharmacist if you suspect your medication may be getting under your skin.

THE MIND/BODY LINK

New research substantiates a connection between stress and psoriasis. "We've explained in the lab how factors produced by nerve fibers in the skin are linked to the earliest phases of inflammation," says George F. Murphy, M.D., a professor of dermatology and pathology at the University of Pennsylvania in Philadelphia who studies skin abnormalities. In a complicated process, nerves cause the inner lining of the blood vessels to stick to white blood cells, which normally travel freely throughout the body. The white blood cells then pass through the walls of the blood vessels into the tissue and cause inflammation. "If we accept this mind/body link, we can think about using stress management to attack the inflammation cascade of events very early, perhaps," Dr. Murphy says.

Stress management can be as simple as time management, says Iona Ginsburg, M.D., a New York City psychiatrist who counsels psoriasis patients. "It makes you feel more competent to handle your responsibilities, decreases your tension and allows you more time to take care of your skin. You have a sense of taking charge, so you feel more in control of this troublesome problem," she says.

John Koo, M.D., a dermatologist and psychiatrist at the Psoriasis Treatment Center, University of California, San Francisco, says many of his patients show more rapid and sustained improvement when they get psychological counseling to address personal problems that are causing them undue stress.

EXTINGUISHING FLARE-UPS

Despite all these precautions, you may still suffer an occasional flare-up. If you do, you'll need to see your physician. Left untended, psoriasis usually doesn't go away. But with appropriate treatment, psoriasis can go into remission for months, years, possibly even for the rest of your life.

What the doctor recommends depends on the extent of your psoriasis and your response to medications. "The treatment really has to be tailored to the individual patient," says Elizabeth Knobler, M.D., director of the psoriasis and phototherapy treatment center at New York City's Columbia Presbyterian Medical Center.

The preventive measures mentioned earlier are also useful in minimizing the severity of a flare-up, but it's likely that you'll need at least one of the following medications to extinguish the flame.

Steroid creams (also known as corticoids, cortisones or corticosteroids), applied daily to affected areas, can help reduce inflammation. They are generally recommended for short-term treatment. Prolonged use can actually damage the skin and exacerbate the condition.

Coal tar is an old-time remedy that reduces inflammation, itching and scaling. Now available in bath and shampoo formulas, as well as in ointments and creams, some of today's products don't have the objectionable color or smell of the original. Some are available over the counter, while others are prescription drugs. They're often used on patients who develop resistance to, or have side effects from, steroids.

PUVA can help. *P* refers to the medication psoralen, a light-sensitizing drug; *UVA* refers to ultraviolet light, a component of natural sunlight. While it's true that sunburn can worsen psoriasis, a controlled dose of ultraviolet light (administered in the doctor's office along with a pill containing psoralen) can actually have a healing effect. The therapy entails about three treatments a week, and exposure is gradually increased to avoid burning. Usually the skin returns to normal within 20 to 30 treatments. PUVA has proved to be very effective in at least 80 percent of the cases. But be aware that this treatment carries all the negative side effects associated with sun exposure—that is, premature skin aging as well as increased risk of skin cancer and cataracts.

A drug called anthralin comes in preparations for both the body and the scalp. Formerly, this treatment had to be administered in a hospital or doctor's office because of its potential to irritate normal skin and permanently stain anything it came in contact with. However, new formulations of the medication have been introduced that significantly reduce these hazards.

Etretinate (Tegison) is a vitamin A derivative, much like Accutane (which has been used to combat acne). The drug is taken orally once a day. Warning: Like its cousin Accutane, etretinate can cause birth defects; don't risk it if you are pregnant. It may also contribute to bone calluses and spurs, dry and fragile skin and high blood cholesterol, so doctors avoid long-term use.

TREATMENT BREAKTHROUGH

FROM GENE REPLACEMENT THERAPY TO VITAMINS

While there are many drugs to relieve the symptoms of psoriasis, there is no drug to cure this skin condition. Apart from the over-the-counter steroids and coal tars, there are powerful prescription drugs such as hydrea, etretinate and methotrexate, each of which can reduce the itching and scaling that characterize this crusty, contumacious skin disease. Unfortunately, none of them is entirely safe, says Alan Menter, M.D., of the Baylor University Medical Center. "Whether there ever will be a drug that's free of toxicity is debatable," he says.

Ideally psoriasis would be treated, even cured, without any drugs at all. Science fiction? Today, yes. But researchers already have "designed" laboratory rats that can serve as genetic models for people with the disease. The researchers hope eventually to identify, and then to repair, the genes that cause psoriasis. "When gene replacement therapy comes into its own, that will be a distinct possibility," Dr. Menter says.

Another promising future cure comes in the form of a vitamin. 1,25-dihdroxyvitamin D_3, which is normally produced in the kidney from a type of vitamin D, can now be made artificially in a laboratory. Used topically or orally, it appears to stop skin cells from growing wildly and to make them mature normally.

Michael F. Holick, Ph.D., M.D., director of the vitamin D laboratory and a professor of medicine at Boston University School of Medicine, says 90 percent of his patients showed a marked decrease in scales and a clearing up of inflammation within two to four weeks when they applied a topical form of 1,25-dihdroxyvitamin D_3 once a day. Sixty-five percent of the patients who took it orally once a day showed similar improvement in two to three months. Unlike current medications, 1,25-dihdroxyvitamin D_3 seems to have fewer side effects. None of the problems associated with the vitamin have turned up in the studies so far. However, psoriasis returns when the treatment is stopped. Standard vitamin D supplements are not effective, Dr. Holick adds, and can be dangerous if taken in high doses.

Methotrexate, taken orally once a week, is a powerful drug that doctors reserve for severe psoriasis cases that resist all other treatment. Primarily an anticancer agent, this drug, when used for psoriasis, is potentially toxic to the liver.

Unfortunately, none of these drugs is entirely safe.

To help control symptoms of psoriasis while minimizing the side effects of these medications, some doctors recommend combined treatment, says Alan Menter, M.D., medical director of the Psoriasis Center at Baylor University Medical Center in Dallas and chairman of the psoriasis subcommittee of the American Academy of Dermatology.

Such a combination of treatments might be to use ultraviolet light with either anthralin or tar; ultraviolet light with methotrexate; or PUVA with etretinate. In some cases, "people can be put in remission for eight months to a year, and sometimes longer," Dr. Menter says.

Of course, *remission* isn't synonymous with *cure,* and flare-ups invariably return. "It is rare that you have a specific drug that will cure a chronic disease," Dr. Menter says. "We can control them, but often we don't cure them."

FIGHTING BACK WITH FISH

Fish oil has shown some promise as an adjunct to current treatments (used alone, its effects are minimal). In a 12-week study at the Skin Research Foundation of California in Santa Monica, 24 psoriasis patients who were being treated with the experimental drug Acitretin were given six 1-gram capsules of fish oil as a daily supplement. All showed more improvement in their condition than a control group that was taking Acitretin alone. Also, the fish oil seems to counter one of the adverse effects of the drug by lowering the levels of certain fats in the blood that the medication tends to raise.

Nicholas J. Lowe, M.D., director of the foundation, says other studies have shown that fish oil enhances the effects of light therapy. The omega-3 acids found in the oil are known to reduce the levels of other acids in the body that cause inflammation, including inflammation associated with psoriasis.

Until more research is done, it wouldn't hurt simply to eat more fish high in omega-3's, such as herring, mackerel and salmon, says Dr. Lowe. It may help keep your skin scales to a minimum.

RABIES

You're following an old deer trail through the woods late one Sunday afternoon when, off to your left, behind a boulder, you catch a glimpse of something brown—an old raccoon, foraging through the bushes for his supper.

You'd like to reach out a hand and offer him some of the berries you've picked for a snack, but you hesitate, as all the headlines about wild animals carrying rabies flood your mind.

Could *this* raccoon have rabies?

ASSESSING THE RISK

Rabies, although rare among humans, is not so uncommon in the animal kingdom, says Makonen Fekadu, D.V.M., the top rabies specialist at the federal Centers for Disease Control (CDC) in Atlanta.

Not all species of wild animals—nor all animals in a species—carry the rabies virus, he adds. Those critters to look out for include, but are not limited to, raccoons along the East Coast, skunks in the north- and south-central states, dogs and coyotes along the border between Texas and Mexico, foxes in New York state and New England and bats throughout the United States.

Other animals—unless they attack you without provocation—should be judged innocent until proven guilty. Domesticated dogs are no longer a serious threat, since rabies vaccinations have virtually wiped out the disease in household pets. In 1990, only 148 dogs in the United States contracted rabies, and none transmitted it to humans. From 1980 to 1991, only 16 cases of human rabies were reported to the CDC, and only 7 of these are believed to have been acquired from animals within the United States.

A FRIGHTENING DISEASE

If so few cases of rabies are found in the United States each year, why does everyone seem to be so afraid of the virus?

Part of the answer may be that rabies is such a deadly disease once symptoms develop. The virus will kill anyone who has been infected unless they begin a series of five vaccinations before the symptoms appear, says Dr. Makonen. Around 30,000 of these postexposure vaccinations are given every year, and a testament to their effectiveness is the rarity of the disease in humans.

Rabies is usually transmitted through a bite or scratch. The virus stays in the area of the wound for several days or months while it multiplies. It's that characteristic that can save your life, explains Dr. Makonen. It gives you an opportunity to get the antirabies vaccinations from your doctor, and it gives the vaccine itself a chance to train your immune system to kill the virus before the virus can spread throughout your body.

Without the vaccination, the virus would eventually move into the nerves, using them as highways to the spinal column and finally to the brain. There are no overt symptoms as this occurs, although those affected by it might begin to feel as though they're getting a cold. Pain, cold, numbness, tingling or burning might also begin at the wound site.

When the virus actually reaches the brain, the possible symptoms include intermittent periods of anxiety, hyperactivity, hallucinations, convulsions and bizarre behaviors, such as biting or an overwhelming fear of water. After rabies symptoms develop, a person with rabies gradually becomes paralyzed and dies of respiratory failure within a few days.

SMART ACTION

There is no way to tell if an animal has rabies just by looking at it. A raccoon walking slowly up the trail is just about as likely to have rabies as the one that's snarling in the bushes. If you're bitten by any animal:

Immediately clean the wound thoroughly with soap and water. Since the rabies virus tends to hang around the wound site, says Dr. Makonen, washing it out with soap and water is the single most effective means of preventing rabies that you have. You should wash even before you seek medical help, he says.

Scratches that do not break the skin rarely cause rabies, and if you are bitten or scratched by a dog or cat that has an up-to-date rabies tag, you are most probably safe. But if there's no current tag, or if you are wounded by another kind of animal, give your local health department a call and find out if the type of animal that hurt you—skunk, raccoon, woodchuck, etc.—is carrying rabies in your area.

If it is, get yourself to a physician on the double to begin your vaccinations. In 1991, three people exposed to rabies decided they didn't need the vaccinations. All three are dead.

DISEASE
FREE

RAYNAUD'S PHENOMENON

Kay pulled on her long johns, flannel pants and heavy wool socks. She pulled on a sweater and insulated vest. She adjusted her ski cap and elbow-length gloves. Her preparations complete, she stepped forward, took a deep breath . . . and ran out to the curb to deposit the garbage can.

"Whew!" she exclaimed, quickly closing the front door behind her. "No problems at all—*this time.*"

THE COLD FACTS

Kay has good reason to fear the cold. She has Raynaud's phenomenon, a mysterious condition that causes the blood vessels in her extremities to clamp down whenever she's chilled: while running to the curb in the dead of winter, or even while picking up a cold soda. But Kay is fortunate that only her fingers are affected.

Raynaud's phenomenon can be caused by diseases—scleroderma, for example—that narrow blood vessels and thus impede blood flow. It can also be caused by constant trauma to the hand from activities like typing and piano playing or from the long-term use of vibrating tools such as chain saws. But in the majority of cases, doctors don't know what causes it, says Jay D. Coffman, M.D., author of *Raynaud's Phenomenon* and a professor of medicine and chief of vascular medicine at Boston University Hospital.

Here's what happens. When the temperature drops, it's normal for blood vessels in your fingers, toes, ears and nose to constrict. This is how your body conserves heat and protects the vital organs. But for people with Raynaud's, this process is greatly exaggerated. "Raynaud's originally was described as 'dead finger' because blood flow to the fingers essentially stops," Dr. Coffman says.

Attacks can last for minutes or hours and usually are accompanied by vivid color changes to the skin—from white to blue to red—as circulation stops and starts again.

Raynaud's rarely is a serious medical problem, and many people don't even discuss it with their doctors. But for others, interrupted blood flow can cause tissue damage, even gangrene. For this reason, anyone with Raynaud's should be under a doctor's care.

HOT TIPS

Although there is no known cure, Raynaud's can be controlled simply by staying warm, Dr. Coffman says. So when the mercury drops:

Bundle up. This is the easiest way to keep your blood vessels—all of them—wide open. It's not enough merely to keep your hands and feet warm, however. "If the back of your neck gets cold, blood vessels in your fingers will constrict to save body heat," says Dr. Coffman. "You have to keep the whole body warm."

Dressing in layers helps trap heat next to your body. So before heading into winter's cold, protect yourself, depending on the weather, by wearing a T-shirt under a shirt under a sweater under a jacket.

Get some lined gloves. Better yet, get lined mittens. These will keep your fingers warm whether you're outside in the snow or inside sipping a cold drink.

Keep your hat on. Hats are very important, because much of the body's heat is lost through the head, Dr. Coffman says. By preventing heat loss from your head, you'll help persuade blood vessels elsewhere in your body to stay open.

Plug yourself in. Sporting goods stores often sell battery-powered socks and a variety of hand warmers that will keep fingers and toes toasty warm, even in the coldest weather.

Insulate yourself. Since cold cans and drinking glasses can trigger attacks, you may want to spend a few dollars for a plastic or foam can holder or an insulating cup. These will keep your hands from getting chilled, even when the drink is icy cold.

Keep the water warm. When you're washing vegetables or salad greens, always let the water run warm before plunging your hands in.

If you smoke, stop. The nicotine in cigarettes can narrow blood vessels, which can further limit blood flow to your fingers and feet, says Dr. Coffman.

Mind your medicines. There are certain drugs—including beta-blockers and some migraine headache medications—that can make the symptoms worse, Dr. Coffman says. Tell your doctor if you're having problems. He may recommend a replacement drug that won't cause side effects.

Prescription relief. Your doctor may also recommend a drug called nifedipine (Adalat, Procardia). Commonly used to control high blood pressure, it's effective for controlling Raynaud's attacks as well. "I have patients who take nifedipine only when they go skiing, and the rest of the time, they do fine without it," says Dr. Coffman. Since nifedipine can cause headaches and other side effects, it's usually used for Raynaud's only when do-it-yourself techniques don't work.

MENTAL HEAT

Perhaps the best way to beat Raynaud's is with your mind, says Robert R. Freedman, Ph.D., a Raynaud's expert and professor of psychiatry at Wayne State University Medical School in Detroit. Studies have shown that people who learn biofeedback can, with their minds, direct warming blood to their fingers—regardless of the temperature outside.

In training sessions at Wayne State, volunteers with Raynaud's were asked to monitor their finger temperatures while listening to a tone. When their temperatures changed, so did the pitch of the tone. Within a few sessions, Dr. Freedman says, they learned to raise their finger temperatures at will. "In every study we've done, the success rate has been 80 percent or better," he says.

The benefits of biofeedback don't end with the ten-week training sessions. Follow-up studies show that some people remain symptom-free as long as three years later. "Virtually all of them say they don't even practice the biofeedback consciously—they just do it automatically," says Dr. Freedman.

To learn these techniques, ask your doctor for a referral to a certified biofeedback professional. If he doesn't know of one, contact the Association for Applied Psychophysiology and Biofeedback at 10200 West 44th Avenue, Suite 304, Wheat Ridge, CO 80033 (they request a self-addressed, stamped envelope).

Another "mind over matter" technique you can practice at home is called Pavlovian conditioning.

You've probably read about the Russian scientist Ivan Petrovich Pavlov, who once "trained" dogs to salivate when they heard a bell ring. Now researchers from the U.S. Army's Cold Research Division say that similar techniques can help people with Raynaud's. Here's how.

Wear the clothes you normally wear indoors. Get two bowls, each large enough to accommodate both hands at once. Fill each bowl with hot (120°F) water. Leave one indoors where it's warm and put the other outside in the cold.

Beginning indoors, immerse both hands in the water and let them soak for several minutes. Then wrap them in a towel (to preserve the heat), go outside, and immerse them in the second bowl for several minutes. By repeating this cycle three to six times a day for several weeks, you can "fool" your blood vessels into staying open, regardless of the temperature outside.

RESTLESS LEGS SYNDROME

They describe their legs as tingling . . . writhing with worms . . . crawling with ants. Or as one sufferer puts it, "a drives-you-nuts kind of thing." Something that gives your limbs an uncontrollable urge to get up and move while the rest of your body is begging for sleep.

Doctors agree that this condition, known as restless legs syndrome, causes some unusual, and extremely uncomfortable, sensations. In fact, it makes doctors uncomfortable, too. That's because they don't know what causes it. They aren't sure how to treat it. They even have trouble describing it.

Just ask Douglas K. Ousterhout, D.D.S., M.D., a plastic and reconstructive surgeon in San Francisco who has had restless legs syndrome since he was a teenager. "You really can't describe what it feels like," says Dr. Ousterhout. "Your legs ache. You want to get up and walk or get up on your toes and get your legs going up and down. That will help, but when you stop moving, it comes right back, of course." Sometimes it comes back for just a few minutes, he adds. Sometimes it lasts for hours.

MILD OR MADDENING

In a way, restless legs syndrome resembles an itch deep inside one or both legs. An itch that often begins in the evening when you're sitting or lying down. An itch that may be mildly annoying during the day but distressingly disturbing at night, when you're trying to sleep. The only solution is to "scratch" the itch, says Lawrence Z. Stern, M.D., professor of neurology at the University of Arizona Health Sciences Center and medical consultant for the Muscular Dystrophy Association. Most of the time, just getting your legs moving will help.

The severity of restless legs syndrome, and the frequency of attacks, varies widely, Dr. Stern says. Some people experience it every night— their legs can sometimes jerk or kick involuntarily. For others—and Dr. Ousterhout is one—it occurs occasionally. In most cases, "it's something people will complain about if their doctor asks them, but it's not the reason they actually go to the doctor," Dr. Stern says. For others, of course, just reading a book, watching a movie or sitting at the dinner table can be torture: They just *have* to walk around. In fact, some people stay up all night because their restless legs won't calm down.

TAKING OUT THE KICK

Eventually your restless legs may take you to the doctor's office for a checkup. When you go, here's what your doctor will probably find: nothing. This is because most people with restless legs have nothing *detectably* wrong. Oh, your doctor may test your blood and, if he's a neurologist, your nervous system. But most people with restless legs have nothing wrong with them that seems to account for their problem—nothing, that is, except an itch too deep to scratch.

Fortunately, there are some things you can do to calm your restless legs.

Hit the track. Regularly exercising your legs, whether by walking, running or doing in-place toe lifts, is probably the best way to ease your restless legs, Dr. Stern says. Dr. Ousterhout agrees. "When I was in high school, I used to go running at night," he remembers. "It was about all I could do that would make it feel better."

Knead your knee. Or whichever part of your leg is giving you grief. While rubbing your legs isn't a *cure* for restless legs, Dr. Stern says, some people say that it helps.

Take a jolt. Don't be alarmed if your doctor sends you home with a rented black box and instructions to plug yourself in. Some researchers believe that TENS treatments—*TENS* stands for transcutaneous electrical nerve stimulation—can significantly relieve the symptoms of restless legs. With TENS, electrodes are placed on the skin over the affected parts of your legs. Small amounts of electricity then are directed into the underlying muscles and nerves. Essentially, your legs become too distracted by the electricity to continue being restless.

A MYSTERY WITH CLUES

Although the cause of restless legs syndrome remains unknown, it is not a medical mystery without some clues, Dr. Stern says. Doctors do know, for example, that restless legs gets worse at night and with advancing age. Pregnant women are prone to it. So are people with kidney problems and rheumatoid arthritis. Restless legs syndrome has also been linked with iron deficiency, diabetes and Parkinson's disease. In fact, a common drug used to treat Parkinson's called levodopa (Sinemet) seems to work for restless legs. In one study, 26 people who took levodopa for two years said their symptoms were much relieved. Other prescription drugs such as clonazepam (Klonopin), carbamazepine (Tegretol), primidone (Mysoline) and bromocriptine (Parlodel) can help.

But many doctors believe the potential side effects of drug therapy may outweigh the benefits of treating this relatively harmless condition, Dr. Stern says. Unless your problem is really severe, your doctor will most likely want to try other therapies before prescribing any medications.

Until more is learned about this malady, it's important for people to know that their restless legs syndrome, while mysterious, isn't imaginary, says Dr. Stern. "I think people often are grateful to learn that restless legs is a recognized clinical entity and that they're not going crazy."

ROCKY MOUNTAIN SPOTTED FEVER

I f you're shooting off to the Rockies for some skiing this winter, don't let fear of Rocky Mountain spotted fever spoil your vacation.

First, the peak season for Rocky Mountain spotted fever is summer—not winter.

Second, even though the disease was first identified in the Rocky Mountain states, it's actually most common in Oklahoma, Tennessee and the Carolinas.

Third, no matter *which* state you are in, and no matter *what* the season, Rocky Mountain spotted fever is hardly anything to worry about. In order to be infected, you first have to get bitten by a tick—and not just any tick. The tick has to be one of three varieties capable of carrying the disease. In addition, your personal tick has to be infected with *Rickettsia rickettsii,* the bacteria that cause Rocky Mountain spotted fever. *And* the tick usually has to hang on to your skin for quite some time before passing on the bacteria. The chances of all of the above happening to you are, well, quite slim. According to government statistics, fewer than 700 Americans a year get the disease.

While this disease is nothing to stay awake worrying about, it's nothing to laugh at either. Rocky Mountain spotted fever can be a nasty disease, starting with flulike symptoms and progressing to delirium, pneumonia and, in some cases, even worse fates. It is treatable, but without treatment, one person in five can die, says John Krebs, a public health scientist with the federal Centers for Disease Control in Atlanta.

STAYING TICK-FREE

The best way to prevent Rocky Mountain spotted fever (as well as other tick-borne illnesses, such as Lyme disease) is to stop ticks from having dinner on you. Experts recommend the following.

Sport the buttoned-down look. Whenever heading into wooded or grassy areas in the summer or spring, don long pants, preferably tucked into high socks, and a long-sleeved shirt to keep the creepy-crawlers away from your (to them) appetizing skin. It also helps to wear light-colored clothing. This makes ticks—which look something like small watermelon seeds—easier to spot and remove before they grab hold.

Remove attached ticks—quickly. A feeding tick is disease waiting to happen. The longer it feeds, the greater the chances it will pass something on to you. "Transmission is unlikely if you remove the tick within 24 hours," says William A. Petri, Jr., M.D., Ph.D., an assistant professor of internal medicine and microbiology at the University of Virginia in Charlottesville.

"The best way to remove a tick is simply to grasp it near the head, preferably with tweezers, and slowly extract it," says Krebs. Try not to crush the tick, since that can spread harmful bacteria. After you've removed the tick, wash the area of the bite with plenty of soap and water. Incidentally, forget about using gasoline, petroleum jelly or other "simple" techniques for removing ticks, says Krebs.

Be repellent. When venturing into a wooded or grassy area on a summer day, particularly in an area known to harbor disease-carrying ticks, apply insect repellents containing DEET to your arms, legs and head. For added protection, you can spray your clothes with repellents containing the chemical permethrin.

Shield your pets. Sure, Fido loves picnics. Unfortunately, ticks love Fido. It is possible for dogs to get Rocky Mountain spotted fever, says Krebs. They may also bring disease-carrying ticks home, where they can hop on you. Protect *all* the members of your family by buckling your pets into tick-and-flea collars before allowing them to frolic in high-risk areas. While some of these collars are quite effective, they are no guarantee that your pets will arrive home tick-free. It's best to also give them a good inspection as they enter the door.

POSTBITE ACTION

Should you get infected, it's essential to get to the doctor as soon as you can. How do you know you've been infected? The first symptoms of Rocky Mountain spotted fever are headache, fever and muscle pain, which usually hit about a week or so after the tick passed you the germ, says Dr. Petri. "People will say it's the worst headache they've ever had, and they'll have muscle aches just about everywhere."

A rash usually appears three to four days after the first flulike symptoms appear. It typically begins on the ankles and wrists, then spreads to the trunk, the palms of the hands and the soles of the feet. Without prompt treatment at that point, the disease can then cause delirium, pneumonia, low blood pressure and vasculitis, an inflammation of the inside of blood vessels that can "affect every organ in your body," Dr. Petri says.

While the rash usually appears early, one person in ten won't get it until the disease is well advanced, and another one in ten won't get it at all. Don't wait for the rash before getting help, Dr. Petri advises. If you're sick and even *suspect* Rocky Mountain spotted fever, you must see a doctor. He'll give you tetracycline, doxycycline or other antibiotics, which should knock out the infection within days.

SEXUALLY TRANSMITTED DISEASES

So you think a sexually transmitted disease could never happen to you? That's what nearly everyone thinks, including the millions of Americans who come down with chlamydia, herpes, gonorrhea, trichomoniasis, genital warts or syphilis every year.

Sexually transmitted diseases (STDs) know no boundaries—if you have sex with another person, you can get infected, no matter what your age, gender, race or income bracket. Some of the diseases can be cured, others, merely controlled. The good news is that STDs are totally preventable. It all depends on you—and your partner.

TRANSMISSION PROHIBITION

Guarding against STDs is in some ways easier than guarding against other diseases—at least you know where you might catch it. But effective prevention doesn't mean you have to join a convent. Instead, consider following this good advice from medical experts.

Stick with one person. A long-term, monogamous sexual relationship with a healthy partner who is also monogamous is the best way to avoid an STD, says Lisa Hirsch, M.D., assistant professor of obstetrics and gynecology and director of outpatient OBGYN services at the University of California, Irvine, Medical Center. "The more sexual partners you have, the more likely it is you'll get infected." Know your partner. It's risky to have sex with someone you've just met or who you won't be able to locate later.

Get examined. "If you're planning to enter a sexual relationship, go see a doctor first and get tested for STDs," advises Beverly A. Sansone, M.D., also an assistant clinical professor of obstetrics and gynecology at University of California, Irvine, Medical Center and medical director of

Planned Parenthood of Orange and San Bernardino counties. "Of course, your partner also has to be examined," she adds.

Avoid misplaced trust. You can ask a prospective partner about his or her sexual history—but don't always expect to get a factual answer, Dr. Hirsch warns. "People are sometimes dishonest in relationships," she says, "or they may have a silent infection like chlamydia, warts or genital herpes and not even know it." You must still take precautions of your own.

THE ABCs OF STDs

Here is a brief guide to some all-too-common sexually transmitted diseases (STDs).

CHLAMYDIA. This low-profile disease doesn't get the publicity it deserves. With about four million victims a year, it is America's most widespread STD. Men often experience painful urination; women may have yellow discharge (or no symptoms at all). It's easily curable with antibiotics.

GONORRHEA. It affects one million Americans a year, and the number is rising. Early signs of infection may be discharge and burning during urination. New strains of the bacteria have become resistant to antibiotics, but the disease is still curable with aggressive medical treatment.

HERPES. There's no cure, but it can be controlled. The herpes virus has already infected approximately 20 million people in the United States. Early symptoms include burning or pain when urinating, pain in the buttocks, legs or genital area and vaginal discharge.

SYPHILIS. An early sign of syphilis is a painless sore in the genital area. Affecting about 74,000 Americans a year, this ancient disease is highly curable with penicillin, tetracycline or doxycycline antibiotics.

GENITAL WARTS. The virus that causes genital warts takes up residence in the private parts of three million Americans a year. You can't cure warts, but you can control them. Your immune system and eliminating stress will do part of the controlling. Medications and laser surgery are often needed to do the rest. Warning: Some types of genital warts may turn into cancer, so *all* should be seen by a doctor.

TRICHOMONIASIS. This parasite is not an equal opportunity attacker. Usually only women suffer its symptoms. Early signs may include discomfort, irritation and discharge from the vagina; in men, painful and frequent urination. It is curable with the antiparasitic medication metronidazole.

Erect the barricades. Latex condoms treated with the spermicide nonoxynol-9 are highly effective in reducing your risk of getting an STD, Dr. Hirsch says. "You have to accept the idea that you *must* use them, all the time, from the very beginning of lovemaking, not just when you're about to have an orgasm," she says. Always use latex condoms; natural-skin condoms are porous, and STD germs pass right through them. You're clear to do away with condoms only after both you and your partner have been found free of any STD and are in a monogamous relationship.

Have an eagle eye. Definitely avoid sex with anyone who has genital sores, a rash, a discharge or any other possible sign of venereal disease. "Develop a high index of suspicion," Dr. Hirsch advises.

Remember that you're not immune. Having had an STD once doesn't mean you're immune to getting the same disease again. You *can* get reinfected, all too easily.

Protect your youngster. "I am appalled at the lack of sex education in schools and our society," says Dr. Hirsch. "The majority of people I see are teenagers, and they're really impressed when I explain to them how they can get chlamydia, gonorrhea, herpes or genital warts. It's like they're hearing it for the first time." If you're a parent concerned about your child's future, realize that there's no substitute for informed parent/child discussions about sexuality, she says.

Just say no. Sex education doesn't mean teaching kids how to have sex, says Dr. Sansone. "In our society, it almost seems expected of 15-year-olds that they should have sex. But they can say no—and they should be encouraged to do so," she says. It's a fact that the earlier a person starts having sex, the more likely it is he or she will contract an STD. It's not the youthful age that causes the disease but the ignorance and lack of education that leads them into unsafe sex, says Dr. Sansone.

IF YOU'RE INFECTED

It happens all the time, and it doesn't mean the end of the world. Not if you know how to handle an STD. The first thing you should know are the most common signs of an STD infection: a sore, blister or rash in the genital area, unusual discharge or irregular menstrual bleeding or spotting. Unexplained flulike symptoms or abdominal pain can also be signs of an infection.

Signs or not, if you think you may have been infected, see a doctor and get tested. Diagnosing some STDs—especially chlamydia and genital warts—can be tricky. "If you are sexually active, it's important to get tested at least every year or more often, depending on your sexual practices," says Dr. Hirsch. Testing may be done by your family doctor, a gynecologist or a state public health clinic.

BE A GOOD PATIENT

You can help the doctor beat your STD infection by following these few measures.

Take all your medication. Antibiotics make you feel better so fast that you might think you don't have to take the full one- or two-week course. *Wrong!* Take all the pills as prescribed, Dr. Sansone says. Otherwise, the infection can return, hardened by the brief skirmish.

Abstain. If you've been infected, don't have sex until you're cured or, if you have herpes or warts, until you're treated and the symptoms disappear.

Use condoms. You can still have sex even if you have herpes or warts—once they're under control—if you use a latex condom. Condoms are the most effective measure for blocking the transmission of these viruses.

TREATMENT BREAKTHROUGH

DRUGS FOR PREVENTION AND CURE

The herpes virus is a clever little bug. It hides out in nerve cells instead of coming out into open space, where the immune system can attack it. It also replicates itself faster than the immune system can stop it. All this makes it difficult to eradicate, yet progress is being made. Researchers are doubtful they'll find a vaccine to cure it, but they expect to find one to prevent its spread in the near future. There are at least seven herpes vaccines in animal or human trials.

On the trichomoniasis front, researchers have found that the mineral iron may promote infection by the parasite along the wall of the vagina, says John Alderete, Ph.D., professor of microbiology at the University of Texas Health Science Center at San Antonio.

Dr. Alderete's lab is involved in a ten-year effort to learn more about the *Trichomonas* parasite and to save women from suffering (men can carry the disease but rarely have symptoms). The iron discovery may lead to new medications, he says. Metronidazole, the current medication used to fight the disease, can cause birth defects, so it is not usually recommended for pregnant women. Doctors also fear that long-term use of the drug may cause cancer.

Working at the genetic level, Dr. Alderete and coresearcher Mike Lehker, Ph.D., hope to find out how iron works in *Trichomonas* and then to devise a safe drug that would come between iron and the parasite, depriving the bug of the glue it needs to hold on in the vagina.

SHINGLES

Varicella zoster, the star virus in childhood chicken pox, sometimes returns years later for an encore performance. After giving you that common childhood disease, it is thought to exit to nerve cells near the brain and spinal cord, where it waits for its cue to reappear. Act II of varicella zoster is quite different from Act I. It's called shingles, and there's little way of knowing when the curtain will rise.

"Up to one million people a year get their first attack of shingles," says Michael Rowbotham, M.D., assistant professor of neurology and anesthesia and associate director of the Pain Management Center at the University of California, San Francisco. "If you've had chicken pox—and you could have had it without knowing it—you have a 40 percent chance of getting shingles at some point in your life." Why some people get it and others don't remains a mystery, although those with an impaired immune system seem to be the best candidates.

ATTACK ON THE NERVES

Herpes zoster, as varicella zoster is called upon its return, circulates along nerve pathways. The virus begins by destroying the nerve cell where it's lain dormant for decades. Then it migrates down the sensory nerves, which carry the sensations of touch and pain, and out to the skin. There will be deep pain in the area under attack—nearly always only one side of the torso, occasionally a leg or arm, sometimes the face or eyes. The pain is often accompanied by fever and fatigue. In a few days, the virus erupts on the skin's surface in blisters.

"The fluid in these blisters is full of live virus, which makes this stage of shingles highly contagious to people who haven't had chicken pox," Dr. Rowbotham says. "After ten days to two weeks, the blisters dry up and scab over and are no longer contagious. If you're an adult who hasn't had chicken pox, you should stay away from someone who has the blisters, because adult chicken pox can be very serious."

For almost 90 percent of the people who get shingles, the battle ends with the healing of the blisters. But those over 50 years old have up to a 50–50 chance of getting postherpetic neuralgia (PHN), a painful condition that can drag on for months or even years.

Those with PHN experience a feeling of numbness where the blisters have healed, yet at the same time, the areas are supersensitive to light touch. This can cause bouts of extreme pain and itching. Oddly, a heavy touch may trigger only numbness. Pain, itching and numbness all are caused by nerve damage, Dr. Rowbotham says.

OUSTER OF THE ZOSTER

There is nothing that can rid the body of the herpes zoster virus, but the antiviral prescription drug acyclovir can help your immune system control it. By far the most popular and effective medical treatment for shingles, acyclovir is inexpensive, readily available and can be taken orally, topically or intravenously, says Dr. Rowbotham. The point of taking acyclovir, he says, is to lessen the severity of the shingles attack. It may also reduce the chance of developing PHN.

Aside from seeing your doctor for medication, there are a few things you can do to help yourself when you have a shingles outbreak.

Treat the sores. Calamine lotion, cool compresses, cornstarch or baking soda plasters can hasten the drying of the sores and give relief from pain and itching. Avoid ointments, which can slow the drying time, and corticosteroid creams, which may suppress the immune system's ability to fight the virus.

Avoid scratching the itch. Scratching can only delay healing and can also spread the virus, says Dr. Rowbotham.

Take a painkiller. Aspirin, acetaminophen or ibuprofen can help reduce the pain from the sores. Take as needed, says Dr. Rowbotham.

Get plenty of rest. Remember, you have an infection, and your body needs rest to recover.

Reach for the Zostrix. If pain persists after the blisters have healed, pick up a tube of nonprescription Zostrix at your drugstore. Made from capsaicin, the stuff that makes hot peppers hot, Zostrix may calm your discomfort.

RELIEVING THE PAIN OF PHN

If you get PHN, you may find it's the most intense pain you've ever had. "But rest assured that PHN tends to get better with time," Dr. Rowbotham says. In the meantime, there are several roads to relief. Some your doctor can prescribe, perhaps starting with an antidepressant.

No, antidepressants are not only for depression. Tricyclic antidepressants—such as amitriptyline, imipramine and nortriptyline—have formidable pain-relieving powers. "They clearly work by enhancing the power of the brain to modulate pain," Dr. Rowbotham says.

Your doctor may also suggest transcutaneous electrical nerve stimulation (TENS). A TENS device, which you can carry around with you, applies a mild electric charge to the skin. The charge interferes with the nerve's transmission of pain. "It can definitely help some people, and it's covered by Medicare," says Dr. Rowbotham.

Here are several other roads to relief you can travel on your own.

Cool the pain. Ice packs numb the nerve endings, preventing them from sending pain signals to the brain, says Dr. Rowbotham. He suggests applying an ice pack to painful areas of your skin for up to 30 minutes at a time, as needed.

Vibrate the pain away. An electric hand massager held against the painful areas may work the same way as TENS and ice—interfering with pain signals, Dr. Rowbotham says.

Exercise. "It's important to stay active," says Dr. Rowbotham. "Staying home in bed won't make PHN go away any faster, and it can make fatigue and depression worse. Regular exercise can help you cope with the pain."

Maintain your positive mental attitude. "Don't blame yourself for getting shingles or PHN," says Dr. Rowbotham. "You didn't do anything wrong. It can strike anybody. It has nothing to do with personality or karma." Instead of wallowing in misery, put the pain on the back burner and focus on the positive aspects of your life—friends, families, activities, work, exercise.

SINUSITIS

Have you ever told a forgetful friend that he has holes in his head? You were only teasing, of course, but you weren't entirely wrong. The truth is, we all have holes in our heads. They're called sinuses, and they're simply empty spaces—one above each eye, one below and two on each side of the nose. The sinuses are lined with membranes that produce mucus.

Mucus is the stuff that prevents your breathing apparatus from getting dry and irritated and that helps to filter dust particles from the air you breathe. When all is well, mucus flows in and out of your sinuses freely.

When you have a head cold, however, or when your nose is all stopped up with allergies, problems may arise. "These conditions can cause an obstruction, blocking off the openings to the sinuses," explains Raymond G. Slavin, M.D., professor of internal medicine and director of the Division of Allergy and Immunology at St. Louis University School of Medicine. Bacteria that normally are harmless may then set up camp in the stagnant mucus. The resulting infection can cause fever, headaches, facial pain and foul-tasting mucus that slides down the back of your throat. Instead of getting better after three or four days, as you would with a simple cold, you feel worse. That's sinusitis.

"It's an incredibly common disease, affecting close to 32 million Americans a year," Dr. Slavin says. Fortunately, it's rarely serious. Better yet, it can often be prevented. Here's how.

SAVE YOUR SINUSES

To prevent sinusitis, you must keep your sinuses open, Dr. Slavin says. To do that, you need to battle congestion. So the next time a cold or allergies have you stuffed up, go on the offensive.

Get steamed. "Steam inhalations are very, very helpful," Dr. Slavin says. Moist heat helps by making the mucus more watery, which helps it drain from the sinuses. One way to work up a good head of steam is to settle in for a long, hot shower or bath. Competition for the bathroom, however, can make this remedy difficult to implement. As an alternative, you might apply a warm washcloth to the nasal area, Dr. Slavin says.

Drink to your condition. Drinking lots of fluids—at least one glass every few hours—helps your body to thin the mucus, says Dr. Slavin. The thinner the mucus, the less likely it is to block up your sinuses. Hot fluids such as chicken soup are even better. The hot, soothing steam helps make the mucus extra watery, which helps it to drain.

If you smoke, stop. Cigarettes dry the delicate mucous membranes inside the nasal passages. This is one reason smokers get more colds and flus than nonsmokers. This, in turn, makes smokers more prone to sinusitis. It's a good idea to stay away from other people's cigarettes, too.

Condition the air. Air conditioners, during allergy season, may help prevent sinusitis by keeping irritating pollen outside. Humidifiers and vaporizers, by adding moisture to the air—and moisture to your nose—can also help by keeping the mucus draining. Both air-conditioning filters and humidifiers must be cleaned scrupulously to avoid the accumulation of mold, Dr. Slavin says.

Visit your pharmacy. "We encourage people who are all clogged up to use a decongestant for a couple of days," says Dr. Slavin. By shrinking swollen nasal tissues and helping sinuses drain, over-the-counter decongestants—sprays or pills—may help keep your plugged-up sinuses clear of infection.

However, Dr. Slavin adds, you shouldn't use decongestant nasal sprays for more than a few days without consulting your doctor. With long-term use, they can irritate the delicate linings in the nose. And when you stop using them, they can cause "rebound" congestion that can be worse than the original problem.

Sniff some saline spray. These over-the-counter nasal sprays, used several times a day, can help clear mucus from your nasal passages, making it easier for your sinuses to drain. At the same time, the salty solution can decrease blood flow to the nose, which helps prevent further congestion. Unlike the decongestant sprays, saline sprays may be used as long as you like.

Don't be a blowhard. Too-powerful nose blowing can actually force bacteria-laden mucus backward from the nasal passages into the sinuses. When you blow, blow gently, Dr. Slavin advises.

Feast on fire. If you've ever dipped a corn chip into a wicked hot sauce, you know that spicy foods can really open your nasal faucets. This is because many spicy foods contain chemicals—capsaicin, for example—that stimulate nerves in the mouth and throat. This in turn triggers a runny nose. So the next time your nose is blocked up, unplug it with your favorite culinary combustibles.

Keep that dental appointment. Bacteria will occasionally migrate from nearby teeth into the sinuses, causing infection there. By keeping your teeth in tip-top shape, you can help prevent dental abscesses *and* the risk of sinusitis.

Keep yourself grounded. Activities such as flying, skydiving and scuba diving cause pressure changes inside your head. Not only can these changes make the mucus slow to drain, they also can make your sinuses feel stuffy. Play it safe and stay on terra firma until your head clears.

Watch (and wash) your hands. Since sinusitis typically follows colds and allergies, you can beat it simply by staying healthy. Since cold-causing viruses often are spread by human hands, keeping your hands clean and away from your nose and mouth can help keep your sinuses clear.

BEATING INFECTION

In many cases, sinusitis disappears on its own, especially if you take good care of yourself. (All of the above tips for sinusitis prevention will also help to treat it.) But sometimes, despite even the best care, sinusitis can linger—for weeks, months, even years. If, after a few weeks, your head still feels like it's stuffed with wet paper towels, then it's time to see your doctor, Dr. Slavin says. And don't worry: Sinusitis is easily treated, most often with antibiotics such as ampicillin and amoxicillin. You should be feeling better in just a few days.

But don't let your sudden good health fool you into thinking you're cured, Dr. Slavin adds. You're not out of the woods yet. After all, there may still be bacteria kicking around in your sinuses. If you stop taking the pills before you're supposed to, you'll be giving these resistant bacteria the opportunity to rally and fight back. If they succeed, you'll get sick all over again. No matter how good you feel, you *must* take the entire prescription, Dr. Slavin says.

While you're taking antibiotics, your doctor may want you to take decongestant pills or sprays at the same time. "We also sometimes prescribe a cortisone nasal spray, which can help reduce inflammation," Dr. Slavin says.

A combination of drugs will usually clear up the worst symptoms. In rare cases, however, your doctor may recommend minor surgery to drain accumulated mucus from the sinuses and to remove infected tissue. Your doctor can do this surgery a number of ways. In most cases, it can be performed through the nostrils with an instrument called a nasal endoscope. It's generally an office procedure done under local anesthesia.

SLEEP DISORDERS

I n our busy lives, what is kinder, more gentle, than sleep? Every night, sleep slips over the horizon to bring restful ease. It is, says Shakespeare, "the death of each day's life . . . balm of hurt minds . . . chief nourisher in life's feast." Obviously, the Bard loved his sleep. But what about people with insomnia, sleep apnea or narcolepsy? For them, sleep is often more stressful than serene, and "life's feast" offers up poor fare indeed.

SLEEP APNEA

The problem wasn't his snoring, says Carl Lander, Jr., of West Newton, Pennsylvania, although he admits his wife had to cover her one good ear before she could sleep. The real problem was *not* snoring: When Carl wasn't snoring, he wasn't breathing. When he wasn't breathing, his oxygen-starved body had to wake him—hundreds of times a night—just to get a gulp of air. Consequently, Carl was always tired in the morning. In fact, he could barely prop open his eyes.

Carl was no more aware of his nightly suffocations than he was of his thunderous, wall-shaking snores. But when he spent the night at a sleep laboratory in 1985, he learned that his chronic exhaustion was caused by a nighttime breathing disorder called sleep-apnea syndrome. "When they tested me in the laboratory, I got about 1 minute of restful sleep in a 7-hour night," he recalls. "Basically, I just wasn't breathing."

RESTLESS NIGHTS, TIRED DAYS

Sleep apneas—the word *apnea* is derived from a Greek word meaning "want of breath"—can last anywhere from 10 seconds to more than 1 minute, says Quentin Regestein, M.D., director of the Sleep Clinic at Boston's Brigham and Women's Hospital. Virtually everyone will have occasional sleep apneas, he says. That's not a problem. It is a problem, as Carl can attest, when they start wrecking your life.

"I used to do sales," says Carl, chairman of the Pittsburgh chapter of AWAKE, a support group for people with sleep-apnea syndrome. "Because I wasn't getting any sleep at night, I was dead tired during the day. Often I fell asleep while I was making my pitch. I fell asleep during a funeral service. I even fell asleep while I was driving—I had at least four car accidents."

But daytime fatigue is only part of the problem, Dr. Regestein says. "When you stop breathing, your heart has to work harder to get oxygen into your blood, and that can cause blood pressure to rise," he explains. "Among people with high blood pressure, about 30 percent have significant sleep apnea; among people with coronary artery disease, it's 10 to 15 percent."

Obviously you can't force yourself to breathe while you're asleep. But there are some things you can do while you're awake.

SAVE YOUR SLEEP

For many people—especially for those with obvious breathing or heart problems—drugs, surgery or special machines may be the only long-term remedy for sleep-apnea syndrome. But if you don't have these problems, says Dr. Regestein, these self-help remedies may be enough to ensure a good night's sleep.

Take off the pounds. Even though thin people sometimes have sleep-apnea syndrome, the majority of sufferers are overweight, Dr. Regestein says. Often they're *very* overweight. The bigger your belly, he explains, the more gravity can work against you. "Your diaphragm becomes broad, flat and less efficient but still has to push against all that weight, and sometimes it just gets plain tired," Dr. Regestein says. Doctors say that a 10 to 15 percent weight loss can result in a *50 percent* reduction in sleep apneas. "It's been shown that sleep apnea can sometimes be remedied entirely by weight loss," says Dr. Regestein.

Beware of B and B. That's booze and barbiturates. You know how relaxed you feel when you take a tranquilizer? Well, your diaphragm gets relaxed, too. In fact, it can get downright lazy, too lazy to breathe, Dr. Regestein says. Your upper airways also relax and fail to widen in your throat when you inhale, and that can cause problems. "You can get an airway obstruction, because the tissue there becomes flabby," he says.

Like sleeping pills, alcohol depresses the central nervous system, Dr. Regestein adds, and people who heft a glass of beer at bedtime will often snore more loudly (and have more apneas) than those who abstain.

JUST A HARMLESS NIGHTTIME STROLL

Joey's parents smiled when he started sliding down the banister. They thought it was funny when he emptied the silverware drawer onto the kitchen floor. They laughed hysterically when he started putting his dad's slippers into the freezer. Then Joey took to urinating in the hallway closet. His parents quit laughing and took him to the doctor. "Relax," said Joey's doctor when they met. "He's not sick—he's just asleep."

For ten-year-old Joey, as for many of his chums, occasional nocturnal perambulations are all in a night's work. In fact, doctors estimate that up to 5 percent of healthy children regularly walk in their sleep, and as many as 30 percent do so at least once in their lives. Even adults will walk in their sleep, although not as often as children, says Quentin Regestein, M.D., director of the Sleep Clinic at Boston's Brigham and Women's Hospital.

"There are a lot of sleepwalkers out there who don't consider it a problem," Dr. Regestein says. "They think it's humorous, a little bit of a joke. Then there are the sleepwalkers who get in their car and start it, or who wander out the door and onto the sidewalk. That's a lot more serious."

Although it's not unheard of for sleepwalkers to mistake second-floor windows for doors, most sleepwalking episodes are harmless, Dr. Regestein says. Sleepers get out of bed, wander around for a few minutes and then return to bed. Some, like Joey, do some odd things, which they rarely remember the following day.

Doctors don't know why people sleepwalk. It seems to run in families, and it occurs less frequently as people age. And folklore to the contrary, it's okay to wake a sleepwalker, Dr. Regestein says. On the other hand, he questions why anybody would *want* to wake them. If your child is sleepwalking, just stay nearby so he won't hurt himself—or mistake a closet for the bathroom.

In those rare cases when sleepwalking is dangerous—for example, when someone is taking to the streets—doctors may prescribe drugs that can help. But most children outgrow it, Dr. Regestein says, and adults simply get used to it. Still, a few precautions are in order. It's a good idea to guard against dangers of falling down stairs or off a balcony. "One guy rigged an electric eye to his doorway that would trigger an alarm if he went out. Some people tie one end of a loose cord to their ankle and the other end to the bed. But it doesn't always help," he adds. "They just start dragging the bed."

Get off your back. If you have sleep apnea, that's the worst position to sleep in. Once again, the culprit is gravity, Dr. Regestein says. Sleeping on your side or your stomach will help you breathe by preventing your tongue from falling back into your throat. To make sure you *stay* off your back, pin a sock with a tennis ball inside to the back of your pajamas, he suggests. When you try to roll over in your sleep—Bump!—the ball will wake you up.

Wear a mask. A relatively new technique called continuous positive airway pressure has revolutionized the treatment of sleep apnea, Dr. Regestein says. While people sleep, a machine pumps air into a face mask they don before going to bed. The increased air pressure "works wonderfully to prevent apneas," he says.

Since Carl started using his machine in 1985, the apnea, snoring and daytime fatigue have virtually disappeared, he says. Sure, the mask wasn't easy to get used to, but compared with the symptoms of apnea, it doesn't bother him at all. "You know, my wife's family always said about me 'Carl? He just sleeps.' But the first Thanksgiving we spent together *after* I had the machine, her uncle said, 'Gee, he really talks!' "

INSOMNIA

Ah, rest! You shut off the light, burrow under the sheets and say good-bye to an exhausting day. You've never been this tired—but your mind is raring to go. "Hey, it's only midnight!" whines your irrepressible brain. "We have *all night* to worry! Speaking of which . . . can you believe what that worm said about your report? . . . Say, it's already 2:14 in the morning! Are you *sure* that clock's working? By the way, you were mighty mean to your poor old hubby. After all, not *every* woman gets a new broom for her anniversary. . . . Look, it's already 3:23, so what do you say we quit this sleep business and have a little snack instead?"

ELUSIVE SLEEP

If this scenario sounds familiar, well, you have plenty of tired company. In fact, insomnia is the most common of all the sleep disorders, and doctors estimate that one-third of the population, every year, spends at least a few nights watching the hands s-l-o-w-l-y turn.

"One way or another, you're going to get the sleep you absolutely need," says psychologist Joyce Walsleben, Ph.D., director of the Sleep Disorders Center at New York University Bellevue Medical Centers. "If you don't sleep at night, your brain will try to sleep during the day, and that can make you miserable."

It can also make you dangerous. Doctors agree that sleep-deprived people—about 17 percent of all adults say they have "serious" insomnia—are far more likely to suffer work injuries and car accidents than their better-rested neighbors.

Just about everyone has an occasional sleepless night—particularly, Dr. Walsleben says, when life's proverbial bucket gets kicked over—when you change jobs, for example, or your husband hands you an anniversary broom for the third year in a row. Once the stress disappears, you'll rest easily once again. But if your insomnia isn't gone in a week or two, Dr. Walsleben says, then it's lasted too long.

IT CAN DRAG ON FOR YEARS

In some cases, people have insomnia for months, years or even decades, Dr. Walsleben says. "I've talked to people who say they haven't slept for the past 14 years," she says. "My first question is 'How did you sleep 15 years ago?' Something must have happened back then that made them stop sleeping." One woman, she remembers, hadn't slept well for 6

PROFILE IN HEALING

NISS RYAN: STAYING AWAKE

When Niss Ryan was a chemistry major at Iowa State University in the 1940s, she could barely keep her eyes open. Among college students, of course, the occasional classroom snooze nearly is *de rigueur,* but Niss was different: She *always* slept.

"I had no idea what was the matter," says Niss, now 67 years old and vice president of Narcolepsy Network, a national support and information service. "I just couldn't stay awake." Not only did Niss sleep her way through classes, she also once slept through a lecture on pottery that she herself was teaching. She was on her feet at the time. "All of sudden I heard people laughing," Niss remembers. "That woke me up, and I realized that I had been talking about my dream."

As with most narcoleptics, Niss also suffers from hallucinations—terrible images that somehow creep from her dreams into her waking mind. "I often thought I heard people trying to break into the house," Niss says. "One time, somebody walked right through the yard and startled me, but I don't think anyone *really* walked through the yard. There are times when you really don't know what is real."

Niss didn't learn what was wrong with her until her first husband, a doctor, made the diagnosis. The stimulants he prescribed helped

---

years. Upon questioning her, Dr. Walsleben discovered that her grown children left home at about the same time she started losing sleep. Subconsciously, she still was waiting for her kids to get home at night, Dr. Walsleben explains.

Of course, the more you worry about getting a good night's sleep, the less likely you are to actually get it, says Timothy Roehrs, Ph.D., director of research at the Sleep Disorders Center at Henry Ford Hospital in Detroit. For example, someone who hasn't slept for four nights will be sweating the fifth night, too—and the *fear* of insomnia virtually guarantees a sleepless night. "Some people can fall asleep while they're sitting in a chair and watching the evening news, but as soon as it's time to go to bed, they begin to worry," Dr. Roehrs says.

Insomnia can be caused by many things, from an aching back to depression to a sleeping disorder such as apnea. If it lasts for more than a few nights, you should see a doctor, Dr. Walsleben says. Most likely, your insomnia isn't caused by a physical problem. It can usually be traced to the way you lead your life—most specifically, your nightlife.

---

her stay awake, Niss says, but they made her feel "strange." To get more relief, Niss investigated alternative treatments. In the early 1980s, a friend suggested she give acupuncture a try.

To her surprise, the treatments seemed to help. Today, Niss says, she's more awake than ever, and the hallucinations and cataplectic attacks have virtually stopped.

Doctors specializing in sleep disorders say it's unlikely that acupuncture had anything to do with Niss's improvement—that perhaps it's the placebo effect or some of the "tricks" she's learned along the way. But Niss is convinced. At times when she stopped the treatments, she says, the symptoms came right back.

Niss doesn't depend only on acupuncture to keep her sleepiness at bay. To stay awake, she doesn't settle in for long sessions of tiring, repetitive tasks. For example, she'll work at the typewriter only until she gets tired. Then she'll do some housework or go for a walk. When she's rested, she'll return to the typewriter.

"I know I will always have narcolepsy, but it is bearable for me now," Niss says. "I no longer take any medication. I usually, but not always, take one nap a day. At night, I usually sleep about 7 1/2 hours—I'd probably sleep more if my husband wouldn't accidentally wake me!"

BEDROOMS ARE FOR SLEEPING

Many people have insomnia because they simply won't let themselves relax, Dr. Walsleben says. But sleep is like love—it needs romancing. Some soothing rituals, she suggests, can help beat the late-night blues.

Adjust the clock. Your body clock, that is. "Your brain is divided into a wake system and a sleep system," says Dr. Walsleben. "At night, you want your sleep system to get stronger. You do that by slowing down, by reducing your anxiety." In other words, don't start your taxes at midnight. If you often bring work home with you, put it aside a few hours before bedtime.

Of course, it's not enough to only protect your sleep system, Dr. Walsleben says. You need to strengthen your wake system, too. You do this simply by being active and organized; the more active and organized you are during the day, the more tired—and ready for sleep—you'll be at night.

Banish stress. Your bedroom is for sleeping—*period.* (You can make an exception for sex, Dr. Walsleben says.) Too many people turn their bedrooms into offices or rumpus rooms. Instead of sleeping, they're worrying about unpaid bills, disobedient children and tyrannical bosses. No wonder they stay awake! When it's time to pull back the covers, Dr. Walsleben says, you should turn down the day's emotional volume, too.

Table your stress—literally. To get stress makers (kids, bosses, money) off your mind, Dr. Walsleben says, put them on paper. "Write your worries down before you go to bed. That will get them out of your head, and you can tell yourself 'They're on the table, I can worry about them in the morning.' "

Be consistent. It's less important what hours you keep, Dr. Walsleben says, than how *regularly* you keep them. Let's say you stay up until 3:00 A.M. watching (for the fourth time) *Psycho III.* You'll be a little sleepy the next day, so perhaps you'll settle down for a 2-hour nap. After that, of course, you'll be wide awake for that night's late movie, *Alien Avengers.* Repeat the cycle a few times, Dr. Walsleben says, and insomnia, not sleep, will be your bed partner. It's okay to stay up late occasionally, but only if you get up at your usual time. Sure, you'll be tired by bedtime, but that's the whole point.

Slow down. "We stay up too late, work very long hours, fly all over the world. As a result, we disturb our sleep/wake system," Dr. Walsleben says. "To slow things down, try taking a nice warm bath early in the evening to relax your muscles. A glass of milk can be very relaxing. And you definitely want to avoid caffeine, cigarettes or other stimulants."

Don't count the hours. Everyone talks about getting 8 hours' sleep, but there's nothing magical about that number, Dr. Walsleben warns. For some people, 5 hours of sleep is enough; others need 10. If you're feeling rested during the day, you're getting enough sleep at night.

NARCOLEPSY

Poor Dagwood Bumstead—he's always exhausted, and he falls asleep at the most inopportune times! When he's not snoozing on the living room couch, he's sneaking a nap at work. And that's when his boss, Mr. Dithers, invariably arrives. Mr. Dithers delivers Dagwood his wake-up kick—and we, the readers of "Blondie," our wake-up laugh. There's something intrinsically funny about Dagwood's droopy travails.

Unless, that is, you happen to have narcolepsy. Then Dagwood's plight suddenly seems less than amusing. This serious, incurable sleep disorder, which can cause sleep attacks, hallucinations and sleep paralysis, may affect as many as 250,000 Americans, many of whom spend their entire lives in a fog of debilitating fatigue, says Michael J. Thorpy, M.D., director of the Sleep-Wake Disorders Center at Montefiore Medical Center in New York City and associate professor of neurology at Albert Einstein College of Medicine.

"With narcolepsy, there's always a background level of sleepiness," explains Dr. Thorpy, author of *The Encyclopedia of Sleep and Sleep Disorders.* "Some children with narcolepsy get lower grades or drop out of school. As adults, they're often unable to keep jobs, because they're sleepy all the time. It can be very hard for them to make friends or develop relationships. They're simply too tired."

Doctors still are mystified by the disease, Dr. Thorpy says. It does seem to run in families, and doctors suspect it's caused by a flaw somewhere in the central nervous system. Narcolepsy also is accompanied by some odd disturbances that can make for some unexpected twists in daily life.

THE NARCOLEPTIC QUARTET

Everyone with narcolepsy suffers from one or more of the following traits, what doctors call the "narcoleptic tetrad." They are:

CATAPLEXY. Triggered by feelings of anger, pleasure or other strong emotions, cataplexy is an abrupt loss of muscle tone that often affects the legs, neck or wrists. Some people merely feel weak when cataplexy strikes; others hit the ground. "I had one patient who had cataplexy mainly during sexual intercourse, and he was very concerned about that," Dr. Thorpy says.

SLEEP ATTACKS. Most of us go to sleep gradually, a little bit at a time. People with narcolepsy, on the other hand, can simply keel over—while reading, watching television or talking with friends. Sleep attacks can strike while you're working—or, even worse, while you're *driving* to work. Automobile accidents are more common among narcoleptics, Dr. Thorpy says.

SLEEP PARALYSIS. Quite common among narcoleptics, sleep paralysis occurs when first going to sleep or in the morning while waking up: Those experiencing an attack may be able to move their eyes, but not much else. They can't even speak. To make things worse, the paralysis sometimes is accompanied by terrible hallucinations. It's like being in a nightmare—and you can't run!

HALLUCINATIONS. These dreamlike images, which occur just before people go to sleep or when they wake up, can seem incredibly real, Dr. Thorpy says. And most of the time, they're incredibly scary. "A lot of people dream of falling through the air or of being buried alive," he says.

STOPPING THE SYMPTOMS

Niss Ryan knows these problems all too well. She is vice president of Narcolepsy Network, a national volunteer organization for people who have narcolepsy. She says some people are so besieged with fatigue, sleep attacks and cataplexy that their lives are turned upside down. "They may experience confusion and may be unable to hold a job," Ryan says. "Some people, however, have learned ways of coping with their symptoms."

Shift gears. Ryan says some tasks—for example, typing and reading—are certain to cause drowsiness after a while. To stay fresh, she frequently alternates sedentary tasks with more vigorous jobs such as housecleaning.

Take frequent naps. "When the sleepiness is overwhelming, the best thing you can do is sleep," Dr. Thorpy says. "Naps can be very refreshing." However, don't sleep for more than 20 minutes, he warns. That can ruin your nighttime sleep.

Listen to your body. The best part about working at home, Ryan says, is that she's free to set her own schedule. For people who have to punch a clock each day, it's not so easy. If your job is really hard on you, Dr. Thorpy says—if, for example, you're required to read hundreds of pages of fine print at late hours—you might want to switch careers.

A Note about Drugs

For some people, Dr. Thorpy says, taking stimulant drugs is the only way to handle the unrelenting fatigue that is always threatening to drag them down. The drugs heighten their arousal system, he explains. "But if you put them in a room and turn out the light, they'll fall asleep just as quickly as they would if they didn't take the drugs."

Even though stimulants will help you stay awake, they won't prevent sleep paralysis or cataplexy, he adds. To relieve these symptoms, tricyclic antidepressants such as clomipramine and protriptyline can be quite effective.

Unfortunately, the drugs used to treat narcolepsy can also cause side effects, and problems such as blurred vision and sexual dysfunction will occasionally occur. In addition, Dr. Thorpy says, "there's always the conflict between the medicine trying to keep you awake and your own body trying to make you go to sleep. That can cause such unpleasant sensations that some people choose not to take any medication at all."

Any cure for narcolepsy is far in the future, Dr. Thorpy says. Until then, people need to learn all they can about this devastating disease. "You've got it for life, and you have to fight your way through it every day," he says.

STRESS

Washers break, roofs leak, bills mount, cars squeak.

Prices rise, stocks fall, checks bounce, kids brawl!

Stress is unavoidable. Always has been, and always will be. But unavoidable doesn't mean unmanageable. The latest research shows that how you react to a stressful event determines its impact on your health. If you let stress bother you, it will—physically, mentally and every which way.

But handle stress intelligently, and you turn the enemy into an ally. Stress can motivate, invigorate and educate. It can be a kick in the pants instead of a slap in the face.

What follows is a selection of proven stress-fighting techniques. There are many to choose from. Once you find the ones that are right for you, you can put stress in its place.

ATTITUDE ADJUSTMENTS

For many of us, stress is caused less by our environments than by our attitudes. Perhaps we expect too much of ourselves or others. Or maybe we suffer from low self-esteem and remain too passive. Either way, stress can result as we fail to get from life what we feel we deserve. The solution?

Change the attitudes that generate stress in the first place. For example:

Be assertive. The secretary who feels like a slave. The salesman who feels frustrated, mired at the bottom of the corporate ladder. What these people lack is respect—from both themselves and others. What they need to turn that around is to be assertive—that is, to be able to communicate needs and feelings.

Be straightforward. Say no politely and firmly—don't make excuses. Admit your feelings. Say "I'm angry" rather than "You are a crumb."

Express your preferences. Say what you want. By asserting yourself, you're putting yourself in control.

Don't try to do it all. How do most top executives do their jobs without buckling under stress? They've learned to delegate. This is nothing more than the fine art of sharing the load. "Stress, for many of us, is a self-inflicted burden in this regard," says psychologist Steven Fahrion, Ph.D., of the Menninger Clinic in Topeka, Kansas. Whether we have too much ego or not enough, we fail to get others to pitch in where they can and should.

This isn't to say you should become a dictator. However, you should consider how your time might best be spent. The idea, experts say, is to delegate what you can so that you're able to spend more time on the things you can't.

Find a safety valve. You come home to the family after work, feeling as friendly as a wolverine, and right away you're dealing with kids and spouses and unpaid bills—more stress, in other words. Next time, blow off some steam first. Take a walk. Soak in the tub. Read the newspaper. Do whatever you have to do to relax. Join the family only when you've calmed down—*not* when you're ready to explode.

Laugh it up. Sure, it's sometimes difficult to force a laugh in tense situations. But that's precisely when you need it most. "We need to revere humor in these high-stress times of ours, not just tolerate it," says Steven Allen, Jr., M.D., the son of comic genius Steve Allen and an assistant professor of family medicine at the State University of New York Health Sciences Center in Syracuse.

One trick for finding humor in the worst of situations is to blow things absolutely, ridiculously out of proportion. Say you're stuck in a traffic jam. Imagine the worst: "These cars will never move. I'll be stuck here for the rest of my life. By the time I get home, my children will have grown up, married and had children. They won't even remember me." When your scenario reaches the point of absurdity, you begin to smile. The situation is put in perspective. Now you can calm down.

PUTTING OFF PROCRASTINATION

Deadlines, at home or the office, can make the calmest person feel stressed out. People who always put things off—and off and off—have two worries: completing the task on time, and suffering from self-disapproval. This double whammy can be terribly stressful, says Neil Fiore, Ph.D., a psychologist in private practice in Berkeley, California, and author of *The Now Habit*.

To pull the plug on procrastination:

Enjoy your playtime. Fill your weekly schedule with time for leisure and friends. You will have less resentment toward work—and less reluctance to get started.

Narrow your focus. Whether you're cleaning your house or designing a city, the big picture can seem overwhelming, too big to tackle. Sometimes it's better to focus on the individual steps. At home, for example, divide tasks into increments: "First I'll pick up the living room . . . then I'll dust." And so on. By keeping your expectations small—and realistic—you may find it easier to get started.

Be lazy for a change. Odd advice for beating procrastination? Perhaps, but some experts say that doing nothing can be an effective starting point when you have the "I can't get started" blues. The sheer boredom of doing nothing may be the impetus you need to kick your rear into gear!

HIGH-OCTANE LIVING

Doctors agree that being physically active—walking, stretching, even working in the garden—is a high-power stress buster. "Just as your mind affects your body, so can your body affect your mind," says Dean Ornish, M.D., author of *Dr. Dean Ornish's Program for Reversing Heart Disease.* When the woes of the world come your way:

Stretch yourself. Literally. Stretching can help you feel more peaceful and relaxed, says Dr. Ornish. As you stretch, imagine the tension

---

RELAXING TOGETHER

Misery may like company, but the desire for comfort likes it even more. "Support groups give their members an opportunity to do something about their problems and to be more than passive victims," says John Renner, M.D., president of the Consumer Health Information Research Institute in Kansas City. "They reduce the sense of isolation that people often feel when afflicted with a serious health dilemma."

Whatever is causing stress in your life—drug or alcohol problems, eating disorders or anything else—there's probably a helpful group out there that would like you for a member. By sharing your problems with like-minded people, you may find your stress levels gradually declining. You may find some new friends as well.

For help in locating a group near you, look in your phone book's Blue Pages. You could also contact the American Self-Help Clearinghouse, St. Clares–Riverside Medical Center, Denville, NJ 07834.

---

leaving your back, neck and other muscles as you gently push them to their comfortable limit.

Walk it off. Yes, you can simply step away from stress—temporarily at least—with what may be the oldest stress reducer of all. Studies by California State University psychologist Robert Thayer, Ph.D., have shown significant reductions in tension after walks lasting only several minutes. Walking not only can provide a needed escape from tension, it also may increase the body's production of mood-elevating brain chemicals called endorphins.

How effective can walking be? A study by Florida's State Department of Health and Rehabilitative Services found that participants in an eight-week walking program were able to reduce the stress they felt at work by 30 percent.

Head for the garden. More lurks out amidst the lettuce leaves than nutrition for the body. There's also nourishment for the soul. "Gardening is a natural, stress-releasing activity without the contrivance and inconvenience of working out at a health club," says Bryant Stamford, Ph.D., a professor of allied health at the University of Louisville and coauthor of *Fitness without Exercise.*

Stress management expert Emmett Miller, M.D., of Menlo Park, California, agrees. "Gardening takes our minds off the unsolvable problems we confront every day. It gives us work to do where we can see progress from minute to minute."

FINDING PEACE

Throughout history, people in all civilizations and from all parts of the world have sought relief from stress. According to Paul Rosch, M.D., of the American Institute of Stress, stress reduction is "a very personal thing, meaning that what works for one person may not work for another." Here are some stress releasers that come with no absolute guarantees but that are worth-a-try options when you need to find a little relief in a big hurry.

Hug your pet. We talk to them, we cuddle them, we confide in them. Research has shown that heart attack victims who have pets live longer. Even watching a tank full of tropical fish may lower blood pressure, at least temporarily. Why are pets so soothing?

"Animals bring out our nurturing instinct," says Linda Hines, executive director of the Delta Society, an organization dedicated to studying human/animal interactions. "They also make us feel safe and unconditionally accepted. We can just be ourselves around our pets."

Keep in mind, however, that pets require constant care. It's a good idea to be sure your pet is housebroken and well trained. "Accidents in the house and annoyed friends and neighbors can be stress makers, not breakers," Hines says.

Let your mind go. According to Herbert Benson, M.D., chief of the Division of Behavioral Medicine at Harvard Medical School, a technique called Relaxation Response can help combat stress and revitalize the mind. First choose a word or phrase—for example, *peace* or *one.* Then sit in a comfortable position, close your eyes, relax your muscles, and allow yourself to breathe slowly and naturally. As you exhale, repeat the word or phrase. After doing this for 10 to 20 minutes once or twice a day, you may notice your stress drifting away along with your exhalations.

Breathe deeply. This infuses the blood with extra oxygen and also stimulates the body to release tranquilizing endorphins. "Deep breathing is one of the simplest yet most effective stress management techniques there is," says Dr. Ornish. "You can do it anywhere, anytime, and it becomes even more effective with practice."

Soothing senses. A magnificent sunset fills you with awe. A great piece of music transports you to distant realms. The smell of a rose overwhelms you with its beauty. What pleases the senses calms the mind as

---

POSITIVE THOUGHTS, POSITIVE FEELINGS

Thoughts cause feelings, and the wrong kinds of thoughts can cause stressful feelings. "We cause ourselves a lot of unnecessary anxiety by seeing the glass as half empty rather than as half full," says Fran Gaal, a psychotherapist in Bethlehem, Pennsylvania.

Do you automatically interpret silence on the part of your spouse to mean anger when it could just as easily mean fatigue? Do you blame yourself when a sudden downpour drenches your wash on the line? Do you dwell on the few times your boss criticized your performance and ignore the innumerable times she's praised you?

We all fall into the negative thinking rut from time to time. We badger ourselves with "should haves" and lose sight of the fact that "good" and "bad" in life is rarely black and white.

"Think in shades of gray," recommends psychiatrist and cognitive therapist David Burns, M.D., "not black or white only." All-or-nothing thinking can lead to anxiety, depression, feelings of inferiority, perfectionism and anger. Allow yourself to fail now and then. It's all part of being human.

---

well. So give yourself time—and opportunity—to indulge your senses. Let your little pleasures bring relief from big problems!

Soak away stress. Hot baths can do more than keep you clean. "It's my daily oasis," says one working mother. "I get in that tub, and my troubles melt." That may sound poetic, but it has some science on its side. Warm baths (between 100° and 102°F) not only relax the muscles but help provide some quiet time as well. So when you need to escape, fill the tub, lie back, and relax.

Mellow out with music. Experts agree that listening to music can work soothing magic. Of course, everyone has different tastes. If listening to Aerosmith helps you relax more than listening to Debussy, that's okay, says Joseph Scartelli, Ph.D., dean of the College of Visual and Performing Arts at Radford University in Radford, Virginia. "Sitting down and forcing yourself to listen to relaxation music that you *don't* like may create stress, not alleviate it," he says.

STROKE

P eople have different opinions about the needs of the human brain. Psychologists say that the brain requires some form of stimulation—even if it's as minimal as watching "Wheel of Fortune." Sleep experts say the brain can't function well unless it gets to dream at night. And some people insist that their brains turn to mush without a large cup of coffee in the morning. But there's no argument about the one thing the brain needs above and beyond anything else: It's *blood*.

Without a constant flow of blood to supply your brain cells with fresh oxygen, those brain cells would quickly die. That is what happens when a blood vessel bringing blood to the brain ruptures or gets clogged. It's called a stroke, and it's America's third largest killer (heart disease and cancer hold the top spots) and a cause of serious impairment in thousands of people. The number of those stricken yearly is about a half million— but it's a number that, happily, is falling every year. In fact, the number of strokes in America has declined by *half* in the past two decades.

Why so? Largely the drop is due to increased knowledge about what causes stroke and what can prevent it. If you're not already privy to this information, it's a "stroke" of good luck that you're reading this chapter!

THE BASICS OF STROKE

Strokes occur in two different ways: *Ischemic* strokes are caused by blood clots that block the supply of blood to areas of the brain. They account for 70 to 80 percent of all strokes. *Hemorrhagic* strokes, the more deadly of the two, are caused by blood vessels that rupture in the brain itself or on the surface of the brain.

Neither kind of stroke is actually a disease—doctors call them "events." The illness behind the event is cardiovascular disease—disease of the blood vessels or the heart, or both. Regardless of what we call a stroke, some people are more susceptible than others. Consider the risk factors for stroke that, for the most part, you *can't* control.

AGE. The older you get, the higher the risk—after you turn 55, the risk doubles every decade.

GENDER. The incidence of stroke is about 30 percent higher in men than in women.

RACE. Blacks have a 60 percent greater chance of death or disability from a stroke than whites.

DIABETES. Even though diabetes can be controlled, the disease may weaken blood vessels, hiking the stroke risk for men by 40 percent and for women by 72 percent.

HEREDITY. If you have a family history of stroke, your own risk is higher than normal.

PRIOR STROKE. It increases the risk of another stroke by several times.

IRREGULAR HEARTBEAT. A condition called atrial fibrillation can cause clots to form that may travel to the brain. It raises the risk of stroke in men by 83 percent and in women by more than 200 percent. Atrial fibrillation often results from a prior heart attack.

FACTORS YOU CAN CONTROL

Now the good part. Let's take a look at those things you *do* have control over that will lessen your chances of having a stroke.

Control high blood pressure. Hypertension (high blood pressure) is the number one risk factor for stroke. So it should be no surprise that controlling high blood pressure has probably had more to do with the decline in death rates from stroke than has any other factor.

High blood pressure can cause and aggravate atherosclerosis—hardening and clogging of arteries that normally are open and flexible and able to adjust to temporary increases in pressure and blood flow. Controlling high blood pressure can often be achieved by eating a healthier diet and losing excess weight. Sometimes drugs can do the trick. The first step, of course, is to have your blood pressure checked. If high, discuss options with your doctor. (For tips on how to control high blood pressure, see "High Blood Pressure" on page 277.)

Avoid heart disease. Even without hypertension, heart disease more than doubles your stroke risk. The three biggies for avoiding heart disease are cigarette smoking (don't), blood cholesterol (keep it low) and blood pressure (the lower, the better). (For a complete heart disease prevention program, see "Heart Disease" on page 249.)

Watch your red blood cell count. The more red cells you have, the thicker your blood, and the more likely you are to form stroke-causing clots, doctors say. If your physician determines that you have this condition, it can be treated by removing blood or by prescribing a blood "thinner" such as aspirin.

Control cholesterol. This fatlike natural blood alcohol strongly contributes to the development of atherosclerosis and heart disease. So if you can reduce your blood cholesterol, you're two steps ahead of stroke. You can keep your cholesterol under control by reducing the cholesterol and saturated fat in your diet. Start by eating more vegetables, fruits and grains—and less meat, dairy products (unless they're low-fat or nonfat varieties) and snack foods. (A complete program for controlling cholesterol can be found in "High Cholesterol" on page 288.)

Stop smoking. Smoking tobacco hikes your risk of stroke by about 70 percent. Part of the reason is that smoking contributes to heart disease and atherosclerosis. It may also make your blood more likely to clot and your blood vessels more likely to constrict. If you don't smoke, don't start. If you do smoke, quit. Researchers from the Framingham Heart Study in Massachusetts say that after four or five clean years, quitters may find that their risk of stroke is no greater than that of someone who has never smoked.

PROFILE IN HEALING

VERONICA McKEEN: *CAN'T* IS A FOUR-LETTER WORD

One day in 1961, Veronica McKeen was in the shower in her home in El Paso, Texas, getting ready to go shopping. As she bathed, several small blood clots broke loose and traveled to the arteries of her brain. There they blocked the flow of blood, and Veronica collapsed. She woke up five days later in the hospital, paralyzed on her left side. She was 23.

"I was in the hospital only two weeks, including the five days I was in a coma," she says. She wasn't given any therapy, and there was no follow-up treatment. "It's hard to believe now," she says, "but that's the way things were in those days."

Things did not go well for the next few years. "I had thought I would just get better, as if I had a cold," McKeen says. She wheeled herself around the house, struggled to walk and battled her mild aphasia (problems with finding the right words). "But after two years, I wasn't getting any better," she says. Depression and anemia set in, along with crying fits and laughing spells. Thus began six years of weekly visits to a psychiatrist, tranquilizers, even shock therapy—and she continued to deteriorate.

By 1970, Veronica hit bottom and found there was nowhere to go but up. "I started realizing I would have to take things into my own

Cut down on drinking. Let's toast to soft drinks and water. Studies show that alcohol increases the risk of both types of stroke, but especially the more deadly hemorrhagic stroke—double for light drinkers, triple for heavy. Alcohol in any form can hike your blood pressure, weaken your heart, thicken your blood and cause arteries to go into blood-restricting spasm. If you must drink, do so in moderation.

Exercise. If you lead a life of ease, sliding into the car even to go to the corner mailbox, you are increasing your risk of heart disease—and you know what *that* means. Exercise can help lower blood pressure, take off excess weight, control cholesterol levels and manage diabetes (another risk factor for stroke). Recent studies have shown that most of the health benefits of exercise come from *moderate* workouts. Brisk walking, for example, is an excellent exercise. You can start by hiking to the mailbox! Of course, it's a good idea to check with your doctor before starting any exercise program.

---

hands," she says. "A very good friend helped. She'd say 'You can,' I'd say 'I can't,' and she'd say 'You *can,* and you *will.*' "

Will: the magic word. A horse lover, Veronica began working at the stables of a nearby racetrack, hobbling around, caring for the horses. Later she wangled herself a job at the betting window. "It helped build my self-confidence," she says. "The more I did it, the more confident I got."

After three years of confidence building, she married a man "who said 'You can, you can, you can,' " she says. "From day one, he told me 'I don't ever want to hear you say 'I can't.' " This new, supportive husband gave her the idea for a 640-mile bicycle ride.

In April 1988, with the Organization for After-Stroke Resources as her backer, she rode from Glendora, California, to Sacramento, stopping at convalescent homes along the way to show strokers they can overcome their disability. "It was eye-opening to the people in those homes, many of whom had just given up," she says.

Veronica now has full use of her left arm; her aphasia has faded, but she still limps slightly. If a doctor tells you "You'll never walk again," get another doctor, she says. "Your recovery depends on you. You don't know what you can do until you try. The sooner you can help yourself, the sooner you get out of that bed or wheelchair, the sooner you can begin to regain your independence."

Shed excess pounds. Obesity is often a prominent partner of heart disease, diabetes, high blood pressure and high cholesterol. Lose weight, and you lower your risk of stroke.

Control diabetes. Statistics show that diabetes increases stroke risk in men by 40 percent and in women by 72 percent. Keeping diabetes under control won't remove the risk altogether, but it boosts the odds in your favor. (For more information on controlling diabetes, see "Diabetes" on page 143.)

TIA: A WARNING SIGN

A transient ischemic attack—TIA—is a not-to-be-ignored warning of an impending ischemic stroke. This "mini-stroke" mimics what a real stroke would do to you: weakness; numbness in the face, arm, hand or leg; loss of the ability to speak clearly or to understand what others are saying to you; dimness or loss of vision in one eye; dizziness or loss of balance. But the symptoms rapidly disappear—in 90 percent of the cases, they fade in less than 6 hours. The importance of the TIA is that 20 to 40 percent of people who have them go on to have a full-blown stroke—their risk is ten times greater than that of those who haven't had a TIA. If you think you've had a TIA, see a doctor immediately.

"The greatest risk of stroke is in the first week after a TIA happens," says Harold P. Adams, M.D., director of the Cerebrovascular Diseases Division at the University of Iowa. But just because you haven't had a TIA doesn't mean you're safe: Only 10 percent of strokes are preceded by a TIA.

THE ROAD BACK FROM A STROKE

Seven out of ten people who have a stroke live through it, although the going can be rough. Survivors may be affected in a large number of ways, from speech problems to difficulty chewing and swallowing. Of the people who survive a stroke, about two-thirds will need some form of rehabilitation, says Michael Reding, M.D., associate professor of neurology at Cornell University Medical College and director of the Stroke Rehabilitation Unit at Burke Rehabilitation Center in New York City.

Through rehabilitation, the brain can develop new pathways that circumvent damaged connections and switches. "Some cells are dead, some that were just outside the damaged area aren't dead but are not functioning," Dr. Reding says. "In the three months after a stroke, these cells will start to recover." As recovery progresses, these still-living cells may take over some of the functions the dead cells used to perform. They'll need practice.

TOP SOURCES OF POTASSIUM

Eating more vegetables and fresh fruit may help protect against stroke. One study found that eating as little as one additional serving a day of these foods might cut the risk of fatal stroke by as much as 40 percent.

What is it about fruits and vegetables that delivers such a giant impact? Potassium. This mineral is known to help control high blood pressure, the greatest risk factor for stroke. Yet scientists believe potassium may have a stroke-protective effect beyond its ability to lower blood pressure.

Your stroke prevention diet should include these foods, the best sources of potassium.

FOOD	PORTION	POTASSIUM (mg.)
Avocado	1	1,204
Potato, baked	1 med.	844
Cantaloupe	1/2	825
Prunes, dried	1/2 cup	600
Watermelon	1 slice	560
Raisins	1/2 cup	545
Orange juice	1 cup	496
Broccoli, raw	1 med. stalk	490
Lima beans, large, boiled	1/2 cup	478
Banana	1	451
Apricots, dried	1/4 cup	448
Squash, winter, baked	1/2 cup	445
Skim milk	1 cup	406
Sweet potato, baked	1 med.	397
Whole milk	1 cup	370
Sardines, Atlantic	1 can	365
Kidney beans, boiled	1/2 cup	355
Sunflower seeds, dried	1/3 cup	331
Apricots, fresh	3	313
Flounder, baked	3 oz.	292
Tomato, raw	1 med.	254
Peach	1	171
Green pepper	1 large	144

"The whole philosophy of rehab is that if you have trouble with some-thing, you keep working at it," Dr. Reding says. "If you have trouble walking, you keep trying to walk. The same goes for dressing or talking. The way you learned to read and write and figure things out in the first place was practice, practice, practice. You have to relearn the basics. That's how the brain learns to adapt to its environment."

Rehab also puts the patient through exercises to keep joints mobile and muscles, tendons and ligaments limber. Exercise provides feedback to the cells that are taking on new roles, Dr. Reding says. Recognize that after a stroke, the patient is likely to get tired even *thinking* about exercise. That's something he needs to work through, says Dr. Reding.

ATTITUDE IS EVERYTHING

"People come out of rehab in all stages," says Frank Shirbroun, Ph.D., executive director of the Organization for After-Stroke Resources (OASR), based in Upland, California. "Most recover many of their skills in the first six months after a stroke, and then a plateau forces them to realize that some of the effects of their stroke are permanent. That's often when depres-sion, hopelessness and decline set in." If you're in that boat, know that you *can* bail out.

Be with your compadres. "Spend time with other survivors and their families," Dr. Shirbroun says. "They can inspire you and ignite your will to get on with life." Hospital social workers, senior centers, stroke survivors' organizations, Alzheimer's and Parkinson's groups and YM/YWCAs are all sources of support group information.

Prove that doctor wrong. "People often don't know what they can do until they try," Dr. Shirbroun says. "You don't have to accept the doctor's verdict that you'll never walk again. It may be physically impossible, but then again, it may not. That's the unknown part of stroke. People can recover far more than many think if they have the will and the access to help. How much a stroke patient can do is very individualized."

The staff at OASR, composed mostly of volunteers, works at convinc-ing stroke survivors and their families that they can get back into society, Dr. Shirbroun says. "Our activities are always in a public facility, like a community center or a school," he says, not shut away in homes and hospitals.

"We try to keep successful survivors in front of our people," says Dr. Shirbroun. "Many of these success stories were once in wheelchairs."

Sing out. About one-fourth of stroke survivors have problems talking. "But often people who can't or won't talk, whether from physical inability or lack of will, can sing," Dr. Shirbroun says.

Play games. "In one of our games aimed at regaining the ability to talk, each person has to say one word that has to do with summer," Dr. Shirbroun says. "One man who had never said one word since his stroke started saying 'bikini' over and over again. He didn't even realize he could say it. Another woman, after her stroke, could only say 'Magic Johnson.' Now she's giving inspirational speeches to other stroke survivors."

Work out. "Even if you're in a wheelchair or relying on a quad-cane, you can exercise," Dr. Shirbroun says. "We have range-of-motion exercises for people in wheelchairs. Because of aquatic exercise, one man was able to get out of his chair, then walk with a quad-cane and finally walk without a cane." The OASR even organizes after-stroke athletic games—bowling,

---

SPEAKING IN TONGUES

Sometimes a stroke can help scientists learn how the brain works. Take the 32-year-old Baltimore man who had a stroke in small arteries deep in his brain. "The area that was damaged was very small but very important," says his doctor, neurologist Dean Tippett, M.D., of the University of Maryland School of Medicine in Baltimore. Important enough to shed light on how the brain produces language.

The man was pure American, born and bred, and spoke no foreign languages. But after a couple of days of slurred speech, he began speaking with a strong Scandinavian accent. "He was pretty clear, and everyone who heard him said he sounded Scandinavian or Nordic," Dr. Tippett says. He added vowel sounds as he spoke, saying things like "How are you today-ah?" When making a statement, his voice would rise in pitch at the end of a sentence, making it sound like a question.

"He stopped forming contractions (for example, saying "don't" instead of "do not"), as if he didn't know the language he was speaking," Dr. Tippett says. "He had to struggle with the English language, as if he were a foreigner. Rather than something being added to his speech, something was actually taken away."

There have been 15 similar cases reported since 1901, Dr. Tippett says, "and each helps us learn the discrete areas responsible for very specific language functions"—like the ability to form contractions. One Swedish woman hit by shrapnel in a German air raid in World War II was in a coma until 1947. "When she awoke," Dr. Tippett says, "she began speaking Swedish with a German accent, which didn't go over well with her fellow townspeople." She retained the unwelcome accent until she died in the 1970s.

basketball, shuffleboard, even card games—played by people who thought they could never again hold and deal a deck of cards, let alone bowl over pins.

See the cup half full, not half empty. All stroke patients fear having another stroke. Depending on your risk factors—gender, blood pressure, heart disease, diabetes—your chances of having another stroke range from 15 to 40 percent. But turn those numbers upside down. "The odds are obviously in your favor," says Dr. Reding. "There's a 60 to 85 percent chance you *won't* have another stroke." And thanks to recent advances in medical knowledge, those odds are getting better all the time.

If you can't find a group, start one. You might be the impetus for saving yourself and others in the same boat from decline. "Too many stroke survivors just plop in front of a TV for the rest of their lives," says Dr. Shirbroun. "And that's a tragedy, because there's a lot of good living still to be done."

TREATMENT BREAKTHROUGH

THE GLUTAMATE CONNECTION

Hospital emergency rooms, intensive care units and probably even ambulances of the near future are going to have new weapons to prevent stroke-caused brain damage. These weapons will target a brain chemical that makes brain cells virtually work themselves into a fatal frenzy in the hours and days following a stroke.

The brain chemical is glutamate. Glutamate normally plays an essential role in making a brain cell fire off messages to neighboring cells, says Stephen Heinemann, Ph.D., professor of neuroscience at the Salk Institute for Biological Studies in San Diego. "It does this by transmitting calcium into brain cells. But after a stroke—when there's a drop in blood supply or oxygen to the cells—glutamate builds up and keeps pumping calcium into the cells," Dr. Heinemann says. "The cells become overstimulated, firing again and again until they die."

So researchers have theorized that if they can block the buildup of glutamate, they can prevent too much calcium from setting off this brain-damaging reaction. No glutamate, no calcium, no cell damage. Cell damage is what often causes severe disabilities in victims of stroke.

When can you expect hospital emergency rooms to have glutamate-blocking drugs to prevent stroke-caused brain damage? "We will be lucky if they are available by the year 2000, but I hope they will be," Dr. Heinemann says.

TEMPOROMANDIBULAR JOINT DISORDER

I f you've got the feeling that you're chewing on a jawbreaker, even though your mouth is full of only marshmallow, you may have a temporomandibular joint disorder. That's quite a mouthful, so most doctors simply call it TMD or TMJ. Whatever you call it, it means you've got a problem with the joints in your jaw, and painful chewing is one result.

Other symptoms of TMD may include headaches, tinnitus (ringing in the ears) and neck pain. You may also hear clicking and popping sounds when you move your mouth.

A BUSY JOINT

Before we talk about things that can cause TMD, let's take a quick tour of the temporomandibular joint itself. To find it, put a finger under your ear and open your mouth. That lumpy thing that you feel moving is the joint. Basically, it's the spot where the top of your jaw attaches to the bottom of your head. Not surprisingly, it gets a nearly constant workout, says Ludwig Leibsohn, D.D.S., president of the Academy of General Dentistry. "Every time you swallow, open your mouth, talk, snore or grind your teeth, that joint is moving," he says.

There are two bones inside the joint. One, the *mandibular condyle,* is the topmost knob of your jawbone. The other, the *mandibular fossa,* is the depression in your skull where the jawbone attaches. And between these two bones is a protective disk called the *meniscus.* This crescent-shaped piece of cartilage provides cushioning and extra support.

Normally the jaw moves smoothly: up and down, side to side and front to back. But when something goes wrong—either inside the joint or in the attaching muscles and ligaments—it no longer moves so easily. Sometimes, says Dr. Leibsohn, it doesn't move at all. That's as bad as TMD can get. Thank goodness, frozen jaws are rare.

USUALLY A MINOR PROBLEM

As many as one in two people may have a temporomandibular joint that calls attention to itself—with occasional pain, stiffness, fatigue or various harmless noises. In most cases, the discomfort (if any) is minimal. Professional treatment rarely is needed.

Until recently, many dentists believed that misaligned teeth, called malocclusions, were to blame for TMD, because they put excessive strain on the hardworking jaw joint. However, studies showed that even when people had extensive (and expensive) dental work to correct their bites, TMD often did not disappear, Dr. Leibsohn says. "People ended up with $30,000 worth of dentistry, and they had the same problem that they had before."

Most dentists today agree there are three primary causes of TMD. These are muscle strain, slipped disks inside the jaw joint and degenerative

---

PROFILE IN HEALING

DOROTHY CARTER: C'EST LA PAIN

Dorothy Carter talks for a living. And as an associate professor of French at Eastern Kentucky University, she does it in two languages. So when her jaw started cramping up during classes, she knew she was in big trouble.

"It started after I had oral surgery," she explains. "As best as I can figure, I simply kept my mouth too wide open for too long. Of course, I'm also a teeth clencher at night, and that didn't help either."

For months, she says, there was pain in her temporomandibular joint, and every day it kept getting worse. "At first it hurt almost all the time—it felt very much as if somebody had taken my lower jaw and was wrenching it sideways. Then the pain worked its way down into my neck; I had trouble even turning my head to back out of the driveway! I was having tension headaches, too."

To make things worse, her jaw just wasn't working right, and sometimes "Comment allez-vous?" came out sounding more like "Co . . . mmmpphh."

Dorothy's doctor prescribed massage, traction, physical therapy

diseases such as arthritis, says Charles S. Greene, D.D.S., a clinical professor of dentistry at Northwestern University Dental School in Chicago.

No matter what the cause of your TMD, if it's giving you pain, you need to do something about it. "Most temporomandibular disorders that cause pain are managed the same way you manage a sore back or a sore shoulder—with a lot of self-care," says Dr. Greene.

RELIEF FOR A SORE JAW

When you have worked your jaw too hard—by chewing gum, clenching your teeth or even talking too much—you essentially have strained and overworked your muscles, Dr. Greene says. "You have to give them some rest to recover—and most of the time, they do." So when your jaw starts hurting:

Try to relax. "More frequently than not, TMD can be traced to some high-tension situation," Dr. Leibsohn says. It makes sense. After all, many people who are under stress clench their jaws, bite their cheeks and grind their teeth at night. Eventually the joint—and the muscles that control it—get tired and sore. The solution, obviously, is to calm down. Your jaw won't

and tranquilizers, but nothing seemed to help. Finally she went to the University of Kentucky's Orofacial Pain Center for help.

"I went twice a week," she says. "I practiced deep breathing and relaxation therapy. Basically, I learned to relax all of my muscles, starting with my toes and working up to my head and jaw. It really helped. I also wear a mouth guard at night to keep me from clenching, and that's helped a lot."

The most important thing, says Dorothy, was learning to let go of stress—stress that kept her teeth clenched and her jaw sore. Now she takes short breaks several times a day. She stretches the muscles in her neck and face. She takes some deep breaths. She calms down. "If I start to tense up when I'm teaching, I will stop and relax a little bit," she says. "I'm much more conscious than I used to be of what the muscles are doing."

Dorothy still has days when moving her jaw, in French *or* English, is slightly painful. But usually it's under control—if she pays attention to what her jaw is telling her. "I find that if I take the time to be aware of what my body is doing, the mind will slow down a little bit, too."

relax unless you do. (For tips on controlling stress, see "Stress" on page 472).

Stop the grind. Some people go to sleep every night, but their *jaws* go back to the same old grind—literally. Nightly teeth grinding, called bruxism, is one of the most common dental problems, and it very frequently contributes to TMD, Dr. Leibsohn says. How can you tell if you're a teeth grinder? One way is to ask your spouse. Or if you wake up every morning with a sore jaw, there's a good chance your jaw is getting less rest than you are. Ask your dentist to take a look. He may recommend that you wear a mouth guard at night to give your jaw a rest.

Lay on the heat. As with any joint injury, applying heat will help increase blood flow, which in turn can help speed the healing time. "I recommend that people wet a washcloth in hot water, wring it out and drape it over the joint. Then put a heating pad over that," says Dr. Leibsohn. He recommends that you apply the heat for up to 20 to 25 minutes at a time, several times throughout the day.

Or put it on ice. While heat is good for long-term pain, you need cold to treat sudden injuries. When you've taken a crack on the jaw—in a car accident, for example, or from a wayward baseball during a Little League game—you want to ice it down, Dr. Greene says. Several times over the course of a day, fill a washcloth with ice cubes and lay it gently on the joint, holding it in place for 10 to 15 minutes. This can help prevent pain and swelling from getting started. After 24 hours, switch to heat for quick-healing relief.

Don't do a Dagwood. In the comic strip "Blondie," Dagwood Bumstead is always wrapping his mouth around triple-decker sandwiches. Clearly, Dagwood *doesn't* have TMD—yet. But pushing your jaw to extremes isn't such a hot idea if you wish to avoid TMD. If you have TMD, making like Dagwood can only make things worse. And if you are prone to gaping yawns, "put one hand under your chin, so you cannot open so widely," suggests Dr. Leibsohn.

Eschew the chew. People who really give their chewing gum a good working-over are likely candidates for TMD, Dr. Leibsohn says. To give your jaw a break, give up the gum. While you're at it, take that pencil out of your mouth, and quit propping the telephone on your shoulder. "These are things that fatigue muscles and can cause neck pain and jaw pain," he says.

Postpone the phone. "If you're one of those people who chats on the phone for 4 hours a night, you're not going to get better," Dr. Greene says. Besides, this might be a good time to polish your writing skills!

BEYOND SELF-HELP

Even though some nine out of ten people with TMD will never need medical treatment, others aren't so lucky, Dr. Greene says. For example, a little stiffness, clicking and popping may slowly progress to excruciating pain. Or perhaps a car accident rearranges the joint in an instant. Or rheumatoid arthritis settles in and causes long-term damage.

Let's say you've always had clicking, and suddenly there's no clicking anymore—because you can't move your jaw. When this happens, you may feel like the Tin Man in *The Wizard of Oz*—before Dorothy came along. Forget the oil can; you need a doctor. Something in your joint—usually the disk—must have shifted.

In some cases, if the joint isn't seriously damaged, chances are that you can be treated with a variety of conservative therapies, says Dr. Greene. These may include anti-inflammatory and muscle relaxant medications, physical therapy treatments, stress management counseling and, in some cases, a plastic splint to wear inside the mouth. This may be all you need to relieve your symptoms and to protect your jaw from further damage.

Unfortunately, not all TMD is so easily treated. Sometimes, if there's been serious damage or degeneration of the jaw, surgery may be needed. Twenty years ago, surgery on the temporomandibular joint was a major proposition, requiring large incisions and plenty of time. It wasn't uncommon for people to spend the better part of a week in the hospital. Surgeons still use open-jaw surgery for some procedures, but more often today, they use a technique called arthroscopy.

With arthroscopy—*arthro-* means "joint," and *-scopy* means "to see"—surgeons can insert lights, scalpels, even video cameras into the joint through an incision that can be smaller in diameter than a pencil. Because there isn't a large, gaping incision to recover from, some people can have the surgery in the morning and return home the same afternoon, says Dr. Greene.

Sometimes an even more conservative procedure may be appropriate, says Dr. Greene. In these cases, the doctor inserts a needle inside the joint to inject fluid that cleans out toxic debris and restores normal motion. This can be done in the doctor's office.

TENDINITIS

A h, spring! Blue skies, warm days and the basketball court all to yourself. You haven't played since high school, yet you pause, just for a moment, to savor the roars of an imaginary crowd: "He has the ball . . . he's going in for the lay-up . . . ladies and gentlemen . . . he's unstoppable!"

Then the day after your moment of glory . . . "Ohhh!" you moan. "Tendinitis—and right after the first game of the season, too!"

You don't have to be a hot-dog basketball player to get tendinitis, a painful inflammation of the tendons that anchor muscle to bone throughout your body. You don't even need a vivid imagination. "If you're physically active, it will crop up sometimes. Tendinitis is very common," says Clifton S. Mereday, Ph.D., chairman of the physical therapy program at State University of New York at Stony Brook.

Tendinitis occurs when stress—either from sudden injuries or, more often, from repetitive overuse—creates microscopic tears in the tendon's muscular fibers. "This causes inflammation, because inflammation is the first step in how the body tries to heal itself," says Joseph D. Zuckerman, M.D., vice chairman of the Department of Orthopedic Surgery and chief of the shoulder service at the Hospital for Joint Diseases Orthopaedic Institute in New York City. "You see it in many people who go out and play basketball or tennis over the weekend and come back with this very painful shoulder."

Indeed, our hardworking shoulders are common sites for tendinitis. So are tendons in the hips, elbows and ankles. "Your muscles and tendons are used to functioning at a certain level, and if you *exceed* that level, you're going to injure them," Dr. Zuckerman says. "To prevent tendinitis," he adds, it's better to go through a gradual training process to increase muscular strength and tendon flexibility."

EXTENDIN' TENDONS

It takes just a little preparation to prevent tendinitis from cramping *your* game. For starters:

Stretch it out. "If your muscles are so tight that they won't permit you to have the motion that you need, you're going to end up pulling or tearing the tendon," says physical therapist Jill N. Samuels, assistant director of East Side Sports Physical Therapy in New York City. "Before you do any kind of activity, you need to stretch. I recommend that people hold the stretch for 20 seconds and repeat it three times."

To help prevent tennis elbow, for example, you need to stretch your forearm muscles. "If you have a table in front of you, put your hands down, elbows straight, and lean forward—that will stretch the undersurface of your forearm," Samuels says. To stretch the other side, just extend your arm straight in front of you and bend the palm down.

Runners and long-distance walkers sometimes have trouble with the Achilles tendon at the back of the heel. To stretch it, lean against a wall with one leg forward and bent and the other leg back and straight. Keep both feet flat on the floor and facing in the same direction. Or stand on a step with your toes near the edge and your heels hanging over the edge. Slowly lower your heels until they are lower than your toes.

Your legs require special care, especially the hamstring tendons at the back of the thighs. "People often pull the hamstring tendons," Samuels says. "A lot of people touch their toes to stretch their hamstrings, but that isn't very effective. Better is to put the foot to be stretched on something (a bench, a step) at waist level and slowly lean forward, lowering your chest toward your thigh."

Take things slowly. "If you want to play serious tennis for an hour and a half, you should work up to it," Dr. Zuckerman advises. In other words, don't start the day with a competitive match. Lob it back and forth for a while. Practice some gentle rallies. *Then* you can work on that perfect passing shot.

DOUSING THE PAIN

When you do get tendinitis, the first thing you need is some downtime to give the tendon a chance to heal. "In the vast majority of cases, once you take it easy and quit doing things that hurt, tendinitis will get better on its own," says Dr. Zuckerman. Dr. Mereday adds, "When it stops hurting so much, that's when you should start stretching and exercising to help it heal." But first:

Quell the swelling. One of the most effective ways to reduce inflammation is to take aspirin or ibuprofen, Dr. Zuckerman says. For more serious cases, your doctor may recommend that you take prescription anti-inflammatory drugs, such as naproxen or indomethacin.

Pack it in ice. Ice has two effects, Dr. Zuckerman says. "It causes the blood vessels to clamp down, and that decreases swelling." It also helps with pain. To be most effective, however, ice should be applied soon after the injury and *before* the swelling starts. Apply for 20 to 30 minutes several times a day. Don't put the ice right on your skin, though—use an ice pack or washcloth.

Follow cold with heat. "Heat tends to increase the blood supply, which helps with healing," Dr. Zuckerman says. But heat should only be used after the initial swelling has gone down—usually within two or three days. At that point, "I often tell patients to use a combination: ice for 10 to 15 minutes, then a heating pad for 10 to 15 minutes."

Rub it down. As with heat, massage can help increase blood flow to inflamed tendons. A cross-friction massage—rubbing the area with a washcloth or other coarse material—can help break up adhesions and collagen formations that may eventually prevent the tendons from moving freely, says Dr. Zuckerman.

Fill the whirlpool. Essentially a whirlpool works like a relaxing whole-body massage. "By increasing blood flow, it helps clear out waste products such as lactic acid and brings in nutrients to the injured area, which speeds up healing," Samuels says.

Stretch away. When the pain begins to fade, start doing some gentle stretches and exercises. Tendons that aren't used after injuries can quickly lose mobility, says Dr. Mereday. "You want to make sure your range of motion is maintained."

THROAT INFECTIONS

A ll kinds of things—like shouting "Hang the ref!" at a ball game or singing (loudly and poorly) "O Sole Mio"—can give you a sore throat. It doesn't mean that you have an infection every time your throat aches. On the other hand, sometimes an aching throat means exactly that.

Throat infections warrant special concern—and special care. One type of infection, strep throat, is caused by a bacterium. If untreated, strep throat can lead to problems like rheumatic fever and rheumatic heart disease, a potentially deadly inflammation of the heart valves. Another kind of throat infection is tonsillitis, which may be caused by a bacterium or a virus. If left to fester, tonsillitis can dole out pain as often and as regularly as Old Faithful spits steam.

The symptoms of both of these infections are similar—soreness, inflammation and pain, which is why you can't diagnose them yourself. So see your doctor without delay if you develop these symptoms.

HOCUS-POCUS STREPTOCOCCUS

Streptococcus here, streptococcus there, streptococcus everywhere! Where would we be without strep? Probably in much better health. Strep's accomplishments in making us sick are legion: One kind infects the urinary tract, another causes bacterial pneumonia, yet another makes teeth decay. And then there's *Streptococcus pyogenes,* the cause of tens of millions of sore throats each year.

How can you tell if there's a strep infection in you or your child's sore throat? The first clue is the age of the sufferer. "Generally, the people most at risk for strep throat are children between the ages of 3 and 12 years old," says Michael Gerber, M.D., associate professor of pediatrics and director of the Division of Pediatric Infectious Diseases at the University of Connecticut School of Medicine. "It's unusual for a child under 3 to get one and even less common after age 12." For adults, the condition is rare.

Strep is worse than most sore throats. "The pain is significant, especially in swallowing," says Dr. Gerber. And in addition to a sore throat, you'll likely notice other symptoms, such as swollen lymph glands in the neck and fever. You may also have a headache, abdominal pain, nausea or vomiting. Generally, you *won't* have coughing, hoarseness, runny nose or sneezing (as you might with a cold or flu bug), says Dr. Gerber.

If you suspect strep, see your doctor or pediatrician. A simple throat culture can identify the bacteria. Once a strep infection is identified, your

THE FRIENDLY FIRE OF RHEUMATIC FEVER

You've survived the sore throat, fever and swollen glands of a strep throat. And now you're back in gear. You're back at work, doing your chores, making runs to the butcher, the baker, the candlestick maker.

But yesterday you had a sharp pain in your side—for a minute there you thought you had appendicitis—and today you seem to be coming down with the flu: Your body's heating up, and the joints in your knees, ankles, elbows and wrists all seem to be taking turns aching, one after the other.

What's going on?

If you had a strep throat within the past few weeks, a good guess might be that you're experiencing the "friendly fire" of rheumatic fever, says Alan L. Bisno, M.D., professor of medicine at the University of Miami and chief of medicine at Miami's Veterans Hospital.

No one knows exactly what causes rheumatic fever, he adds, but scientists suspect that the immune system warrior that shot down your strep throat bug a few weeks back is now shooting out your joints. And although the warrior is a friend, the result of his friendly fire is an inflammation wherever he shoots.

The inflammation in your knees isn't going to hurt you beyond a few aches and pains, explains Dr. Bisno. But if that immune system warrior decides to take a shot at your heart, you could be in a whole heap of trouble.

"We say that rheumatic fever licks the joints but bites the heart," says Dr. Bisno. That's because the aggravation to your joints goes away, but the heart can suffer permanent damage. Forty to 50 percent of those who develop rheumatic fever will go on to develop inflammation of the heart that can flare into a major conflagration at any time. And the resultant fire damage around your heart valves can

doctor can help you knock it out with antibiotics. Caution, however: Antibiotics are effective only if given time to work, says Pat Gilmer, M.D., an ear, nose and throat specialist with the University of Oklahoma Health Sciences Center in Oklahoma City. People taking antibiotics often feel so much better in a day or so that they're tempted to not take the full supply. But if you don't take *all* the medication, the strep throat can develop into an even more serious infection. Or the bug can come back and get you again in a few days, says Dr. Gilmer.

cause heart failure during the initial bout of rheumatic fever, during a subsequent recurrence or—without any warning symptoms at all—even ten years down the line. There's no way to predict when or if it will happen.

One thing doctors can predict is that unfortunately, once you've had rheumatic fever, you're more prone to get it again. Scientists aren't sure why, says Dr. Bisno, but they suspect that people who develop rheumatic fever to begin with may have a genetic predisposition to an immune system that first attacks the strep and then turns and attacks its host.

That's why even after massive doses of aspirin have doused the initial inflammation, your doctor will probably put you on continuous antibiotics for a good chunk of your life. Your doctor may prescribe a shot every four weeks or pills every day.

How long must you stay on antibiotics? That depends, says Dr. Bisno.

Some people stay on antibiotics their entire lives. Others, depending on their age and occupation, might not. Older folks, for example, seem to run into fewer strep bugs than kids. So unless they're working around kids all the time—as a schoolteacher, perhaps, or a nurse—they might at some point be able to discontinue medication. It's a gamble and a guess. But it's the best way to protect your heart once the disease develops.

To reduce the odds that you'll develop rheumatic fever to begin with, says Dr. Bisno, promptly treat every strep infection with antibiotics. You can't go running to the doctor for a strep test every time you have a sore throat, of course. But whenever you have a sore throat and fever without any other symptoms—no runny nose, no sneezes and coughs—go and get the test, says Dr. Bisno. A sore throat that occurs by itself and not as part of a group of symptoms could very well be strep.

TONSILLITIS: YOU DON'T NEED THIS

Tonsils are made to get infected. These two roundish glands in the back of the throat spend the first few years of your life trapping incoming germs and developing antibodies to help you fight future infections. But the tonsils' usefulness wears off at about age three.

In many people, the tonsils keep right on trapping germs and getting infected. Tonsils attract both viruses and bacteria (including strep), and you can see the results with a flashlight—swelling and sometimes a white coating. Infected tonsils cause pain, fever and swollen glands. You may also have bad breath and recurrent ear problems as the infection travels upward along the eustachian tubes.

Short of surgery, there's no realistic way to prevent tonsillitis, says Barry C. Baron, M.D., associate clinical professor of otolaryngology at the University of California, San Francisco, Medical Center and an otolaryngologist (ear and throat doctor) in private practice at the California Pacific

---

TREATMENT BREAKTHROUGH

ATTACK ON THE M PROTEIN

A vaccine for strep throat may be in the making. "We're much closer than we've ever been," says Michael Gerber, M.D., associate professor of pediatrics and director of the Division of Pediatric Infectious Diseases at the University of Connecticut School of Medicine. Scientists are discovering the genetic building blocks of the M protein—a part of the strep bacteria that shields it from the human body's protective white blood cells.

Adults don't get strep throat nearly as often as children do, and that may be the key to a successful vaccine. Researchers at Rockefeller University figured that repeated exposure to the strep bacteria in childhood protects adults against later infections. Over time, they reasoned, adults build up antibodies that can deal with the M protein and cut through it to clobber the strep. The researchers concocted a vaccine designed to slice through the M protein and tried it on mice. The vaccinated mice didn't get strep throat; they developed antibodies that overcame the strep bacteria, M protein and all.

This means that instead of having to build up immunity gradually, people may someday be able to get a vaccine that immunizes them against strep. Perhaps strep throat will even become a thing of the past. "I think we'll see a strep vaccine for human use available in the near future," says Dr. Gerber.

Medical Center in San Francisco. If strep is the cause of tonsillitis, antibiotics can knock it out. But if your tonsils are swollen due to a viral illness, "only time will provide a cure," says Dr. Baron.

Many people suffer repeated bouts of tonsillitis. The infections may never be totally cured with antibiotics, leading to symptoms that bounce back. For these people—anyone with four or more bouts of tonsillitis a year—surgery is the best treatment, says Dr. Baron. More than 400,000 tonsillectomies are performed every year. That is not as many as in pre-antibiotic days but is a number that attests to the operation's success.

One study showed that children who have their tonsils removed actually have improved health and no impairment of their immunity. Adults, too, are good candidates for tonsillectomy. The operation is usually fairly simple, and you may be discharged the same day. You'll never suffer tonsillitis again.

AN INFECTED THROAT'S ANTIDOTES

For strep throat or tonsillitis, you can help ease your discomfort and speed your recovery by following these suggestions from the experts.

Stay in bed. Bed rest is a key part of treatment, at least at the peak of your misery, says Dr. Gilmer. Kids should stay home from school to avoid spreading the infection to classmates.

Drink lots of fluids. They can soothe your raw throat. Warm tea with honey is good. Stay away from acidic drinks like citrus juices, which can irritate a sensitive throat.

Gargle with warm saltwater. One-quarter teaspoon of salt in 1/2 cup of warm water matches the natural moisture, salt and temperature balance of your throat. Gargle every hour or so.

Take a painkiller. Aspirin, ibuprofen (Advil, Motrin) or acetaminophen (Tylenol, Anacin-3) will help reduce your pain to tolerable levels, says Dr. Gerber. Aspirin should not be given to children with the flu because of the risk of Reye's syndrome, a life-threatening neurological disease. It's safe, however, for strep throat. That's another reason to see a doctor to make sure it really is strep.

Build up a head of steam. Humidifiers and vaporizers can moisten and soothe the inflamed, dry throat that accompanies a strep infection. Or try filling your washbowl with hot water, draping a towel over your head to catch the steam and inhaling for a few minutes.

Give your throat a spray or a suck. Over-the-counter throat sprays and lozenges, such as Chloraseptic and Sucrets, have ingredients that temporarily deaden pain, says Dr. Gerber. Stay away from products that contain aspirin, because aspirin taken this way can irritate an already inflamed throat.

THYROID DISEASE

Butterfly-shaped and wrapped around your windpipe just below the Adam's apple, the thyroid gland weighs less than an ounce. But its hormones, especially thyroxin, are vital to your physical and mental health. Your metabolism, heartbeat, body temperature, digestion and even how you think depend on the hormones secreted by the thyroid.

When your thyroid isn't working right, you feel it. If it's too slow—a condition called hypothyroidism—you feel like you've taken the world's best sleeping pill. If it's too fast—a condition called hyperthyroidism—you feel like you just drank 20 cups of espresso. Fortunately, "almost anything that goes wrong with the thyroid is reversible," says Edward Ruby, M.D., assistant professor of medicine at Thomas Jefferson University Hospital in Philadelphia.

HYPOTHYROIDISM

The easiest type of thyroid disease to reverse is hypothyroidism—which is lucky for the five million afflicted Americans, most of whom, for unknown reasons, are women. The trick is to know you have it. Even doctors are sometimes fooled. "It's not the kind of thing where you wake up one day and say 'I'm really sick,'" Dr. Ruby says. "Hypothyroidism comes on very subtly and gradually, over months or even years, so you and your doctor may attribute the symptoms to aging. One of the symptoms is the accumulation of fluid under the eyes, and I've even known some patients who had cosmetic surgery to get rid of the bags when in fact they had hypothyroidism."

Another risk is being diagnosed as having a mental illness. Undoubtedly, some patients in mental institutions actually have hypothyroidism, says Dr. Ruby. They may be seen as depressed, or even as mentally retarded, because the disease causes mental sluggishness.

Many cases of hypothyroidism are caused by an autoimmune disease. The immune system makes antibodies that mistakenly attack and damage thyroid cells. No one knows why this happens, but the condition tends to run in families, so genetics seems to play a role. As time goes on, the constantly inflamed thyroid is less and less able to make enough hormone. The symptoms may barely be noticeable at first and are easy to attribute to other conditions. Symptoms include constant fatigue, weak or aching muscles, heightened sensitivity to cold, constipation, weight gain even when eating less, and an inability to concentrate.

GIVING YOUR THYROID A BOOST

A blood test called a TSH (thyroid-stimulating hormone) test will tell you if you have a thyroid problem or not. Should your problem be hypothyroidism, "treating it is fairly easy," Dr. Ruby says. "You just replace what's missing—thyroxin. You take a little hormone pill once a day for the rest of your life."

Thyroid hormone replacement is fairly safe, but the dosage has to be considered carefully. "There's a risk in building up the hormone levels in the blood too quickly, which can lead to hyperthyroidism," says Dr. Ruby.

Again, it's the highly accurate TSH test that helps pinpoint the optimum dose. Your doctor will measure your TSH level to make sure you're getting just the right amount of hormone.

HYPERTHYROIDISM

George and Barbara Bush are only two of the estimated two million Americans with overactive thyroids. Hyperthyroidism is also an immune system disorder, but instead of the thyroid shutting down, it churns out too much hormone.

Common symptoms of hyperthyroidism include bulging eyes, frequent loose stools, heightened sensitivity to heat, excessive sweating, weight loss without dieting, fatigue and muscle weakness, insomnia, hand tremors and nervousness and irritability that, Dr. Ruby says, "can approach mania." Most seriously, hyperthyroidism can cause very dangerous rapid and irregular heartbeats.

COOLING DOWN YOUR THYROID

Treating hyperthyroidism "is a different kettle of fish," Dr. Ruby says. "It's more difficult to plan the therapy." Much depends on how severe the disorder is and how it's affecting your heart.

If you're not in imminent danger of a heart attack, radioactive iodine treatment "is the easiest, safest and most common treatment for hyperthyroidism," says Dr. Ruby. Radioactive iodine treatment takes advantage of the thyroid gland's natural affinity for iodine. You drink a solution of radioactive iodine, which then makes a beeline for the thyroid. There, over the next 12 weeks, the radioactivity destroys the hormone-producing cells. This treatment has been used for 40 years, says Dr. Ruby.

Some doctors prefer to give just enough radioactive iodine to get the thyroid gland back to normal, but judging that exact dosage can be difficult. Other doctors prefer to give enough iodine to wipe out the thyroid altogether. Of course, once your thyroid is destroyed, you become hypothyroid (and then must take that little hormone pill once a day).

The radioactive iodine treatment is effective 80 percent of the time on the first try, Dr. Ruby says. Half of the successful treatments return overactive thyroids to normal; the other half create hypothyroidism. In 20 percent of the cases, the person needs more treatment.

Drug treatment is an option, but the most common drugs used, methimazole and propylthiouracil, have two major shortcomings: Some people get rashes or hives, and the drugs take time to work. Some people are so at risk from a rapid heart rate that it's dangerous to wait for these drugs to work alone, says Dr. Ruby. Other medications such as propranolol and sodium iodide have to be added.

Surgery—"a last resort"—removes 90 to 95 percent of the thyroid gland, says Dr. Ruby. Usually the goal is to return hormone levels to normal. It shows how overactive a thyroid gland can be when 95 percent is surgically removed, yet hormone production becomes normal.

DISEASE
FREE

TIC DOULOUREUX

People with tic douloureux say it's the worst pain they've ever had. Women, who make up a slight majority of the sufferers, say the pain is even worse than childbirth. "One of my patients said it was like a firecracker going off inside her cheek," says Gerhard H. Fromm, M.D., professor of neurology at the University of Pittsburgh School of Medicine.

It's no wonder this condition is painful. The source of the pain is the same nerve that controls touch and pain in the teeth, tongue, gums, jaw and the entire face. This nerve, called the trigeminal nerve, gives the disorder its official name, trigeminal neuralgia. The pain gives it its common name—*douloureux* is French for "painful." *Tic douloureux* means "painful twitch." Even the slightest stimulation to the face—shaving, talking, a smile, a frown, a kiss, a soft breeze, a hot or cold beverage or brushing the teeth—can set off that firecracker.

Despite its intensity, however, the pain of tic douloureux is almost always completely manageable. Although there are no home remedies, there are several good medical options available to you and your doctor.

A CURSE OF THE AGED

Tic douloureux has a distinctive signature that goes beyond facial pain. It's highly associated with aging, the pain has a hair trigger, it comes and goes, and it tends to get worse over time.

The trigeminal nerve emerges from the brain at the back of the skull, and that's where the problem starts. "A blood vessel may begin pressing on the nerve, and that can cause the pain," says Dr. Fromm. Why does it happen? No one knows for sure, but aging plays a major role. As we grow older, hardening blood vessels lose their flexibility; and women especially are prone to osteoporosis, which can soften the skull bones, allowing the skull to settle from its own weight. The bottom line: The trigeminal nerve can get squashed by blood vessel and bone.

Each year, about 11,000 Americans get their first attack. Most tend to be 50 years or older. Normally the pain flashes through just one side of the face like a bolt of lightning and lasts 1 or 2 minutes. Months may pass without another attack, but the victim lives in perpetual fear of another onslaught. As time passes, the disorder progresses. Attacks grow more frequent and more painful and involve wider areas of the face.

Those with tic douloureux have a difficult time living normal lives and may have to quit their jobs. The pain and fear can play havoc with marital relations—a kiss can cause intense pain. Brushing the teeth, let alone visits to the dentist, are out—so teeth and gums may deteriorate. "It's the kind of disease that won't kill you, but it at times makes you feel like you want to die," says Claire Patterson, former sufferer and founder of the Trigeminal Neuralgia Association.

PROFILE IN HEALING

CLAIRE PATTERSON: SURGERY TOOK AWAY THE PAIN

One morning in 1978, while putting on her makeup, "I felt a little electric shock at the end of my nose," recalls Claire Patterson. It was the first symptom of what turned out to be trigeminal neuralgia—tic douloureux. There began a nine-year saga of pain and medication, more pain and more medication and a gradual worsening of the condition.

When it was bad, "my husband couldn't even kiss me on the cheek, or I'd be on the floor in agony," Claire says. "I kept working, I was functional, though I don't know how I did it, because the side effects from the medication were terrible." In her career in public relations and fund-raising, she had to have her wits about her, but the drugs she was given to control the disease made her drowsy and confused. "Even when the pain would disappear for days, I was always on a tightrope, wondering if I would get an attack while making a presentation," she says. "Just when you think it's gone, it comes back."

Each time a remission ended, the pain would return worse and more widespread. "In the final year, I was having attacks even from swallowing," she says. By the summer of 1987, she was on three drugs to control the attacks and wound up in the hospital emergency room with a toxic reaction. The only option left was surgery. At the

CONQUERING THE PAIN

Back around the middle of the 1800s, a doctor wrote that tic douloureux attacks reminded him of epileptic seizures in their abruptness, intensity and brevity. So when the first epilepsy drug, phenytoin (Dilantin), came along in the 1940s, doctors tried it on tic douloureux. It worked. People quickly become resistant to Dilantin, however. (It also has some strong side effects, including fatigue and rashes.) Currently, carbamazepine (Tegretol) is the most prescribed drug. It's often given along with baclofen (Lioresal), a drug developed by Dr. Fromm and his team at the University of Pittsburgh.

Your nerves have a feedback system, kind of like the heating system in your house. When the temperature reaches a certain point, a thermostat cuts off the heat. "The drugs work the same way—when an impulse to the nerve reaches a certain point, the drugs cut off sensitivity before the impulse becomes painful," says Dr. Fromm.

University of Pittsburgh Presbyterian Hospital Medical Center, neurosurgeon Peter Jannetta, M.D., was pioneering microvascular decompression—brain surgery to separate the offending blood vessel from the trigeminal nerve.

"He found that my cerebral artery was wrapped around the nerve," Claire says. "It was like a telephone switchboard up there." At 50 years old and in good health, she was a good candidate for the surgery—and she came through with flying colors. "I was out of bed in 24 hours and home in six days, and I haven't had an attack since," she says. It took a while for her to relax and know everything was going to be all right—to know that brushing her teeth or kissing her husband wouldn't trigger excruciating pain.

Claire founded the Trigeminal Neuralgia Association to provide emotional support for those with the disease and to let them know what their options are. "They have to know that they're not malingerers, not complainers, not wimps," she says. "The disease disrupts your entire life—people have to quit their jobs, their marriages suffer, and they live in constant fear of an attack, so they can't plan anything." But as Claire discovered after nine long years—it doesn't have to be that way.

She says that others can contact the association by writing to the Trigeminal Neuralgia Association, P.O. Box 785, Barnegat Light, NJ 08006.

For most people, the drugs kill the pain within two days. Only 5 to 10 percent of people don't respond or can't tolerate the side effects, which, for the newer drugs, may include dizziness, drowsiness or nausea. (Tegretol also stands accused of lowering white blood cell counts. This would happen very rarely, but your doctor should regularly check your blood.) "After you're pain-free for a time, you may be able to cut back on the dosage or quit the medication altogether," says Dr. Fromm. But while you're on the drugs, it's essential that you take them as prescribed and communicate with your doctor about the side effects and the pain relief. The goal should be to keep the dosage as low as possible.

THE SURGICAL SOLUTION

For the small number of people who can't be helped by medication, there are two highly effective surgical techniques available—the success rate of either is approximately 80 percent.

One procedure, called radio-frequency rhizotomy, takes place just beneath the skin. The surgeon cauterizes the small roots of the trigeminal nerve. Injections of glycerol—a type of alcohol—can also do the job. The goal is to slightly damage the trigeminal nerve's pain fibers without harming the touch fibers. You're out of the hospital in a couple of days, free of pain. "But this treatment doesn't really clear it up permanently," Dr. Fromm cautions. "The pain is apt to return eventually." Because of this, the treatment is usually best for people who are unable, because of health or age, to undergo major surgery.

"Major surgery" is the procedure called microvascular decompression, involving a week-long hospital stay. Although the risks are greater, so are the results, Dr. Fromm says. Using microscopes and miniature instruments, the surgeon goes into the skull and moves the offending blood vessel away from the nerve.

The key to successful surgery—any kind, but especially the more involved surgery—is a highly skilled, highly experienced surgeon. "Be sure to get a surgeon who has done a lot of these operations," Dr. Fromm advises. "One or two a year isn't enough."

For a very few, probably around 10 percent, even microvascular decompression won't work. The last resort is neuronectomy—the actual cutting of the trigeminal nerve's pain fibers, causing permanent loss of sensation in the face and mouth.

TOXIC SHOCK SYNDROME

I n 1980, the federal Centers for Disease Control (CDC) in Atlanta began receiving reports of a mysterious, sometimes deadly disease striking hundreds of women. The women, investigators soon learned, had several things in common. Most were between the ages of 18 and 52. Most were having their periods when they became ill. And most were using high-absorbency tampons.

Experts called the disease toxic shock syndrome. While not a new disease, investigators eventually linked the sudden outbreak of cases to the use of high-absorbency tampons and especially to one particular brand of super-absorbent tampon. In fact, when these super-absorbent tampons were removed from the market, the incidence of toxic shock syndrome declined as quickly as it had appeared. But it has not disappeared.

What is this dangerous disease, and what does it have to do with tampons?

A SHOCK TO THE SYSTEM

Toxic shock syndrome occurs when a strain of staphylococcus bacteria—or, more precisely, poisons produced by staph—gets inside the body. It may follow skin infections, childbirth or surgical procedures, but in a majority of cases, it gets in through the vagina—usually during menstruation when tampons are used.

In the early stages, toxic shock syndrome may cause fever, vomiting, diarrhea and muscle aches, says Ken Zangwill, M.D., a medical epidemiologist at the CDC. Without medical attention, however, toxic shock syndrome can be, quite literally, toxic. Approximately 6 percent of these cases are fatal, says Dr. Zangwill.

The bacteria that cause toxic shock are common. "Staph may be found on the skin, in the nose and throat and in other mucous membranes," says

Dr. Zangwill. It's not entirely clear why staph infections, which usually are mild, will on occasion produce toxic shock syndrome.

The link with menstruation isn't entirely clear either, Dr. Zangwill says. It's possible that tampons, by drying the inside of the vagina, create a favorable environment for staph. It has also been suggested that inserting and removing tampons may very slightly damage the vaginal lining. "This could potentially allow the organism to penetrate and get into the body," says Dr. Zangwill.

REDUCING THE RISKS

Though toxic shock syndrome can be extremely serious, the risks of actually getting it are extremely low, says Dr. Zangwill. "Toxic shock is a rare disease, even among tampon users."

To lower the risks still further:

Abandon tampons. Since toxic shock syndrome usually occurs in tampon users, switching to sanitary napkins—which don't irritate the vagina—will help prevent it. Even using tampons less often can help, says Dr. Zangwill. For example, some women use tampons during the day, then switch to sanitary napkins at night.

Avoid "super" tampons. According to the CDC, each 1-gram increase in tampon absorbency increases the risk for toxic shock by 37 percent. In other words, a "super" tampon that absorbs 9 grams of fluid can be *111 percent* more risky than a "slender," which absorbs no more than 6 grams. Doctors recommend women use the least absorbent tampon that still is adequate for their needs.

The Food and Drug Administration requires tampon manufacturers to list absorbency ranges on the outside of packages. If you're not sure which tampons are right for you, ask your doctor or pharmacist for help.

ACTION ALERT

If you do suspect toxic shock, fast action can be a lifesaver. That's why it's so important to watch out for symptoms. If while menstruating you have a high fever (more than 102°F) and are vomiting and having diarrhea, remove the tampon and see your doctor *immediately.*

Toxic shock syndrome always requires hospitalization, Dr. Zangwill says. Since the disease usually is accompanied by severe fluid losses through vomiting and diarrhea, most people will require fluid replacement therapy. They'll also get antibiotics.

When leaving the hospital, most people take with them a 10- to 14-day supply of antibiotics. After two weeks, the infection—and the danger—should be gone.

TRAVELER'S DIARRHEA

Have you ever spent an entire vacation waltzing from toilet to toilet? Even seasoned travelers get traveler's diarrhea. Why, even Peace Corps workers, who are used to living in remote, far-off places, have frequent bouts with it. But Peace Corps volunteers typically spend months in foreign countries—they have time to be sick *and* do their jobs. On the other hand, tourists like you usually only have a week or two to explore a foreign land—that's about the same amount of time it takes to shake off a good bout of this affliction. The last thing you want to do is spend your precious, hard-earned vacation days getting acquainted with hotel plumbing!

While there's no way to guarantee you won't spend at least a few hours—or maybe even a few days—requesting a seat near the rest room, there's no reason that traveler's diarrhea should hold you hostage there. Prevention is a matter of recognizing unfriendly invaders.

GETTING A RAW DEAL

Traveler's diarrhea can be caused by viruses and parasites, but more often the villains are bacteria, says Herbert L. DuPont, M.D., professor of medical sciences and director of the Center for Infectious Diseases at the University of Texas Medical School and School of Public Health at Houston. Make that *hungry* bacteria. They live everywhere—on tables, floors and kitchen counters—and they flock to any meats, sauces and vegetables that happen to be nearby. They're especially partial to raw foods and water and just about anything served at room temperature.

Those appetizing hot salsas that commonly grace tables in certain southern climates, for example, are popular gathering spots for germs, Dr. DuPont says. Exposed to room temperatures for hours at a time, they provide bacteria a perfect environment in which to live, prosper, breed and produce their toxins. With every tacoful of sauce you eat, a few thousand—

or a few million—organisms with names like *Escherichia coli,* shigella and salmonella get a free ride to your insides. Some burrow into the delicate lining of your intestines. Others may produce a poison that makes you sick. In either case, your gastrointestinal tract doesn't take kindly to this intrusion. After a few hours (or perhaps a few days), you get the message that an eviction is in the works. And that's when you get diarrhea.

PREVENTIVE MEDICINE: WHEN IT'S NOT A GOOD IDEA

Doctors have long known that antibiotics such as doxycycline, trimethoprim and norfloxacin can *prevent* traveler's diarrhea. In fact, researchers have found that these antibiotics, taken for the duration of your trip, can prevent the problem in as many as nine out of ten people.

But many doctors are reluctant to prescribe antibiotics solely as a preventive for traveler's diarrhea. Why?

For one thing, antibiotics are only effective against bacteria; they're useless against viruses or parasites. All three organisms can cause diarrhea, but there's no telling which one is likely to get you.

And when it comes to killing bacteria, antibiotics aren't 100 percent effective; some survivors will invariably remain. So even though you might not get sick right away, these hardy few will lie in wait in your gut, multiplying rapidly and biding their time. Then weeks or even months later, they might attack with a vengeance.

Finally, antibiotics carry side effects. Some types can make you extremely sensitive to sunlight—risky business for vacationers headed for the sun. They can also cause allergic reactions. Some types can stain children's teeth.

"Generally, it's better to avoid drugs until you actually get sick," says Herbert L. DuPont, M.D., an infectious disease specialist at the University of Texas Medical School and School of Public Health at Houston. "When traveler's diarrhea does strike, *then* take an antibiotic. You should start feeling better within a day."

Occasionally doctors will recommend antibiotics as a preventive for people who simply can't afford to get sick, even for a day—for example, businesspeople on a deadline, athletes traveling to a competition or those with serious health problems.

For the most part, however, doctors believe that traveler's diarrhea simply is too benign—too short-lived and free of long-term consequences—to justify even the minor risks of taking antibiotics.

IT'S ANYWHERE, IT'S EVERYWHERE

Traveler's diarrhea occurs in all parts of the world, Dr. DuPont says, although some countries are riskier than others. Bacteria flourish in regions where sanitary waste disposal, food storage and personal hygiene are less than ideal. And the less attention paid to these things, the greater your chances of getting ill.

Familiarity often confers a degree of safety. That's why you can share a meal with the local in the town you're visiting but only *you* end up with diarrhea. Their intestines consider the bacteria friendly—heck, they grew up with it. But forget about developing an immunity to the bacteria in a particular region, even if you're a seasoned traveler. Sure, people and bacteria can learn to live in peace with each other. But such relationships, like good marriages, can take a lifetime to develop. A one-week cruise in the Caribbean just won't do it.

Some people will develop diarrhea worse than others; some won't develop it at all. That's because some are more resistant to the infection than others. "If you travel to Mexico, the chance of getting traveler's diarrhea is about 40 percent," Dr. DuPont says. "If you travel to the northern Mediterranean, it's about 10 percent." Just the same, foreigners visiting the United States are also at risk. But Americans traveling in America can get it, too. This is because traveler's diarrhea is caused not only by bacteria but also by travel itself. After all, if you normally feed your intestines home cooking and then bombard them with mashed potatoes from roadside greasy spoons, they're not going to thank you for it. In addition, the stress and excitement of travel can put your bowels in an uproar. "If you travel from Houston to Philadelphia, your chances of getting sick are somewhere between 2 and 5 percent," Dr. DuPont says.

THE TRAVELER'S LITTLE BLACK BAG

For a person on the go, this urge to go can be more than a minor inconvenience. But diarrhea rarely sidelines a traveler all vacation long. Symptoms of traveler's diarrhea often abate after 24 hours. But even one day of chills, diarrhea and vomiting can feel like a very long time when time is limited. Besides, vacations are too short to spend in bed—or in the bathroom.

That's why some people opt to stop the problem even before it starts by packing an antidiarrhea arsenal along with the bathing suit and sunblock.

But preventive medication is no guarantee that you won't get sick,

MICROBES ARE FOREVER

The ancient Greeks got it when they sailed to Troy to fight for the lovely Helen. Hannibal (and his elephants) got it when they trudged across the Alps. Mr. and Mrs. Whippit got it when they honeymooned in Tijuana—and they never even left the hotel. With these odds, it seems that tomorrow's space travelers, whatever galaxy they go to, will probably get it, too. Doctors agree that traveler's diarrhea, like travel itself, probably is eternal.

"Even if you have immunity to all the bugs in your area, you won't have immunity to all the bugs in another area," says Ban Mishu, M.D., a medical epidemiologist with the federal Centers for Disease Control in Atlanta.

There was a time, soon after the first penicillins were developed, that travelers felt unassailable. Even though they couldn't avoid all the menacing organisms, they reasoned, they could bombard the most notorious—bacteria—with antibiotics. And they did. But in the long run, it didn't work. Why? Because bacteria are always changing. All the efforts that you make to protect yourself from one strain of bacteria can be canceled when the bacterium changes its coat, so to speak.

Doctors always are developing new antibiotics to destroy new strains of bacteria. But in time—a few decades, a few years or even just a few months—bacteria can mutate and become resistant to new antibodies. And scientists scurry back to the drawing board.

Even when antibiotics remain effective, they can "cause" traveler's diarrhea by skewing the balance between competing organisms, Dr. Mishu says. Twenty years ago, for example, many egg-borne infections were caused by a bug called *Salmonella typhimurium*, which made a lot of people sick. When the egg producers successfully waged war on it, people *quit* getting sick from eating contaminated eggs—for a while. Then in the early 1980s, there was a sudden increase in *another* type of bacteria, called *Salmonella enteritidis*. "Getting rid of one strain only gives another strain the opportunity to get stronger," Dr. Mishu explains.

The war between humans and microbes will never end. Bacteria change, the environment changes, *we* change. "I don't think there will ever be a time when we're risk-free, when there will be an antibiotic that will retain its potency for all the bugs it might come into contact with," says Dr. Mishu.

warn doctors. Some germs are more resistant to medications than others. If, however, you want to err on the side of caution, ask your doctor about these preventives.

Make bismuth your business. Some doctors recommend taking two tablets of Pepto-Bismol—bismuth subsalicylate—four times a day. It can be taken safely for up to three weeks of traveling. Be forewarned, however, that the drug can darken the tongue and stools. It can even cause a mild ringing in the ears, called tinnitus. These side effects should disappear when you stop taking the drug.

And don't be concerned should you run out or forget to take the drug along. It is readily available across the United States.

Bring antibiotics—just in case. Because most cases of traveler's diarrhea are caused by bacteria, an antibiotic can be an effective defensive weapon, Dr. DuPont says. But not every antibiotic will work against all bacteria. Also, drugs in foreign countries aren't always as safe as those in the United States. Before you leave, tell your doctor where you're headed. He'll do his best to prescribe an appropriate antibiotic—just in case.

Know when you can slow the flow. Drugs like Imodium A-D are the most effective agents to control diarrhea and are safe for use if you don't have more severe symptoms, such as fever or bloody stools. (In such cases, you'll need an antibiotic.)

While passing one or two soft stools may be normal for travelers, you can easily argue that even mild diarrhea is hardly the best thing for you when you're about to embark on a daylong sight-seeing trip by bus or you have only one day left for the beach. Under such circumstances, it's fine to keep diarrhea under control, says Dr. DuPont. But don't prolong the use of these drugs, because they treat only the symptoms, not the condition. Such drugs can stop diarrhea by slowing contractions in the bowel. As soon as it's convenient, doctors say, stop taking the drugs, so that nature can run its course.

Pack a water protector. Boiling is an effective way to rid water of impurities, but few have the time, place or inclination to stand watch over a pot just for a glass of water. But iodine liquid or tablets, which you can buy stateside at many pharmacies and sporting goods stores, are just as effective. Water conditions vary from place to place, so ask your doctor about any special instructions for safe water consumption.

CULINARY CAUTIONS

Of course, all the bismuth and boiling in the world won't do you a whole lot of good if you view your vacation as a no-holds-barred eating escape. Just like you, the germs that cause traveler's diarrhea have their favorite foods and hangouts. The salad bar and beach bar top the list. You can save your gut a heap of turmoil, says Dr. DuPont, by following a few simple caveats.

If you can't cook it, don't eat it. Stay away from uncooked vegetables and undercooked meats and shellfish. Most bacteria can't survive high heat, so make sure your supper arrives piping hot. If it's served at room temperature, it might not be safe. Exceptions to this might include sugary toppings and citrus fruits. Don't be afraid to pour syrup on your pancakes— "syrups and jellies are safe because of their high sugar content," Dr. DuPont says. "Citrus fruits are also safe because of their ascorbic acid content."

If you can't peel it, don't eat it. Fruits such as avocados and melons usually are safe, because bacteria can't penetrate the peel. When you throw away the peel, you toss the bacteria, too. But bacteria *can* migrate from the peel to the pulp while you skin it. To be safe, scrub the whole fruit with a mild bleach solution (ten drops of bleach per quart of water) before you peel it.

Drink only bottled beverages. Water purification systems are not as sophisticated in most countries as they are in the United States, so bottled water is quite common. Tap or stream water carries its own kinds of bacteria, viruses and parasites—*Giardia,* for example—that can cause severe diarrhea. To be safe, stick with bottled water or soft drinks, Dr. DuPont says, even for brushing your teeth. And learn to do without ice in your drinks, unless you're sure it was made from purified water.

Steer clear of street food. Those tacos, burritos and stuffed potatoes sold by those price-is-right street vendors may be easy on the pocketbook, but you may be biting off more than you bargained for. Street food is notorious for harboring diarrhea-causing organisms. While poorly maintained restaurants go out of business, street vendors simply move to another corner.

Never say "I never." Don't get overconfident, even if you've survived a dozen trips without getting sick. "You have to be as diligent on the last day of your trip as you are on the first day," warns Theresa van der Vlugt, M.D., director of medical services for the Peace Corps in Washington, D.C. "Being wise about what you put in your mouth—that's what it comes down to."

GETTING BACK ON TRACK

Prevention has its limits. Given time, even the most careful and most frequent travelers will come down with a touch of traveler's diarrhea, Dr. van der Vlugt says. At best, the biggest inconvenience will be frequent trips to the bathroom. At worst, you'll spend several days in bed. No matter how slight or severe your symptoms, doctors caution, diarrhea shouldn't be taken lightly.

The organisms that cause travelers to get diarrhea emit a toxin that can stimulate secretion of fluids in your intestines and impair absorption of fluid from the food and liquids you eat. All the water that would normally be absorbed is lost through diarrhea, and that puts you at risk for dehydration. At particular risk are young children and the elderly.

The answer?

Replace what's lost. Diarrhea, particularly prolonged bouts, can really take it out of you—literally. It's crucial to keep replacing lost fluids and minerals, Dr. DuPont says. "What we recommend is flavored mineral water and saltine crackers," he says. Drink it slowly but frequently throughout the day. The water replaces lost fluids, and the crackers are a good way to fill up on salt. Crackers are also easy on the system if your stomach is feeling upset.

Give it time—but not too much time. Doctors say that traveler's diarrhea usually is self-limiting. That is, it goes away on its own and, in most cases, is nothing to worry about. But sometimes intestinal infections can be serious. If you start noticing bloody stools, or if you feel lousy for two weeks or longer after coming home, see a doctor.

For most vacationers, traveler's diarrhea is usually nothing more than an inconvenience. If you're extremely careful—and a little bit lucky—you can often escape unscathed, Dr. van der Vlugt says. "A Peace Corps volunteer could not expect to live in a village and not acquire an illness. But tourists eating in a hotel restaurant? I see no reason why they need to be ill."

TUBERCULOSIS

T uberculosis is back.

The deadly respiratory disease that took so many lives during the first half of the 20th century was soundly trounced back when potent antibiotics were developed. Scientists now report that the disease has launched a comeback.

Its comeback, first reported in 1986, is targeting mainly older folks who had TB as children and people who have tested positive for the human immunodeficiency virus (HIV)—the virus that can lead to AIDS.

These two groups of people are particularly susceptible to TB because of their weakened immune systems, explains Jo Ellen Schweinle, M.D., an infectious diseases researcher at Yale University School of Medicine. The immune system is less effective in older people, and it's gradually being destroyed in those with HIV.

Unfortunately, adds Dr. Schweinle, since TB is transmitted by droplets of respiratory secretions exhaled by one person and inhaled by another, the increased incidence of TB puts everyone in jeopardy.

ATTACKING THE LUNGS

"Any time you have people walking around with TB, you're at risk," says Dr. Schweinle. An otherwise healthy individual inhales the TB bacteria and deposits them in his lung. His immune system goes on the alert and sends in a battalion of defensive warrior cells to do battle. If his immune system is successful, it will wall off the bacteria and prevent their spread. If it is not, the bacteria will kill the lung tissue. The spot where the bacteria landed will soften into a substance that feels like cream cheese. Eventually the spot liquefies, and the infected person coughs it up, leaving a hole where once there were healthy cells. It's not long before that "cream cheese" begins to turn the lungs into Swiss cheese.

Fortunately, the immune system still has a chance to heal the lung and plug the hole, and in most cases, doctors say, that's exactly what it does. The TB bacteria then become dormant until old age or a potent disease such as influenza, cancer or pneumonia reactivates them.

How do you know you've got TB? Unexplained fever, persistent cough, weight loss and recurrent night sweats are frequently the only clues you'll have, says George M. Lordi, M.D., an associate professor of medicine at the University of Medicine and Dentistry of New Jersey in Newark. But those symptoms—especially if you've been exposed to someone with a nagging cough—should be enough to have your doctor order a skin test, a chest x-ray and, if indicated, a microscopic examination of your sputum.

If your skin test is positive, says Dr. Lordi, your doctor should go ahead with preventive treatment *even* if your x-ray and sputum show no evidence of the disease. You have the tuberculosis infection if your skin test is positive, says Dr. Lordi. And although it may not be the active disease, it should be treated with preventive therapy now, so that it doesn't flare up in later years, when your immune system is not quite so efficient.

HEADING FOR A KNOCKOUT

No matter how tuberculosis is contracted, the disease is treatable, says Dr. Lordi. Doctors can attack the disease with a one-two punch of chemotherapy and antibiotics.

A person will usually be noninfectious 14 days after treatment begins, adds Dr. Lordi. Within two to three months, most patients will have negative sputum tests. Medication should be continued for between six and nine months, depending on response. Otherwise, the disease will reappear in a stronger and more virulent form that is harder to treat.

THE IMPORTANCE OF STRONG IMMUNITY

Fortunately, it's not all that easy to develop tuberculosis if you have a strong immune system, says Dr. Schweinle. So you should pamper your immune system. Eat right and stay calm, she advises. A balanced diet will give your immune system the nutrients it needs to stay on its toes, and staying calm will eliminate the immune-suppressing effects of stress. Dr. Schweinle says avoiding crowds will reduce your exposure to the immune-taxing infectious diseases that thrive on human sociability.

If your immune system is on the alert, chances are nine out of ten that even if you're exposed, the disease will pass you by.

ULCERS

Ulcers were once as much a mystique as they were a disease. To tell the world you had craterlike little sores in your digestive system was to say that you were a hardworking, hard-living, no-nonsense kind of person. No goofing off in your life. No, sir. You were someone with responsibilities, one who didn't shy from stress, a corporate shark in wool pinstripes.

Well, it turns out that what we once thought was so simply isn't so. Ulcers and stress have a Hollywood-style marriage: Sometimes you find them together, sometimes you don't. Some Wall Street moguls never get ulcers, while some Easy Street loafers have ulcers galore.

That's not to say that stress never plays a part in creating ulcers. It may. But as we turn to the experts for tips on beating this common ailment, it's clear that there are *many* reasons for ulcers and *many* ways to attack them.

WHO GETS THEM—AND WHY?

Anyone can get an ulcer—and about one in ten Americans does. Ulcers may form just about anywhere in the digestive system, but most commonly, they rear their ugly little heads in the duodenum, the top part of the small intestine. Your first sign of an ulcer might be a gnawing or burning pain in your upper abdomen—often when you haven't eaten for a while. The pain often subsides when you pop an antacid or grab a bite to eat.

Ulcers form when powerful digestive juices start to burn through the delicate pink lining of your digestive organs. Either the acid is too strong or the mucus lining that *usually* does a terrific job of protecting your organs goes on strike, or both. But how does such an imbalance occur? And why does one person get ulcers while another doesn't?

"We simply don't know," says Gregory F. Bonner, M.D., staff gastro-enterologist with the Cleveland Clinic Florida in Fort Lauderdale. He explains that while many factors may encourage ulcers, by far the most susceptible among us are those who have had ulcers before. The little devils are notorious repeat offenders. They also run through families. And they have a special affinity for people who regularly take aspirin, ibuprofen or any other nonsteroidal anti-inflammatory drugs (which include most pain relievers and arthritis drugs), says Dr. Bonner.

If you suspect you have an ulcer, don't suffer in silence. Untreated ulcers can cause serious illness or even death. On the other hand, if treated, your chances for a quick and complete recovery are excellent. Most com-

---

PROFILE IN HEALING

HELEN WILSON: WINNING THE BATTLE

Helen Wilson's ulcers today are nothing but a memory—an *awful* memory. "I'd be hungry, but I couldn't eat. I'd have these bad pains in my stomach, stinging kinds of pains that would last sometimes for about an hour. And I'd wake up during the night with the pain—just about every night," says the 68-year-old resident of Los Angeles.

Helen's first battle with ulcers came in the 1970s, but there have been a number of episodes since—of both the duodenal (in the intestine) and the gastric (in the stomach) varieties. "The doctors at first gave me the drug Tagamet, which I'd take for about three to four months. The ulcers would go away, but then within a month they would usually come back," she says.

What caused her ulcers in the first place, and what made them return, no one can say for sure. But she and her doctors have some good ideas. Topping the list: her genes. "It seems like ulcers run in my family. My son has them, too," says Helen. Years of smoking were undoubtedly another factor. "About a pack a day," she says. And stress also likely played a role. "I used to get upset a lot at my husband when he was drinking. When I'd get upset, that's when the pain would start."

Today, Helen Wilson feels that her life is much less stressful. Mr. Wilson no longer has a drinking habit, and Mrs. Wilson no longer has the responsibility of raising three children and two grandchildren. As another favor to her digestive system, she quit smoking in 1987. And on advice from her son, experimenting with his own recurring ulcers, she also gave up greasy foods like bacon and gravy. Meanwhile, her doctors have attacked her ulcers with newer medications, such as Zantac.

All these changes in her life seem to have made a difference. She happily reports that she's been free of ulcers since 1991.

monly, treatment consists of a medication that suppresses the production of digestive acid long enough for the ulcer to heal. The most often prescribed medications are called H_2 blockers. For some patients, other drugs that either neutralize acid or coat the stomach may be just as effective.

Treatment for ulcers is so fast and effective that many doctors won't even bother with fancy diagnoses before beginning treatment. "We'll treat most people empirically," says Dr. Bonner. That is, if you describe to your doctor something that sounds like an ulcer, he may just go right ahead and prescribe medication. If, however, you are over 50 years old or the medication doesn't relieve your pain within two weeks, your doctor will likely recommend testing. The two common tests for ulcers are the upper GI (gastrointestinal) series, an x-ray of your digestive organs, and an endoscopy, in which the doctor looks into your gut via your throat by inserting a tube with a little television camera at the end of it.

HABITS THAT HEAD OFF ULCERS

The tricky part about ulcers isn't diagnosing or treating them—that's relatively easy. The tricky part is keeping ulcers from recurring. Within one year of being exorcised, *70 to 80 percent* of ulcers come back to haunt their victims' insides. But you can go a long way toward protecting yourself by following the ulcer-busting tips recommended here.

Discard your cigarettes. If you smoke, you now have one more reason to quit. Actually, you have *three* new reasons to quit: "People who smoke get more ulcers. People who smoke have ulcers that heal more slowly. And people who smoke get their ulcers back more quickly," says Thomas O. G. Kovacs, M.D., director of the Peptic Ulcer Clinic at the Center for Ulcer Research and Education (CURE), part of the Division of Gastroenterology at the University of California, Los Angeles. What the exact link between smoking and ulcers is no one can say. One theory is that the nicotine in tobacco somehow hinders the pancreas from doing its usual job of neutralizing acid in the small intestine.

Check your medicines. If you're one of the millions of Americans who regularly take aspirin or other nonsteroidal anti-inflammatory drugs, understand that recent studies have shown that these can cause ulcers. They also slow the healing of ulcers. What do you do if you need these drugs? Talk to your doctor about possible substitutes. If you must take a nonsteroidal anti-inflammatory drug, there are others drugs you can take in addition to counter its negative effects on the protective lining of your stomach and intestines.

Think about what you put in your mouth. The whole business of what people with ulcers can and cannot eat "has reached mythical proportions," says Dr. Kovacs. Once upon a time, eating a bland diet with lots of

NAILING DOWN BACTERIA

In the world of ulcers, the future looks bright—especially when seen through a microscope. For deep within the bodies of ulcer patients, a tiny discovery has been made. Doctors now know that a bacterium called *Helicobacter pylori* is playing some kind of important role. Figuring out exactly what that role is "may give us a cure for ulcers," says ulcer authority Thomas O. G. Kovacs, M.D., of the University of California, Los Angeles.

For the moment, *H. pylori* has scientists stumped. Most people (but not all) who have ulcers turn out to be infected with *H. pylori*. At least a half-dozen studies have shown that by killing the bacteria while an ulcer is healing, you significantly reduce the chances of an ulcer coming back. One Dutch study, for example, fed bacteria-killing medications to 17 people with healing ulcers (healing with the help of traditional drugs)—and *not one* suffered a relapse within the following year. (Normally, 70 to 80 percent of them could expect to see their ulcers return.)

But despite the obvious connection between the bacteria and the disease, scientists can't yet say that one causes the other. Hapless researchers who have swallowed huge amounts of *H. pylori* have wound up with gastritis—but no ulcers. And in some countries like Peru, where nearly everyone is infected with *H. pylori,* people suffer no more from ulcers than do people in countries where comparatively few carry the bacteria.

"It may be that the bacteria make people more susceptible to ulcers, either by disrupting the protective factors in the digestive system or by affecting acid production," says Dr. Kovacs. Whatever the mechanism, one thing is clear: The only good *H. pylori* is a dead one. The problem is that killing them isn't easy. It takes large doses of two, generally three, different medications (antibiotics and bismuth), each with its own side effects.

So for now, most doctors are ignoring the *H. pylori* bacteria, because dealing with the bacteria is so difficult and because treating ulcers with antacid medications is so effective. In addition, one of the drugs used to kill *H. pylori* in laboratory studies does not have U.S. government approval for use on the public. But in the near future, things may change, says Dr. Kovacs. "A simpler way to kill the bacteria may revolutionize the treatment of ulcers."

milk (which was thought to coat the stomach) was the primary form of ulcer therapy. Unfortunately, few people got better. In truth, milk is bad for ulcers, because it encourages acid secretion. And spicy foods, it turns out, don't matter much at all. Studies from India have shown that people eating mountains of hot chilis see their ulcers heal at the same rate as anyone else's. Most doctors today will tell you that you needn't limit your diet—unless a particular food bothers you. Individuals will differ.

You should perhaps pay the most attention not to what you eat but to what you *drink*. Coffee, caffeinated or not, boosts acid output. But don't despair, coffee lovers. You may not need to quit—rather, try to limit yourself to no more than a cup or two a day, says Dr. Kovacs. Alcohol should also be consumed only in moderation.

Keep calm. No, stress no longer plays the leading role in the world of ulcers. Research has linked stress and ulcers, but the evidence that one causes the other is anything but firm. If corporate sharks do get more ulcers, some researchers speculate that it may have more to do with excessive use of coffee, alcohol and aspirin than with any direct effect of stress. All the same, if you're prone to ulcers, try to relax more, and perhaps seek stress reduction counseling. It can only help—but don't expect miracles.

WHEN PROBLEMS PERSIST

Ulcer medications today are so good that "at the end of eight weeks, 90 percent of all ulcers will be healed, no matter what drug you're using," says Dr. Bonner. But if your ulcer is the tenacious type, a new drug called omeprazole should do the trick. It's even more powerful at reducing acid secretion than the popular H_2 blockers.

Omeprazole has set a stunning track record in several European studies, healing *nearly 100 percent* of all ulcers in as short as two to four weeks. But since the long-term effects of taking this new drug are still unknown, most doctors are using it only if more traditional drugs have been tried without success.

Another new, still experimental drug therapy, one that may greatly reduce your chances of relapse, is the use of powerful antibiotics.

Surgery for ulcers was once a common thing. In recent years, however, the number of operations for ulcers has dropped considerably. Fewer than 5 percent of all ulcer patients today will ever face a scalpel. Who are the unlucky few?

Those with serious complications, such as bleeding or perforation of the intestinal or stomach wall. There are several different types of operations, depending on the problem. The pros and cons of ulcer surgery—as with any kind of surgery—need to be weighed carefully.

Urinary Tract Infections

They danced in Greek *tavernas,* raced from the bulls in Pamplona and nibbled goat cheese in Corsica. Altogether a perfect honeymoon—until the new Mrs. Drabble started going to the bathroom 15 times a day. She went twice during breakfast, three times during lunch and six times during supper—and that was before her evening espresso! "My dear, let us talk of love," crooned the dashing Mr. Drabble, thinking only of romance as the full moon rose and reflected in the sparkling sea. "Excuse me," sighed Mrs. Drabble, eyeing the ladies' room. "I'll be right back!"

MARAUDING MICROBES

Urinary tract infections (UTIs) often come at the worst times, says Joshua Hoffman, M.D., an internist in private practice in Sacramento, California. It's very common for infection-causing bacteria in and around the vagina to be "massaged" into the urethra, the tube that extends to the bladder, during intercourse. That's why doctors sometimes refer to UTIs as "honeymoon cystitis."

More than 80 percent of all UTIs are caused by bacteria that originate in the intestine and live quite comfortably and, most of the time, harmlessly in the area near the anus. Trouble begins when they migrate—during sex, for example—into the urethra. In women, the anus and the urethra are close together, so it's relatively easy for bacteria to make the trip. Men, with their extra inches of anatomy, rarely are affected. That's why UTIs often are considered a woman's problem.

Of course, you don't have to be on your honeymoon, or even be sexually active, to experience the aching, burning and frequent urination that commonly accompany a UTI. At least one out of three women will eventually contract a UTI, and women who are particularly susceptible get three, four, even five a year, Dr. Hoffman says.

UTIs can occur anywhere in your urinary tract. An infection in your bladder is called cystitis; in your urethra, urethritis; in your kidneys, pyelonephritis. While pyelonephritis can be quite serious (see "Kidney In-

---

ANTIBIOTICS TO THE RESCUE

Antibiotics are so effective at curing a urinary tract infection (UTI) that some doctors are prescribing them as a preventive for some women plagued with recurrent attacks.

According to researchers at the University of Washington School of Medicine in Seattle, daily antibiotics can be highly effective in preventing UTIs, even when taken for as long as five years. What's more, they don't appear to cause antibiotic-resistant strains of bacteria, which often is a risk with the long-term use of antibiotics.

Another study done by researchers at the same school found that while some women may benefit from taking antibiotics every day, others can take them only as needed—after intercourse, for example, when they're more at risk for contracting an infection. In the study, researchers looked at two groups of women prone to UTIs. One group took antibiotics after they had intercourse. The other took placebos (blank pills). Of the 16 women who took postcoital antibiotics, only 2 (12.5 percent) developed a UTI. Of the 11 women taking placebos, 9 (81.8 percent) developed infections.

Doctors typically are cautious about the long-term use of antibiotics. For one thing, bacteria adapt to their environment. They can also change very quickly—sometimes in days or even hours. When bacteria are exposed to antibiotics in less-than-lethal doses, they can develop particularly virulent strains that are hard to kill. What's more, antibiotics can sometimes cause unpleasant, even dangerous, side effects.

But the bacteria that cause UTIs usually are fairly predictable and easy to get rid of. Used in low doses both to treat UTIs and to prevent them, antibiotics are quite safe, says Sacramento, California, internist Joshua Hoffman, M.D. "Antibiotics are concentrated in the urine, which is why urinary tract infections are easy to prevent," Dr. Hoffman says. "You can use small doses of antibiotics, which turn out to be a very large concentration in the bladder, and that knocks the bacteria out."

---

fections" on page 326), most UTIs are easily treated, Dr. Hoffman says. Even if you do nothing, your body's natural defenses will usually clear things up. Call your doctor if your condition doesn't improve within 24 to 48 hours, says Dr. Hoffman.

BEATING THE BUGS

If you've had one UTI, you'd prefer never to have another. Women with recurrent UTIs can stop the vicious cycle with preventive maintenance, says Dr. Hoffman. Here's how.

Flush them out. It's entirely normal to wake up in the morning with bacteria in your bladder, Dr. Hoffman says. You don't even know they're there. But if you start the day without urinating, those few invaders have time to multiply rapidly. A few hundred can turn into thousands in no time. Flushing them out will prevent them from gathering enough forces for a successful attack. But a good defense means more than emptying your bladder when you wake up. You have to keep the flow going all day long.

"There are a few bugs in your urinary tract almost all the time, but when you urinate, you wash them out," Dr. Hoffman explains. To keep your bladder—and urethra and kidneys—bacteria-free, you have to keep fluids moving. The more water you drink, the more you urinate. The more you urinate, the lower your chances for picking up an infection.

You should drink at least six to eight glasses of water a day. Water and fruit juices are preferred over most other liquids such as soft drinks, which can contain salt that inhibits urination.

A caution: If you're already taking antibiotics for a UTI, too much water can make them less effective. Ask your doctor how much water you should drink during and after your therapy.

Infectious interruptus. Because bacteria always are in and around the vagina, it's difficult to prevent them from getting into the urethra during intercourse. But you can flush them out by going to the bathroom after sex, Dr. Hoffman suggests.

Wipe away. Left to themselves, the bacteria in the periurethral area—that is, in the area near the urethra—like to stay at home. But if you push them toward the urethra, you're courting a UTI. "After a bowel movement, wipe the rectal area toward the *back* and the urethral area separately toward the *front*," Dr. Hoffman says.

Be a bad host. If your urine is sweet and nice, it'll attract bacteria. If you make it acidy and inhospitable, bacteria will hit the road. "High doses of vitamin C can help acidify urine," Dr. Hoffman says. "In combination with lots of fluids, that may help prevent some UTIs."

If you have problems with recurrent UTIs, you might want to ask your doctor about vitamin C therapy. Although vitamin C is not toxic, high dosage of any vitamin should be taken only under the supervision of a doctor. Long-term use of high doses of vitamin C can cause digestive problems such as diarrhea. You can get plenty of extra vitamin C naturally by increasing your intake of citrus fruits and certain green vegetables such as broccoli and kale.

The cranberry connection. Some doctors believe there may be some merit to this folk remedy, although no one has come up with a universally acceptable answer as to why it may work. One theory suggests that cranberry juice may contain chemicals that prevent infection-causing bacteria from clinging to the urinary tract. Some say it simply helps boost vitamin C intake. At the very least, it will boost your fluid intake and help flush bacteria from your system, Dr. Hoffman says.

Diaphragm dangers. Some women who use a diaphragm are particularly prone to UTIs, perhaps because it gives bacteria two more chances—during insertion and removal—to get inside. If you get frequent infections, ask your doctor if another type of birth control might be more appropriate for you.

VARICOSE VEINS

Do your legs start aching in the afternoon?

Do you always wear long pants, even at the beach?

Do you stare at your legs and wonder "Where's Route 66?"

Welcome to the world of varicose veins, that twisting topography of swollen, congested blood vessels that twist and hump like interstate highways on a road map. Caused by structural weaknesses inside, varicose veins are proof that gravity only goes one way—*down*.

AN UPHILL BATTLE

Basically a varicose vein is a blood vessel that doesn't quite have the oomph to push its cargo—blood—back into circulation. Here's what happens. When blood exits your heart through the arteries, it shoots right along, assisted both by gravity and by the heart's pumping action. The return trip through the veins, however, is more arduous. Not only do your veins exert less pressure, but also much of the journey, particularly from the feet and legs, is uphill.

To help the blood move upward, your veins are lined with tiny one-way valves. The valves open to let blood through, then snap shut as it passes. This system allows the blood to move in stages, its weight supported by the valves. Sometimes, however, the valves fail. (Or in some cases, they're congenitally absent.) When this happens, the rising column of blood comes crashing down. "Instead of carrying blood away from the skin and muscles and to the heart, the vein now is carrying blood in a *reverse* flow," explains Mitchel P. Goldman, M.D., an assistant clinical professor of dermatology at the University of California, San Diego, and the author of a textbook on the treatment of varicose veins. Since the blood has trouble going upward, it tends to pool at the bottom of the vein. When this happens, the vein becomes varicose—distended, in other words.

Varicose veins are extremely common, affecting one in five adults, Dr. Goldman says. Women are five times more vulnerable than men, and the veins often crop up during and after pregnancy. Varicose veins rarely are a serious problem, although the impaired circulation, if left untreated, can cause ulcers to develop on the lower legs. But they can make the legs achy and tired. They also can make them *look* bad. Even with surgery, there isn't a cure for varicose veins, Dr. Goldman says. But with a few simple tricks, you can relieve some of the ache—and, in some cases, help prevent them from forming.

KEEP THE BLOOD MOVING

Your heart is a real powerhouse, pumping approximately 1½ gallons of blood every *minute*. But varicose veins don't get enough of that action. For your blood to keep moving, it needs some extra help. For example:

Walk your dogs. Unlike arteries, veins depend on your muscles to move blood along. Every time you stand up, take a walk or flex your toes, the muscles in your legs squeeze the veins, actually *squirting* the blood upward. The more you move your legs, the more pressure you exert on your veins—and the less blood you have just sitting there. Every now and then, shift your weight from foot to foot. Wiggle your toes. Move your feet, heel to toe, to get a really good stretch.

Flatten those heels. "When you wear high heels, you do not activate your calf muscles properly, which allows blood to collect in the veins," Dr. Goldman says. Flat heels can give your muscles (and your veins) the help they need. Of course, flats are a bit more comfortable, too.

Prop them up. Since your blood, like Isaac Newton's apple, has a powerful tendency to go downhill, it naturally gravitates to your legs—and your varicose veins. You can reverse the flow simply by raising your legs above the level of your heart. During the day, put your feet up now and then to let the blood drain out.

Keep your weight down. This can help in two ways. First, when you're overweight, you have more blood, and this puts additional strain on your veins. Second, leaner people have more muscle, and muscle, remember, helps move the blood along. In other words, too much cushion means not enough pushin'.

Fill up on fiber. "If you're straining to have a bowel movement, you're going to put a lot of pressure on the pelvic veins, which impedes the blood flow back to your heart," Dr. Goldman says. Try to eat several helpings of fruits, vegetables and whole grains a day. This will help the stools pass more easily and will take some of the pressure off your veins.

Stay out of hot water. In fact, you should avoid all high temperatures, whether from saunas, hot tubs or sunbaked beaches. Heat dilates your veins, which in turn lowers the pressure that pushes the blood uphill, Dr. Goldman says.

Loosen up. Those tight-fitting pants, girdles and panty hose that flatter your figure can *flatten* the veins between your heart and your legs, Dr. Goldman says. Do your bloodstream a favor and stick to looser, more comfortable clothes.

Wrap them up. While tight clothes can make your varicose veins worse, graduated compression stockings, which apply *prescribed* amounts of pressure, can help prevent them. For stockings to work, however, they should be fitted to your legs by a doctor, Dr. Goldman says.

In fact, most people with varicose veins don't need medical treatment, he adds. But when your legs really are hurting, or you're so self-conscious that you refuse to wear shorts in July, then it might be time to consider more serious measures.

GOING FOR THE CURE

If the idea of surgery scares you stiff, think how Galen's patients must have felt. Galen, a Greek physician who practiced medicine some 1,800 years ago, suggested that varicose veins be removed—with hooks! Today's techniques are more sophisticated, thank goodness, and surgery—with a scalpel or, in many cases, with injections—often is the best bet for varicose veins, Dr. Goldman says.

When you have surgery, the problem veins simply are removed. "The legs have thousands and thousands of veins, and most of them are connected to each other," Dr. Goldman explains. "By eliminating the useless veins, you're going to improve the circulation to the others." Once removed, varicose veins don't come back. However, *other* veins may eventually become varicose, he adds.

With surgery, of course, there always are risks—from bleeding, infection and other complications. There's also the risk of scarring, which in some cases can be as unsightly as the veins are. To avoid these risks, many doctors now are removing varicose veins with a procedure called sclerotherapy, or injection therapy, Dr. Goldman says. With injection therapy, the doctor injects an irritating solution into the vein, which then collapses and eventually disappears.

With smaller veins, one injection may be enough; larger veins may require two, three or even four injections, Dr. Goldman says. After each treatment, the legs are wrapped with graduated compression stockings to prevent the collapsed veins from opening up again. Should a vein reopen, another injection will close it again.

Most varicose veins are "100 percent" curable, Dr. Goldman says. "Particularly for smaller veins, I can't see the treatments getting much better than they are now."

VISION PROBLEMS

There ought to be a law against what aging can do to your eyes. Getting older seems to be a major player in three of the four leading causes of blindness—glaucoma, macular degeneration and cataracts (the fourth is diabetes). If eyes are truly the window of the soul, how is your soul supposed to see out if the blinds are drawn? Why should you have to play peekaboo with the beauty of life?

The odds are that you don't. The human eye is an intricately complex and delicate organ. Its components are tiny and fragile. Yet thanks to remarkable advances in ophthalmology in the past 20 years—from sunglasses to eyedrops to laser surgery—the risks of blindness are relatively slight. And for many aging people, the new treatments can also curb some of the vision problems that used to be a matter of course. Among the most notable are cataracts.

CATARACTS

Right behind your iris and pupil is the lens, a transparent, elastic material that does exactly what its name implies—focuses the light entering the eye. Tiny muscles can narrow or thicken the lens as needed. A cataract is a clouding of the lens, blocking the passage of light through it. Aging is a major cause. Half of all Americans between the ages of 65 and 74, and 70 percent of those 75 and older, have some degree of cataract formation. The most common symptom is fuzzy, blurry or double vision that gets worse in the evening. No matter how many new eyeglass prescriptions you get, they may not help.

The great news about cataracts is twofold: Even if you do develop cataracts, there's only a 15 percent chance they will interfere with your normal activities, and even if cataracts do cause you trouble, surgery can help most of the time.

STOP TROUBLE BEFORE IT STARTS

No one really knows what causes most cataracts. But researchers found that fishermen on the Chesapeake Bay had much greater chances of developing cataracts than miners in West Virginia.

"There is evidence that ultraviolet and blue light increases the risk of developing at least one type of cataract over your lifetime," says Walter Stark, M.D., professor of ophthalmology at Johns Hopkins University and director of the Corneal and Cataract Service of the Wilmer Eye Institute at the Johns Hopkins Hospital in Baltimore. That's why protecting your eyes from the sun is your best insurance against cataracts.

Wear shades and a hat. The American Academy of Ophthalmology (AAO) recommends that you wear sunglasses that block ultraviolet light whenever you're outdoors. Studies show that regular use of sunglasses can reduce the risk of cataracts and slow their growth if you're developing them. Look for the designation Z80.3 on the sunglasses: It indicates that they filter out 95% of the harmful rays. A broad-brimmed hat can also help, according to the AAO.

Get a daily dose of vitamins C and E. Another theory on cataracts says that they are caused, at least in part, by the oxidation of the lens by so-called free radicals. The body's own defenses against oxidation decrease with age. Vitamins C and E and the minerals zinc and selenium are known antioxidants and are believed to help the body neutralize free radicals, thus helping to prevent cataracts from forming.

You can get lots of these nutrients by eating plenty of fruits and vegetables. You can also take supplements, but not all doctors recommend them. "I don't routinely prescribe them, but I don't object either," says Michael Klein, M.D., associate professor of ophthalmology at Oregon Health Sciences University in Portland. If you decide to take supplements, Dr. Klein stresses that you consult your doctor. Vitamins and minerals can be toxic in high dosages.

GETTING A NEW LENS ON LIFE

Sun protection, vitamins and glasses have their place, but if glasses do not give adequate vision, the only avenue left may be to surgically remove the cataracts. Cataract surgery is one of the most common types of surgery in America—each year, about 1.2 million operations are performed—and "99.9 percent" of the time, the surgeon implants a synthetic lens to replace your old, cloudy one, Dr. Stark says.

Cataract surgery is so common that "some people tend to trivialize it," Dr. Stark says, "but it is major surgery." Do you really need surgery? Maybe not. "A cataract is not a malignancy," he says. "It will not hurt the eye. There's no harm in putting off surgery. It does not have to be removed unless the reduced vision interferes with your life. If you can still see well enough to do everything you want to do, then you do not need surgery."

Cataract surgery also may not be enough to restore your vision, even though it's successful 95 percent of the time. "You may have a moderate cataract but severe macular degeneration, and cataract surgery will not help you," Dr. Stark says. "On the other hand, you may have a severe cataract and severe macular degeneration, and cataract surgery may help restore some of your vision."

You can usually have cataract surgery as an outpatient. You'll go to the hospital, where the surgeon will make a small slit in the eye and slide out the lens. Then the new synthetic lens will be inserted and the incisions will be closed. The operation to remove the lens takes only 45 to 60 minutes, but preoperative and postoperative procedures boost the total time to about 10 hours, Dr. Stark says. You can go home the same day.

Recovery is usually swift, he says. "You can do pretty much what you want to do the day after, using common sense," he says. "The main thing is not to get hit or bumped in the eye. You can go back to work as soon you want, but you should avoid strenuous activity or contact sports for a few weeks."

In about 30 to 40 percent of the cases, another operation is needed within five years, Dr. Stark says. And this is where lasers come in. In the first operation, he says, the doctor "put the new lens in the old lens capsule. Over time, the capsule itself becomes hazy"—in effect, forming its own version of a cataract. The doctor can use a special laser to fire light through the lens and into the capsule, punching a tiny hole in the capsule and clearing up your vision.

GLAUCOMA

Glaucoma is called the "sneak thief of sight" because it doesn't affect your central vision at first, says Cynthia Bradford, M.D., assistant professor of ophthalmology at the University of Oklahoma Health Sciences Center in Oklahoma City. "It creeps in from the side. If you first learn you have glaucoma by noticing you can't see as far as you once could, you already have very significant damage. When you lose this peripheral vision, it can't be restored. Your vision can be 20/20 straight ahead, but only straight ahead—tunnel vision, like peeking through a straw."

A normal eye is filled with fluid, and that fluid drains through tissues between the iris and cornea (the clear membrane covering the iris). In the most common form of glaucoma, the drains get backed up—no one knows why—and the fluid either flows out more slowly or stops flowing completely. The fluid buildup increases pressure throughout the eye, damaging the tiny blood vessels that feed the retina and optic nerve. Without nutrients, the cells of the optic nerve begin to die, and your vision begins to die, too.

Glaucoma is a leading cause of blindness in America—about one of every seven legally blind Americans has lost his or her vision to this progressive eye disease, and nearly a million have become visually impaired. Heredity plays a significant role in glaucoma: Your risk is far greater than normal if others in your family have had the disease. If you are black or have diabetes, anemia or atherosclerosis, your risk is also considerably higher.

KEEPING A WATCHFUL EYE

There is no cure for glaucoma; it can only be controlled. But controlling it can save your sight. "It's very amenable to treatment," Dr. Bradford says, and the key to successful control is early diagnosis. "By the time the doctor can *see* any damage, the actual damage to the optic nerve is significant. It's like not weighing yourself until you've gained 200 pounds." Once you've lost some vision, you can lose your remaining vision even faster, she says.

Thankfully, an ophthalmologist doesn't actually have to see damage to detect glaucoma. There are seven or eight different tests that reveal pressure, vision loss and nerve damage, Dr. Bradford says. "You put all the tests together and decide whether there's enough suspicion for glaucoma damage to put the person in treatment."

One crucial test is measuring the pressure inside your eye. Just because your fluid pressure is high doesn't mean you have eye damage, Dr. Bradford says. "Some people can have higher than normal pressure yet never have glaucoma damage," she says. "Others get damage at lower pressures."

The key to early diagnosis is a yearly eye exam if you're over 40 years old, Dr. Bradford says. "If everybody in your family gets glaucoma at age 20, you should be checked earlier," she says. "I've had people come in nearly blind from glaucoma at age 40, and they say, 'Yes, Dad went blind from glaucoma at 42.'"

GETTING THE DROP ON IT

Medication in the form of eyedrops is the first line of treatment, Dr. Bradford says. A class of drugs called beta-blockers is often the first medication prescribed. In eyedrop form, they're known by such brand names as Timoptic, Betagan and Betoptic.

The main problem with medication is side effects, sometimes so severe that people refuse—or "forget"—to take it, Dr. Bradford says. Glaucoma patients are supposed to drop the medication in their eyes up to four times a day to keep the pressure steady. But in one study, one-fourth of the patients missed an entire day of medication each month, and 30 percent used their entire daily dosage in a short period instead of spreading it throughout the day.

"Any medication can have side effects, and even physicians forget potential side effects from eyedrops," Dr. Bradford says. "Most people don't have any trouble at all, but younger people will often get very lethargic—they'll say, 'I just can't get going,' and they'll quit doing everything because they get so tired. Older people can get a dramatic slowing of the

---

TREATMENT BREAKTHROUGH

TECHNIQUES TO HELP PREVENT BLINDNESS

We asked vision experts to look into the future for insight as to what's possible for the prevention of blindness. Here's what they had to say.

GLAUCOMA. Researchers are studying the use of computers for early diagnosis of glaucoma, says ophthalmologist Cynthia Bradford, M.D., of the University Oklahoma Health Sciences Center in Oklahoma City. "You take a picture of the optic nerve and have the computer analyze it," she says. "Then you repeat the process six months later and see if the computer can be more sensitive in picking up any changes in the optic nerve." She also thinks lasers will become even more popular, allowing people who don't respond to medication to get surgery sooner.

CATARACTS. "The instruments used in cataract surgery will get smaller and smaller," Dr. Bradford says. "And eventually the solid lens implant will give way to a substance that's injected through a little hole. It will be able to focus just like your natural lens. There are a lot of bugs to be worked out still, but it could be wonderful, and people will line up for that one."

MACULAR DEGENERATION. Ophthalmologist Wayne Fung, M.D., is working on using a natural immune system chemical called interferon alpha-2a as a treatment for the wet (and most serious) form of macular degeneration. In this disease, the eye for some reason goes overboard in producing masses of tiny blood vessels, which bleed and form scar tissue under the retina. Dr. Fung believes that the

---

heart rate, so they need their pulse checked before they're put on the drops. In fact, some patients' heart rates drop so much it can put them at risk for heart failure." Other side effects can include hallucinations, male impotence and exacerbation of asthma.

Other antiglaucoma drugs also have side effects, "so you still have to be careful," Dr. Bradford says. "I tell my patients to let me know if they're having problems and to let other physicians know they're on the eyedrops." Also be sure to ask your doctor or pharmacist *exactly* how to take the drops, how much and how often. It's not a guessing game.

One antiglaucoma drug, pilocarpine, now comes in a wafer form, so you don't have to remember to use drops and can't take it improperly. The contact lens–size wafer, called Ocusert, slips under either your upper or

distressed macular cells are telling the body to make the abnormal blood vessels. He also thinks that this type of interferon can nullify the messages the distressed cells are sending. Another possibility is that interferon "turns off" the cells that are sending the distress signal. Injections of this type of interferon can reverse or at least slow down this abnormal growth of blood vessels and can clear up the bleeding, Dr. Fung says.

Other advances could come in the form of chemicals that can be applied directly to the retina to loosen the scars of macular degeneration, Dr. Fung says, "without dissolving the retina." The scars could then be peeled off, smoothing out the retina and restoring sight.

EYE TRANSPLANTS? Not much chance of eye transplants anytime in the near future, says Dr. Fung. "We can't transplant nerve tissue, and the retina and optic nerve are extensions of the brain. It's the same reason we can't transplant spinal cords." Some neurologists are now trying to grow retinas in test tubes using natural body substances called nerve growth factors (NGF). "In macular degeneration, the outermost colored layer of the retina gives out," Dr. Fung says. "Researchers are trying to apply NGF to this layer to see if it can be regenerated."

Another, so far unlikely, development is a visual aid like a miniature camera inside a glass eye. The miniaturization is attainable, Dr. Fung says, "but there's no way to transfer the image to the brain." Again, nerve tissue is involved, and man has not been able to duplicate it.

your lower eyelid and works steadily for a week. The main disadvantages are that it's more expensive, you may have trouble adjusting to the feeling of something under your lid and it can fall out, especially when you're sleeping.

"It's very frightening to be told you have glaucoma," Dr. Bradford says. "But it's like being told you have high blood pressure. If you take the drops and have follow-up exams, you should do fine and keep your vision. You're not going to go blind."

TURNING ON THE FAUCET

With the kind of side effects that come with medication, it's no wonder that many people with glaucoma ask for surgery. In fact, British ophthalmologists favor surgery over medication, Dr. Bradford says. In America, laser surgery is the second choice if medication fails. Called laser trabeculoplasty, or LTP, the surgeon focuses the laser light on the eye and makes about 50 tiny burns in the drainage area, where the cornea and iris meet. "It doesn't punch a hole in the area," Dr. Bradford says. "It just shrinks one area with scar tissue, that pulls open other areas, and the fluid can drain out." It's an outpatient procedure with little pain.

If more conventional surgery fails to control your glaucoma, your doctor may decide to give you some high-tech plumbing called the Molteno implant. It's a small plastic plate that's attached to a 3/4-inch-long silicone drainage tube. The surgeon sews the plate onto the white of your eye and inserts one end of the tube into your eyeball and the other end behind the eye. The excess fluid will drain out to the back of your eyeball, where your body will absorb it.

This little faucet can be installed in a 40-minute hospital operation. You'll use antibiotic-steroid eyedrops for about six weeks after the surgery. Your eye should lose the redness and regain its normal vision in about two weeks.

"There are certain people for whom other methods to control glaucoma have failed," Dr. Bradford says. "That's when the Molteno implant might be used. There are risks with it, too. Any time you put a prosthetic piece in the body, you risk infection or failure of the piece. Certainly there are people who have had their vision saved by the Molteno implant."

MACULAR DEGENERATION

Macular degeneration ranks second to glaucoma as a cause of legal blindness in America, although there's only a 4 in 100,000 chance you'll go blind from it. Yet it's the number one cause of new cases of blindness in people over 65 years old—its official name is age-related macular degeneration. And the likelihood you'll develop it is higher if your family has a history of it.

There's no known cause for the disease and no known way to prevent it, Dr. Klein says. "If you live long enough, you're going to have some macular degeneration, but it doesn't necessarily have to influence your sight to a significant degree," he says. Approximately 10 in 100 people over the age of 60 will have some vision loss from macular degeneration, he says.

The macula is the central area of the retina, which lines the back of the eye. It is responsible for sharp central vision, necessary for reading, driving and recognizing faces and fine details. With increasing age, this tissue can break down and lead to vision loss. The major symptoms are a blurring of central vision, development of a blind spot and distortion of straight lines into wavy lines. The degeneration usually affects both eyes to some degree, but only one eye might suffer significant vision loss.

Macular degeneration is usually classified into two general types—dry, and wet. The dry type is the most common, accounting for 80 to 90 percent of the cases, Dr. Klein says. Its symptoms evolve so slowly that you may not notice them, except to become aware that "Hmm, I can't see as well as I used to." It's usually not enough loss to become legally blind, but it can interfere with driving and reading, he says. "One theory suggests that it's caused by exposure to light over a lifetime, especially the shorter wavelengths like blue and ultraviolet," Dr. Klein says. "The retina has to react to this light, and the tissues lose their ability to handle the waste products this reaction produces. Free radicals accumulate and destroy the tissues."

The wet, or exudative, form is less common and much more serious. It comes on quickly and progresses rapidly—usually over a matter of weeks. New blood vessels start growing beneath the macula—again, no one knows why, although the body might be trying to repair the macula. These blood vessels bleed and leak and form scar tissue. "The wet form is responsible for approximately 90 percent of legal blindness caused by macular degeneration," Dr. Klein says. "And it's the one form that is sometimes treatable by lasers." Early diagnosis is important to be able to treat it with lasers—if you're at risk, you need at least annual eye checkups, he says. Often the first sign is a distortion or blurring of vision in one eye when you read or look at objects with straight lines.

Having the dry type doesn't protect you from getting the wet type, Dr. Klein cautions. "If you have the dry type, you have to be aware of precipitous changes," he says, "especially a rapid development of blurriness or developing a central blind spot over a period of days or weeks." These symptoms could herald the onset of the wet type. If this happens, see a doctor immediately.

DELAYING DEGENERATION

There are no effective medical treatments for the dry type of macular degeneration, and it may get worse with time. But since one prominent theory involves oxidation and free radicals, "if somehow we can help the eye get rid of those waste products, maybe we can help macular degeneration," says Dr. Klein. That's why some doctors prescribe antioxidants—supplements like vitamins C and E and beta-carotene. Other often-recommended supplements are the trace minerals zinc and selenium, which are important in the retina's metabolism.

There is some evidence that at least zinc can be of some benefit. A study at the Louisiana State Eye Center found that patients who took 100 to 200 milligrams of zinc twice a day had less vision loss and less deterioration of their retinas than patients who took a placebo. The researchers,

---

HELPING YOURSELF: ATTITUDE AND VISION AIDS

"People think that if you're blind, you don't see. We don't consider anybody blind who has usable vision, because they're not totally blind," says Lorraine Marchi, executive director of the National Association for Visually Handicapped. The legal definition of *blind* refers merely to distance and side vision, not what you can see up close, she says. And low-vision aids and self-help techniques can help you make the most of your vision. If you have any vision left at all, Marchi says, you can read if you want to.

"It's a re-education of the brain, that's all it is—learning how to use that residual vision properly, and not being afraid to do away with all those darned old wives' tales," Marchi says. "In fact, the more you use your reduced vision, the better the brain interprets what it sees. Actually, your vision can improve, maybe not on the eye chart but because your brain becomes accustomed to a new way of seeing."

What you need is motivation. "We find that the people who are going to benefit from vision aids are those who have motivation," Marchi says. "The motivation comes from being able to understand what the problem is. We have a 97 percent success rate with our people, because we explain everything to them."

however, warned that the study was small—only 151 people—and that excess zinc can have dangerous side effects. Large amounts of vitamin E can also have side effects. For these reasons, self-treatment with nutritional therapy is not recommended.

DETACHED RETINA

No one can describe a detached retina in quite the same way as ophthalmologist Wayne Fung, M.D. Imagine a basketball, Dr. Fung suggests, a basketball inflated with gelatin. Now imagine that gelatin melting, from the center outward. Imagine that the only firm part of the gelatin left is an outer shell—the rest has turned to liquid. Now imagine that outer shell finally collapsing inward.

That's about what happens to your eyes as you age. The basketball is your eyeball. The gelatin is the vitreous humor, a gel that fills the eyeball and that's as firm at birth as an ice-cold batch of gelatin. "By the time you

---

Vision aids can help those with glaucoma, macular degeneration and other eye diseases. If you've lost your peripheral vision to glaucoma but medication and surgery have brought the damage under control, you can take advantage of mobility training, says ophthalmologist Cynthia Bradford, M.D., of the University of Oklahoma Health Sciences Center in Oklahoma City. "You have to learn how to get around," she says. It could include something as simple as learning to turn your head to see where you're going or using a cane.

Low-vision aids include simple things like:

TELESCOPIC LENSES. They can be built right into a pair of glasses. One type looks like a tiny camera viewfinder perched on top of your glasses.

CLOSED-CIRCUIT TELEVISION. It lets you read print enlarged up to 60 times on a TV screen.

FIELD ENHANCER. This is a special prism that increases the peripheral vision of someone with glaucoma.

ADJUSTABLE LAMPS AND HIGH-INTENSITY LIGHT BULBS. These increase the amount of light in a room.

LARGE-PRINT PUBLICATIONS. There are many books and magazines that come in large-print editions. There are even large-print telephone dials, calculators (couldn't we all use those!) and needle threaders.

---

reach 30 or 40 years old, the vitreous humor begins to melt like gelatin sitting on the kitchen counter," says Dr. Fung, consultant to the Retina Clinic at the California Pacific Medical Center in San Francisco. As it melts, "floaters" appear; they're tiny, unmelted pieces of the gel that appear as little spots or strings in your vision—literally, spots before your eyes.

Finally, the solid outer layer of the gel caves in. Voilà—no more gelatin in contact with your retina. You feel nothing. There are no symptoms. "It happens safely in 9,999 of 10,000 people," Dr. Fung says.

But if you're 1 in 10,000 people, you get a detached retina. The retina is the crux of your vision. It's literally an extension of the brain that lines the inner surface of the eyeball and transmits visual signals to the brain's vision centers. What happens is that the collapsing gel, rather than peeling cleanly away from the retina, instead pulls a chunk of the retina with it, leaving a hole. "The now-liquefied gel flows through the hole and collects beneath the retina like water behind wallpaper," Dr. Fung says.

As the fluid accumulates beneath the retina, it detaches the retina from the wall of the eye. It's painless, but you do get visual symptoms. "You may notice a gray or dark curtain coming in from the top, bottom or side of one eye, depending on where the hole is," Dr. Fung says. "When the hole first forms, you may see a shower of hundreds of black dots and a lot of strings"—like floaters run amok. *But these aren't floaters.* "Blood from the torn retina is bleeding into the eye," he says. "Some people have described it as black ink being dropped into clear water or hundreds of blackbirds flushing out of a tree."

If you see these symptoms, get to an ophthalmologist immediately; your vision is in danger.

Only 10 percent of detached retinas are caused by injury—like Sugar Ray Leonard's head getting bounced around the ring. No one knows why the retina detaches in the other 90 percent of the cases. One in 10,000 are slim odds, but if you've had cataract surgery, Dr. Fung notes, your risk climbs to 8 in 1,000 or as high as 7 in 100 if the surgery was complicated. That's because, he says, "the surgery can make the vitreous become liquid much more quickly, and it tends to cave in rather suddenly." But microsurgery for cataracts has vastly reduced the risk of a detached retina.

SURGERY TO THE RESCUE

Treatment for a detached retina keys on the hole or holes. "We can't patch the retina, because we have no good glues that the human body will tolerate," Dr. Fung says. "No, we don't take out the eye [he wants that in]. When my patients ask me that, I say, 'If I could do that, I'd take your eye home tonight, and after dinner, I'd take it down to the shop and fix it, and you could pick it up in the morning.'"

In a surgical procedure called the scleral buckle, the surgeon first finds the hole. If he uses cryosurgery, he freezes the wall of the eyeball at the place where it adjoins the hole in the retina. Or he may use a laser to burn the area from inside the eye. Either method makes the body's immune system inflame the area, sealing up the hole with a scab—"using the body's own glue," Dr. Fung says. Then he sews in tiny, sterile sponges that force the outer wall inward to meet the retina. The success rate of a scleral buckle is about 90 percent, and you're usually out of the hospital the following day. You'll have some pain for a few days, but you should be able to return to work in about a week.

A newer technique is the pneumatic retinopexy. The hole in the retina has to be in the upper half of the eyeball for this method to work. That's because the surgeon injects an expandable gas into the eyeball, and as the gas expands inside the eye, the gas bubble naturally moves up. The surgeon then has you sit up and positions your head so that the expanding gas blocks the hole. Sometimes a laser will be used to reinforce the seal. The body absorbs the fluid that has built up beneath the retina, and the retina gradually settles back into place. The entire procedure can be done right in the doctor's office in 30 to 60 minutes. You do have to be careful for the next few days, holding your head in the position the surgeon suggests in order to keep the gas bubble over the hole.

"You don't have to walk on eggshells, but the hole does have to be in the upper part of the eye, because we can't expect someone to stand on their head for 8 hours a day," Dr. Fung says. Again, the success rate is about 90 percent.

YEAST INFECTIONS

Sandra loves her summer job as lifeguard at the local pool. Perched above the azure water, she savors the squeals of liberated school-children and the warm sunshine grazing her bare shoulders.

On many days, however, Sandra is just itching to climb down and change into her shorts. "It happens every summer when I sit around in a wet bathing suit," she says. "I wind up with a vaginal yeast infection that itches like mad."

For Sandra's friend Rose, yeast infections often occur in winter, when her sinuses kick up. "I take antibiotics to knock out the sinus infection and get a yeast infection in return," says Rose.

The fungus that causes vaginal yeast infections doesn't care if the weather outside is arctic or tropical. What *Candida albicans* craves is the warm, moist environment of your body cavities. Any clothing that traps heat and moisture and prevents ventilation of the genitals—a wet bathing suit, panty hose, skintight jeans, synthetic leotards—creates the ideal breeding ground for candida.

Even if your clothes are breezier and baggier than Bozo's, however, you may not be safe from the yeast beast.

If you are one of the three in four women who will experience a yeast infection at least once, you're *not* likely to miss it. Besides the awful itch, symptoms include a cottage cheese–like discharge, a yeasty odor and burning during urination and intercourse.

WHAT MAKES YEAST FEAST

Candida is no stranger to your body. It's normally present in minute amounts in the vagina as well as in the mouth and intestines of both sexes.

Ordinarily this troublemaker is kept in check by the "lactobacilli gang"—your body's friendly bacteria. These good guys create a vaginal environment that fungi hate. Candida is also kept in check by your immune system.

Any number of factors can upset this balanced vaginal system, permitting candida to breed to infection-size proportions. For instance, hormonal changes occurring during pregnancy, premenstruation or menopause can alter the vaginal environment and increase glycogen (blood sugar). This sugary environment provides a veritable feast for yeast.

Similarly, women who are diabetic and have unusually high blood sugar levels are prime candidates for yeast infections.

In addition, certain outside elements that contact the vagina may irritate delicate tissues and allow yeasts already present to proliferate. Among them: chemical douches, deodorant mini pads, perfumed toilet paper, spermicides, tampons, even your sexual partner.

And that's not all. The incidence of yeast infections is rising faster than a yeast cake in a hot oven. Some experts blame the overuse of broad-spectrum antibiotics. "Some people use them as if they were drinking water," says Jack Sobel, M.D., professor of medicine and chief of infectious diseases at Wayne State University School of Medicine in Detroit. These popular drugs do their job with devasting force: They wipe out bad bacteria as well as the good bacteria that keep yeast in line.

HOW TO FOIL A FUNGUS

By paying attention to your personal habits, you can avoid becoming another yeast infection victim, says Marjorie Crandall, Ph.D., a microbiologist and candida researcher who left a faculty position at Harbor-UCLA Medical Center to found the Yeast Consulting Services in Torrance, California. After suffering vaginal yeast infections for nearly two decades, Dr. Crandall learned strategies to outwit the fungus. Here's her advice and tips from other experts.

Let your panties breathe. Whenever possible, wear loose, cotton clothing that allows air to circulate and moisture to evaporate, says Dr. Crandall. Change out of sweaty leotards after your workout. Avoid skin-tight jeans, girdles and other snug clothing. Wear only cotton-crotch panty hose and underwear. At night, sleep without panties.

Say no to pigment and perfume. Dyed and scented personal products can irritate delicate tissues and provide easy entry for fungi, says Dr. Crandall. Stay away from feminine hygiene sprays, colored toilet paper, tampons and deodorant sanitary pads. Even wearing colored panties may be asking for trouble. Likewise, don't use scented detergents or fabric softeners with your panties in either the washer or dryer.

Wash with water only. Wash your genitals daily, but don't use soap.

"The harsh detergents in soap remove natural oils secreted by the skin, which protect you against infection," says Dr. Crandall. Don't use bubble baths, salts or oils in the tub. Be sure to dry thoroughly.

Practice the right way to wipe. "Wipe from front to back after a bowel movement to prevent intestinal bacteria from migrating to the vagina," says Lila E. Nachtigall, M.D., associate professor of obstetrics and gynecology at New York University School of Medicine in New York City.

Use unscented lubricants. Use plain, water-based vaginal lubricants to prevent uncomfortable friction during intercourse that can irritate tissues. Look for Replens, a combination lubricant/moisturizer that comes in a vaginal suppository. This product lowers the pH, increasing the acidity of the vagina, which may help control unfriendly organisms, says Dr. Nachtigall.

HOW TO KNOCK A FUNGUS COLD

If you're itching to get relief for a yeast infection, you'll find it at your local drugstore.

Antifungal vaginal products containing clotrimazole (available as vaginal tablets or creams) are effective candida killers. Before you plunk down $15 or so on one of these products, however, see your doctor for proper diagnostic tests. Examining vaginal discharge under a microscope is the only sure way to tell if you have a yeast infection or an imposter.

Once you get a proper diagnosis, follow the directions for the antifungal agent. Initial relief should come in about three days. But it will take about a week to wipe out the enemy in most cases, says Dr. Crandall. (Some women may need to use medication for a longer time in order to prevent recurrences.)

In the meantime, you can soothe the itch with a douche made from baking soda (1 tablespoon to 1 quart of warm water).

DEFENSE FOR THE YEAST-PRONE

For some women, vaginal yeast infections are like dust on the furniture: They keep wiping it out, only to have the infection return. If your body likes to harbor yeast, you may have to develop a long-term defense strategy. This should include all the tips given earlier, plus a few more.

If you take antibiotics, be vigilant. "You can usually prevent an infection if you start using the antifungal medication as soon as you take your first antibiotic capsule," says Steven Witkin, Ph.D., associate professor in the Immunology Division, Department of Obstetrics and Gynecology at Cornell University Medical College in New York City.

Take the yogurt treatment. Inserting yogurt vaginally is an old home remedy that has never been scientifically proven. But eating yogurt has, according to a study at the Long Island Jewish Medical Center.

Fifteen women with a history of five or more yeast infections a year ate a cup of yogurt daily. The number of infections fell from an average of three during the first six months to less than one infection after a year.

The yogurt contained active cultures of *Lactobacillus acidophilus*. Possibly these friendly bacteria migrate to the vagina, where they destroy the candida. "While this information is preliminary, it couldn't hurt to try it," says Eileen Hilton, M.D., who conducted the study. Use only yogurt with active cultures of *L. acidophilus*. If you can't find it, you can make the yogurt from acidophilus milk.

Check your partner. If you're sexually active, it's possible that the infection has been passing back and forth between you and your mate like a football. "If you're getting recurrent vaginitis, have your partner checked for yeast and have him use a condom," says Raymond Kaufman, M.D., professor and chairman of obstetrics and gynecology at Baylor College of Medicine in Houston.

Look for the allergy connection. If infections still recur, you may be allergic to the condom or spermicide. "Twenty-five percent of women with recurrent yeast infections have an allergy to things like the semen and spermicides," says Dr. Witkin. This allergic reaction releases histamines that block infection-fighting immune cells, allowing yeast to grow uncontrollably. If you suspect your yeast infections are linked to condom use, switch brands.

INDEX

Note: Page references in boldface indicate tables.

Alcohol (continued)
    lupus and, 340
    motion sickness and, 380
    osteoporosis and, 397
    psoriasis and, 436–37
    sleep apnea and, 463
    stroke and, 481
    ulcers and, 522
Allergens, 10, 54
Allergies, 9–16. See also Asthma
    earache and, 154
    food, 14, 16
    immunotherapy for, 12, 14, 15
    insect venom, 12–14
    prevention, 11, 14
    testing, 10
    treatment, 12, 13, 15
    yeast infections and, 545
Allopurinol, 226
Alpha blockers, 431
Alpha glucosidase inhibitors, 148
Alprazolam, 429
Altitude sickness, 17–18
Alzheimer's disease, 19–22
    normal memory loss vs., 352,
        352
    Parkinson's disease vs., 410
Amantadine, 317–18, 422–23
Amenorrhea, 369–70
American Lupus Society, 338, 339
American Self-Help Clearing-
    house, 474
Amitriptyline
    for back problems, 67
    for fibromyalgia, 201
    for migraines, 238
    for postherpetic neuralgia,
        458
Amoxicillin, 229, 461
Ampicillin, 461
Anal ailments, 23–28
    abscess, 26–27

fissures, 23–26
hemorrhoids, 263–66
itching, 27–28
Analgesics, for arthritis, 49
Anal stretching, for fissures, 25–26
Androgenetic alopecia, 230
Anemia
    iron-deficiency (see Iron-defi-
        ciency anemia)
    pernicious, 34
Angina, 250, 256
Angioplasty, 257, 259
Angiotensin converting enzyme
    (ACE) inhibitors, 287
Anorexia, 158, 159, 162–63
Antacids, 221, 222, 276
Anthralin, 438, 440
Antibiotics
    for acne, 3
    for conjunctivitis, 181
    for earache, 153–54
    for emphysema, 167
    for food poisoning, 206
    for keratitis, 185
    for Lyme disease, 344
    for meningitis, 360
    for pelvic inflammatory dis-
        ease, 417–18
    for periodontitis, 229
    for pneumonia, 422, 423, 424
    for prostatitis, 432
    for rheumatic fever, 497
    for Rocky Mountain spotted
        fever, 451
    for sexually transmitted dis-
        eases, 455
    for sinusitis, 461
    for strep throat, 497
    for syphilis, 453
    for traveler's diarrhea, 510,
        512, 513
    for ulcers, 521, 522

Clothing
    Raynaud's phenomenon and,
      444
    varicose veins and, 529
    yeast infections and, 542, 543
Clotrimazole, 544
Coal tar, 141, 438, 440
Cochlear implant, 245
Coffee. *See also* Caffeine
    anal itching and, 27
    for constipation, 129
    fibrocystic breasts and, 192
    gastritis from, 222
    high blood pressure from, 286
    hot flashes and, 365
    osteoporosis and, 397–99
    PMS and, 428
    ulcers and, 522
Colchicine, 225
Cold air, bronchial spasms from,
    52
Colds, 116–24
    airplane ear and, 156
    lupus and, 340
    medications, **118–19,** 121
    treatment, 117–24
Cold sores, 91–93
Cold treatment. *See also* Cryosur-
    gery
    for arthritis, 47
    for back problems, 67
    for bursitis, 76
    for carpal tunnel syndrome,
      97
    for endometriosis, 172
    for headaches, 239
    for muscle pain, 383–84
    for neck pain, 391
    for postherpetic neuralgia,
      458
    for tendinitis, 495
    for TMJ disorder, 490

Colitis, ulcerative, 309, 310, 311,
    314
Collagen, for acne scars, 2
Colon cancer, 82, 85–86, 87, 89, 90
    inflammatory bowel disease
      and, 312–13, 314
Colonic diverticula, 149
Computerized psychotherapy, 137
Condoms, 454, 455, 545
Congestion, cold-related, medica-
    tions for, **118**
Conjunctivitis, 180–81
Constipation, 125–30
    anal fissures and, 24
    bowel movement habits and,
      125, 128–29
    coffee for, 129
    fiber for, 126–28
    hemorrhoids from, 264
    hernia and, 271–72
    laxatives for, 129–30
Contact lenses, keratitis and, 185
Contact ulcers, on vocal cords, 333
Continuous positive airway pres-
    sure, for sleep apnea, 465
Contraception. *See also specific*
    types
    cervical dysplasia and, 104
Corgard, 238
Corns and calluses, 210–11
Coronary bypass surgery. *See* By-
    pass surgery
Corticosteroids. *See* Steroids
Cortisone. *See also* Hydrocortisone
    for arthritis, 49, 50–51
    bone problems from, 396
    for sinusitis, 461
Cosmetics, acne and, 3
Coughing
    from bronchitis, 72, 73, 74
    cold-related, medications for,
      118–19

Fluoxetine, 138, 429
Flying, ear pain from, 155–56
Folate, canker sores and, 93
Food. *See also* Diet
  cravings, iron deficiency and, 31
  traveler's diarrhea and, 513–14
Food allergies, 14, 16
Food poisoning, 203–7
  causes and types, 203–4
  poisonous mushrooms and botulism, 205
  prevention, 206–7
  treatment, 204–6
Foot care, for diabetes, 147
Foot problems, 208–15
  athlete's foot, 208–9
  bunions, 209–10
  corns and calluses, 210–11
  heel pain, 213–14
  ingrown nails, 214
  odor, 214–15
  plantar warts, 211–13
Fruits
  calcium in, 395
  cancer and, 86, 88
  for constipation, 126–27
  iron in, 35
  potassium in, **484**
  traveler's diarrhea and, 514
Fungicides, 209, 544
Furosemide, 396

G
Gallbladder surgery, 218, 219
Gallstones, 216–19
Gamma globulin, 269
Gardening, for stress reduction, 475
Gas
  inflammatory bowel disease and, 312

irritable bowel syndrome and, 321, 323
  lactose intolerance and, 328, 329
Gastritis, 220–22
Gastroenteritis. *See* Food poisoning
Gaviscon, for heartburn, 276
Gene replacement therapy, for psoriasis, 439
Genetics
  asthma and, 57
  blood pressure and, 278
  heart disease and, 249
  inflammatory bowel disease and, 312
  lactose intolerance and, 329
  lupus and, 338
Genital warts, 453, 454
German measles (rubella) vaccination, 106, **107**
Giardia, 514
Ginger, for motion sickness, 380
Gingivitis, 227
Glaucoma, 532–36, 539
Glucose
  diabetes and, 143–44, 145
  for memory, 350
Glutamate, stroke and, 486
Gluten, celiac disease and, 99–102
Gonadotropin-releasing hormones (GnRH-a), 173, 198
Gonorrhea, 453
Gout, 223–26
Grains, celiac disease and, 99–102
Greens, calcium in, 395
Griseofulvin, 209
Growth factors, for osteoporosis, 398
Gum disease, 227–29

H

Hair loss, 230–33
Hair transplants, 231–33
Hallucinations, from narcolepsy, 466, 470
Hallux valgus, 209–10
Hand pain, from carpal tunnel syndrome, 95–98
Hand washing, for colds, 122
Hay fever, 10
Headaches, 234–41
    causes, 234–37
    cluster, 234–35
    cold-related, medications for, **119**
    migraine, 234–35, 235–36, 238, 240–41
    tension, 234, 236–38
    treatment, 236, 237–41
Head injuries, hearing loss from, 243
Hearing aids, 245, 246, 247–48
Hearing loss, 242–48
    causes, 242–44
    tinnitus, 244–47
    treatment, 247–48
Heart attack, 250, 251, 252, 253, 254
    atrial fibrillation from, 479
    cholesterol and, 288, 296
    high blood pressure and, 279
Heartbeat, irregular, 479
Heartburn, 220, 274–76
Heart disease, 249–59
    atherosclerosis, 250, 479, 480
    lifestyle changes and, 252–53, 256
    menopause and, 361–62, 364, 365
    prevention, 250–55
    from rheumatic fever, 496–97
    statistics, 249
    stroke and, 478, 479
    surgery, 252, 253, 257–59
    treatment, 255–57
Heart infections, 260–62
Heat, varicose veins and, 528
Heat treatment
    for arthritis, 46–47
    for back problems, 67
    for blepharitis, 183
    for carpal tunnel syndrome, 98
    for conjunctivitis, 181
    electrosurgery for plantar warts, 213
    for endometriosis, 172
    for fibromyalgia, 202
    for headaches, 239
    for muscle pain, 384–85
    for neck pain, 391
    for phlebitis, 420
    for Raynaud's phenomenon, 444, 445
    for stress reduction, 477
    for tendinitis, 495
    for TMJ disorder, 490
Heel pain, 213–14
Helicobacter pylori, 521
Hemophilus, 180
Hemophilus influenzae
    meningitis from, 359, 360
    vaccination, 106, **107**
Hemorrhagic strokes, 478, 481
Hemorrhoidectomy, 266
Hemorrhoids, 263–66
Hepatitis, 267–70
    vaccination for hepatitis B, **107**
Herbal tea, for relaxation, 366
Herbicides, cancer and, 87
Hernia
    abdominal, 271–73
    hiatal, 274–76

Herpes, genital, 453, 455

Herpes simplex virus, 91–92, 184

Herpes zoster virus, 456, 457

Hiatal hernia, 274–76

High blood pressure, 277–87
    alcohol, caffeine, and smoking and, 285–86
    diet for, 279, 282–85
    lifestyle change for, 403
    medications, 286–87
    readings, 277–78, 284–85
    risk factors, 278
    sodium and, 280–81, 282
    stroke and, 479
    weight control and exercise for, 278–82

HIV. *See* Human immunodeficiency virus

Home, allergens in, 11, 55–56

Hormone replacement therapy, 363–65, 367

Hormones
    cancer and, 90
    carpal tunnel syndrome and, 96, 98
    fibrocystic breasts and, 191, 192, 193
    fibroids and, 196, 198
    hair loss and, 232
    heart disease and, 255
    lupus and, 339
    menopause and, 362
    menstrual problems and, 370, 371

Hot baths, for stress reduction, 477

Hot flashes, 361, 362, 363
    treatment, 365–66

H_2 receptor blockers, 276, 520, 522

Human immunodeficiency virus (HIV), 5–6, 7, 8, 516

Human papillomavirus, 104

Humidifiers
    for bronchitis, 74
    for colds, 122
    eczema and, 140
    for influenza, 319
    for laryngitis, 333
    Legionnaires' disease and, 336
    for sinusitis, 460
    for throat infections, 499

Humor, for stress reduction, 473

Hydrea, 439

Hydrocortisone. *See also* Cortisone
    for anal itching, 28
    bone problems from, 396
    for eczema, 141, 142
    hemorrhoids and, 265–66

Hyperglycemia, 143

Hypertension. *See* High blood pressure

Hyperthyroidism, 501–2

Hyperventilation syndrome, 189

Hypoglycemia, 148

Hypothyroidism, 500–501

Hysterectomy, 169, 170–71, 196

Hysteroscopy, for fibroids, 197

I

Ibuprofen
    for arthritis, 49
    for back problems, 67
    for bursitis, 76
    for endometriosis, 172
    for phlebitis, 420
    for PMS, 429
    for tendinitis, 494
    for throat infections, 499
    ulcers and, 519

ICAM, for colds, 123

Ice treatment. *See* Cold treatment

Imagery
    for canker sores, 94

for irritable bowel syndrome,
324
Imipramine, 458
Immune system
allergies and, 9–16
cancer and, 88–89
chronic fatigue syndrome
and, 111, 112
colds and, 117, 118, 120
endometriosis and, 169
mononucleosis and, 375
rheumatoid arthritis and, 45,
46
thyroid disease and, 501
tuberculosis and, 516–17
Immunizations. *See* Vaccines
Immunotherapy
for allergies, 12, 14, 15
for cancer, 90
for inflammatory bowel disease, 311, 313
for plantar warts, 213
Imodium, 313
Imodium A-D, 325, 513
Impotence, 299–303
causes, 299–300, 301
penile implants for, 302–3
treatment, 300–303
Impotence World Services and Impotents Anonymous, 303
Incontinence, 304–7
Inderal. *See* Propranolol
Indigestion, 220
Indomethacin, 221, 495
Infections. *See also specific types*
in children, 106–9
Infertility, 416, 417, 418
Inflammatory bowel disease,
308–15
cancer and, 312–13, 314
nature of, 308–10
treatment, 311–15

Influenza, 316–19, 340
Infrared photocoagulation, for
hemorrhoids, 266
Ingrown nails, 214
Injection therapy, for varicose
veins, 529
Insect venom, allergy to, 12–14, 15
Insomnia, 465–69
Insulin, diabetes and, 143, 144,
145, 147–48
Interferon, 90, 534–35
Intra-cellular adhesive molecule
(ICAM), for colds, 123
Intraductal papillomas, 193
Intrauterine devices (IUDs), en-
dometriosis and, 170–71
Iodine, radioactive, for hyperthy-
roidism, 502
Iron
canker sores and, 93
food sources, 30–35, **32–33**
for trichomoniasis, 455
types, 30–31
Iron-deficiency anemia
causes and risk factors, 29–30
diet for, 31–35
menstruation and, 29–30, 373
supplements for, 35
Irritable bowel syndrome, 320–25
diet and, 321–22, 323, 324–25
emotions and, 322, 324
gas and, 321, 323
symptoms, 320–21
Ischemic strokes, 478
Isotretinoin, 3, 4
Itching, anal, 27–28
IUDs, endometriosis and, 170–71

J
Jaw problems. *See* Temporomandi-
bular joint disorder (TMD/
TMJ)

Tinactin, 209
Tinnitus, 244–47
TMD/TMJ. *See* Temporomandibu-
lar joint disorder
Tobacco. *See also* Smoking
cancer and, 79
Toenails, ingrown, 214
Toes, gout and, 223, 225
Toilet paper, anal itching and, 27,
28
Tolnaftate, 209
Tonsillectomy, 499
Tonsillitis, 497–98
Toothbrushing, gum disease and,
228
Toxic shock syndrome, 507–8
Tranquilizers, 463
Transcutaneous electrical nerve
stimulation (TENS)
for back problems, 67–68
for postherpetic neuralgia,
458
for restless legs syndrome,
447
Transient ischemic attack,
482
Transurethral resection of pros-
tate, 431
Traveler's diarrhea, 509–15
causes, 509–11
culinary cautions, 513–14
preventive medication, 510,
511, 513
recovery, 514–15
Tretinoin, 3
Trichomonas, 455
Trichomoniasis, 453, 455
Tricomin, 232
Tricyclic antidepressants. *See* Antidepressants
Trigeminal neuralgia (tic douloureux), 503–6

Trigeminal Neuralgia Association,
505
Triglycerides, 295
Trimethoprim, 510
Trusses, 272
Tuberculosis, 516–17

U
Ulcerative colitis. *See* Colitis, ulcerative
Ulcers, 518–22
causes and risk factors,
518–19
recurrence prevention, 520,
522
treatment, 519–21
on vocal cords, 333
Urethritis, 524
Uric acid, gout and, 223, 224, 226
Urinary incontinence, 304–7
Urinary tract infections, 523–26
Uterine cancer, 370

V
Vaccines
for AIDS, 7, 8
for allergies, 15
for bacterial meningitis, 360
for childhood infectious diseases, 106–8, 109
immunization schedule,
107
for colds, 123
for hepatitis, 269, 270
for herpes, 455
for influenza, 317, 318
for Lyme disease, 343
for pneumonia, 424
for rabies, 442
for strep throat, 498
Vaginal discomfort, from menopause, 362, 363, 366

Vaginal yeast infections, 542–46
Valproate, 178
Vaporizers
    for bronchitis, 74
    for influenza, 319
    for sinusitis, 460
    for throat infections, 499
Varicella. *See* Chicken pox
Varicose veins, 419, 527–29
Vegetables
    calcium in, 395
    cancer and, 86, 88
    for constipation, 126
    iron in, 33
    potassium in, **484**
    traveler's diarrhea and, 514
Vegetarian diet, for high choles-
    terol, 294–96
Vein inflammation (phlebitis),
    419–20
Veins, varicose, 419, 527–29
Viral meningitis, 358–59
Viruses. *See also specific types*
    cold, 123
Vision aids, 539
Vision problems, 530–41
    attitude and vision aids,
        538–39
    blindness prevention, 534–35
    cataracts, 530–32, 534
    detached retina, 539–41
    eye transplants for, 535
    glaucoma, 532–36, 539
    macular degeneration, 532,
        534–35, 536–39
Visualization
    for canker sores, 94
    for irritable bowel syndrome,
        324
Vitamin A, 84–85, 120
Vitamin B complex, 93, 350
Vitamin B$_6$, 429

Vitamin B$_{12}$, 34
Vitamin C
    cancer and, 80–81
    cataracts and, 531
    for colds, 120, 122, 124
    for emphysema, 165
    food sources, **80–81**
    for high blood pressure,
        284–85
    iron absorption and, 35
    for macular degeneration, 538
    for Parkinson's disease, 412
    for urinary tract infections,
        525–26
Vitamin D, 395–97, 439
Vitamin E
    cataracts and, 531
    for emphysema, 165
    for fibrocystic breasts, 192
    for hot flashes, 365–66
    for macular degeneration,
        538, 539
    for Parkinson's disease, 412
    for vaginal dryness, 366
Vocal cord inflammation, 332–34
Vocal polyps, 333
Vomiting, from food poisoning,
    204, 206

W

Walking
    for back problems, 63
    for diabetes, 145
    for stress reduction, 475
Warts
    genital, 453, 454
    plantar, 211–13
Water, constipation and, 128
Weight control. *See also* Obesity;
    Overweight
    for arthritis, 45
    for back problems, 64

cancer and, 86–87
diabetes and, 144
for endometriosis, 170
fatigue and, 187, 190
for fibroids, 196
for gallstones, 217
gout and, 224–25
heart disease and, 252
for hemorrhoids, 265
hiatal hernia and, 275
for high blood pressure, 278–82
for impotence, 300
for sleep apnea, 463
stroke and, 482
for varicose veins, 528
Weight lifting
for arthritis, 48
bursitis and, 76
osteoporosis and, 399
Whiplash, 390
Whirlpool bath, for tendinitis, 495
Whooping cough (pertussis) vaccination, 106, **107**

Work. *See also* Occupational hazards
stress and, 473–74
Wrist, carpal tunnel syndrome and, 95–98

Y

Yeast infections, 542–45
Yoga, for heart disease, 256–57
Yogurt
canker sores and, 93
lactose intolerance and, 330
for yeast infections, 544–45
Yohimbine, 301

Z

Zantac, 276, 519
Zinc
cataracts and, 531
for macular degeneration, 538–39
for phlebitis, 420
Zostrix, 457